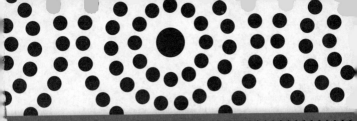

pocket posh® dining out calorie counter

your guide to thousands of foods from your favorite restaurants

Pamela M. Nisevich Bede, MS, RD, CSSD, LD

Andrews McMeel Publishing, LLC

Kansas City • Sydney • London

Produced by

DOWNTOWN
BOOKWORKS INC.

President	Julie Merberg
Senior Vice President	Patty Brown
Layout by	Jennifer Richman/Richman Creative Group
Special Thanks	LeeAnn Pemberton, Sarah Parvis, Jennifer Sharp, Jason Bede, Jenna Bell

Pocket Posh® Dining Out Calorie Counter copyright © 2011 by Downtown Bookworks Inc. All rights reserved. Printed in China. No part of this book may be used or reproduced in any manner whatsoever without written permission except in the case of reprints in the context of reviews.

Andrews McMeel Publishing, LLC
an Andrews McMeel Universal company
1130 Walnut Street, Kansas City, Missouri 64106

www.andrewsmcmeel.com

11 12 13 14 15 LEO 10 9 8 7 6 5 4 3 2

ISBN: 978-1-4494-0340-9

Library of Congress Control Number: 2010937882

Illustration by **robinzingone**®

Preface	IV
Introduction	V

FOOD COUNTS

Applebee's	2	Jimmy John's	175
Arby's	7	KFC	176
Arthur Treacher's / Nathan's Famous	10	Little Caesars	180
A&W	12	Lone Star	181
Auntie Anne's	16	Long John Silver's	184
Baja Fresh	17	LongHorn Steakhouse	186
Baskin-Robbins	22	McDonald's	193
Blimpie	24	Mrs. Fields	203
Bob Evans	28	Noodles & Company	204
Boston Market	34	Nothing But Noodles	206
Bruegger's Bagels	36	O'Charleys	208
Buffalo Wild Wings	41	Olive Garden	216
Burger King	45	On the Border	221
California Pizza Kitchen (CPK)	48	Outback Steakhouse	228
Captain D's Seafood Kitchen	53	P. F. CHANG'S	230
Carl's Jr.	55	Panda Express	237
Chevys Fresh Mex	58	Panera Bread	238
Chick-fil-A	62	Papa John's	244
Chili's	63	Papa Murphy's	245
Chipotle Mexican Grill	70	Pizza Hut	246
Cold Stone Creamery	71	Popeyes Louisiana Kitchen	250
Corner Bakery Café	75	Potbelly	251
Church's Chicken	85	Quiznos	254
Dairy Queen	87	Red Lobster	260
Denny's	96	Red Robin	280
Domino's Pizza	105	Romano's Macaroni Grill	280
Don Pablo's	106	Ruby Tuesday	283
Dunkin' Donuts	111	Skyline Chili	291
Einstein Bros.	122	SONIC Drive-In	294
Fazolis	129	Starbucks Coffee	297
Five Guys	132	Subway	302
Friendly's	133	Taco Bell	304
Godfather's Pizza	138	TGI Friday's	309
Hardee's	144	Wendy's	310
IHOP	148	Whataburger	313
In-N-Out Burger	161	White Castle	315
Jack in the Box	162	Misc. Beverages	319
Jamba Juice	163	Adult Beverages	323
Jason's Deli	170		

preface

For many people, dining out is a favorite way to relax and socialize with friends. For others, it is simply necessitated by a busy lifestyle. Dining out can certainly be a delicious and healthy treat, but when you aren't in charge of cooking the food yourself, it is more difficult to tell how food is prepared. That's what makes this book an invaluable companion. Encased within the cover is helpful information for all of us who are working towards making wiser selections for health and wellness. While eating healthy can be a challenge, especially with so many menu and restaurant options, remember this one thought: Each day you have multiple opportunities to impact your health. With each meal you select and every bite you take, you are providing your body with the fuel it needs to thrive. That said, there are many different types of fuel. This book will provide you with the information you need in order to determine which menu items are "prime" fuel, and which ones should be left behind.

When considering what to enjoy at your next meal, take a moment to consult this pocket guide. Allow it to help you make better choices when dining out or waiting to place an order at the drive-thru window. It is my hope that you will use this book to help you keep track of what you eat as well as the power to make healthier choices for your waistline and your overall health and well-being.

Eating right is possible whether you're eating at your favorite fast-food location or taking the time to enjoy fine dining with family and friends. The benefits of a healthy diet are real, and I am honored that you've chosen this book as an important part of getting there.

Here's to a healthier you!

Pamela M. Nisevich Bede, MS, RD, CSSD, LD

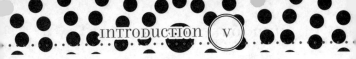
introduction

Healthy Weight Fundamentals

Many diners who seek out the help of nutrition guides such as this one are looking to either improve their health and well-being or looking to winnow their waistline. Research tells us that reaching and maintaining a healthy weight is about balancing calories-in with calories-out. Calories are a way to think about the amount of energy you get from food and the amount of energy your body burns during exercise. When thinking about how many calories to consume, keep the following in mind:

• Protein and carbohydrates provide 4 calories per gram.

• Fat provides 9 calories per gram, which means that high-fat foods often pack a huge calorie punch.

• Walking for 5 minutes burns about 15 calories; sleeping burns about 1 calorie per minute.

To lose weight, you have to burn more calories than you take in. While this may not be groundbreaking news, it certainly can be challenging to put into action. In addition to keeping track of calories by using this pocket guide, here are thirteen tips to living and dining out in a healthy way:

1. Healthy eating starts with you! Many of us who struggle with weight and making better food choices should remember one thing: Packing on the pounds doesn't happen overnight, but progress towards better health can be made every minute. To move towards better health, begin by holding yourself accountable. Use this book to track your progress and assess how far you've come and where you'd like to be in 1 week's time, 1 month's time, 3 months' time, and so on. Keep track of your progress in a diet-and-exercise journal. See how you're doing compared to your goals, making adjustments where there is room for improvement. Simply being more aware of what you're eating each day is doing something right for your health.

2. Leave the Clean-Plate Club behind. It's okay to leave some food behind, especially when you're dining out. Throughout the years, portions at many restaurants have grown significantly. As you'll see in this guide, an average restaurant meal can run 1000 or more calories. Choose a smaller portion size, order a side salad instead of fries, and don't super-size anything! Remember: Bigger only seems better, so don't get lulled into super-sized deals (and waistlines!). Apart from ordering smaller menu items (kid's meals and senior sizes anyone?), or taking home leftovers, try out the "plate method": Fill half of your plate with veggies (your choice, but aim for bright colors and green veggies), and the other half of your plate with lean protein and a starch, such as a small baked potato, brown rice, or whole wheat spaghetti.

3. Start smart. Learn what to look for on the menu. There are always key terms included on the menu that will help steer you away from poor choices and towards healthier ones. Apply the breaks when it comes to words like au gratin, battered, buttered, breaded, creamed, crispy, deep-fried, pan-fried, or golden. Instead, aim for baked, broiled, fresh, grilled, poached, lean, roasted, or steamed selections.

4. Watch those portions! It's time to downsize portions and avoid the urge to double-up (unless it's veggies). By simply adding in extra servings of meat, cheese, bacon, and sauces can easily double the calories of any sandwich. A typical restaurant portion provides enough food for 2 to 3 meals. So to battle the bulge while still getting the most bang for your buck, consider splitting a meal with someone you are dining with, or simply ask for a to-go box when ordering and dish out half of the entrée as soon as it arrives at the table.

5. Eat those fruits and veggies. I've never met a person who was successful in both losing weight and eating healthy by avoiding produce. Fruits and vegetables offer lots of vita-mins, minerals, and nutrients without adding excess calories, sugars, fat, or salt to your diet. Fresh, roasted, and sautéed are healthier ways to enjoy these types of foods.

6. Be a creative consumer. Dining out should be an enjoyable experience, one that leaves you feeling refreshed and taken care of. As a restaurant patron, feel free to mix up the offerings on your plate by requesting a healthier side (swap those fries for some steamed veggies), or simply beef up your sandwich by adding in various types of veggies. You can add more than just lettuce, tomato, and onions. Add sliced carrots, chopped bell peppers, sliced mushrooms, and more.

7. Opt for good carbs. The secret to carbohydrates is to select healthier, more nutrient-dense carbs like those that come from high-fiber foods, such as whole grains, low-fat dairy, beans, vegetables, and fresh fruit, over refined grains and fried potatoes.

8. Go for the WHOLE grain—and avoid the bread basket. When dining out, opt for fiber-rich whole grains by ordering foods that contain the word "whole," as most bread products are wheat products. If you prefer the taste of refined grains, and know that whole grains are a healthier choice, start with a compromise. Mix whole grains with refined grains to slowly transition towards eating all whole grains. Lastly, make dining out a creative experi-ence by trying "new" grain choices such as protein-packed quinoa, brown rice, or whole wheat pastas.

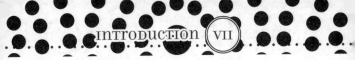

9. Aim for heart healthy fats and oils. While fat often gets a bad rap, it is vital for good health. Just keep in mind the type and amount of fat that is in your food. Remember to choose foods that contain oils instead of solid fats (like lard and butter), and foods that contain heart-healthy vegetable sources (like vegetable oil-based spreads, vegetable oils, and avocado) instead of highly saturated animal fats. Lastly, remember your portion control when it comes to fats. While fat is important to any healthy diet, it packs a big calorie punch. So go easy on the sour cream topping, the extra butter for dipping, and the additional side of salad dressing.

10. Proteins to prefer. Pick healthy proteins from plant sources, such as beans, nuts, and soy products, as these items are rich in protein while being low in fat. Seafood also offers good protein choices while offering heart-healthy oils. If including poultry or meat, choose lean types and roast, bake, broil, poach, or sauté (no deep-fried chicken wings, please!). As for cuts of meat, oftentimes meats ending with loin, such as sirloin and tenderloin, are leaner choices. Lastly, remove the following from your diet: gristle, poultry skin, and marbling, as these items equal saturated fat and calories.

11. Avoid drinking your calories. Many restaurant drink options can pack as many calories as the entrées. So avoid those unfulfilling calories by choosing unsweetened teas, coffees, and water instead. Added bonus? Not only is tap water inexpensive, it also won't cost you anything in terms of calories. So drink up for best health!

12. Get moving. Make it a goal to move more every day—especially on days when you dine out. Look for opportunities to work physical activity into your day. If it's hard to find time to get to the gym, join a sports team or take a dance class. Look for other ways to move more. Take the stairs, go for a walk, lift weights during commercial breaks—where there's a will, there's a way. Set up an appointment with yourself for exercise (and keep it!). Designate a special time of the day for your workout and let everyone know that this is your time. If you have children at home, set up an appointment for them, too. Aim for activity after school and before homework.

13. Mindfully remember the big picture. Enjoy your delicious dinner with family and friends by savoring each bite and eating slowly, just like your mama told you! Thinking of eating out in the context of your whole diet and plan ahead. If you know you are going to order your favorite heavy meal at dinner, go lighter at lunch (and take an extra stroll around the block). If you are a habitual fast-food junkie, it's quite alright to forgo fries and a soft drink in favor of a salad and water. Actually, I encourage it. Your waistline will thank you!

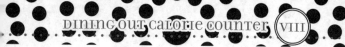
Tips for Healthy Dining Out

What to Remember When Dining Out at Burger Joints
Burger Joints: Less Healthy Choices
- Double-patty hamburger with cheese, mayo, special sauce, and bacon
- Fried chicken or fish sandwich
- Salad with toppings such as bacon, cheese, and ranch dressing
- Breakfast burrito with steak
- French fries
- Milkshake
- Chicken nuggets or tenders

Burger Joints: Healthier Choices
- Regular, single-patty hamburger without mayo or cheese
- Grilled chicken sandwich
- Veggie burger
- Garden salad with grilled chicken and low-fat dressing
- Egg on a muffin
- Baked potato or side salad
- Yogurt parfait
- Grilled chicken strips
- Limit cheese, mayo, and special sauces

What to Remember When Dining Out at Chicken Chains
Chicken Chains: Less Healthy Choices
- Fried chicken, original or extra-crispy
- Teriyaki wings or popcorn chicken
- Wings in general
- Caesar salad
- Chicken and biscuit bowl
- Extra gravy and sauces

Chicken Chains: Healthier Choices
- Skinless chicken breast without breading
- Honey BBQ chicken sandwich
- Garden salad
- Mashed potatoes
- Limit gravy and sauces
- Choose the bun, not the biscuit
- Choose grilled chicken, but lose the skin

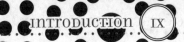

What to Remember When Dining Out at Taco Locales
Taco Locales: Less Healthy Choices

- Crispy shell chicken taco
- Refried beans
- Steak chalupa
- Crunch wraps or gordita-style burritos
- Nachos with refried beans
- Extra sour cream or cheese

Taco Locales: Healthier Choices

- Grilled chicken soft taco
- Black beans or vegetarian refried beans
- Shrimp ensalada
- Grilled fresco-style steak burrito
- Veggie and bean burrito
- Limit sour cream or cheese
- Always ask for extra veggies
- Go for guacamole, but watch the portion size of this heart-healthy fat

What to Remember When Dining Out at Sub and Sandwich Shops
Sub and Sandwich Shops: Less Healthy Choices

- Foot-long sub
- High-fat meats such as pepperoni, tuna salad, bacon, meatballs, or steak
- Extra higher-fat (cheddar, American) cheese
- Extra mayo and special sauces
- Think twice before choosing wraps, which are often higher in fat and calories than other breads

Sub and Sandwich Shops: Healthier Choices

- Six-inch sub
- Customize it. Skip the "as is" sub with all toppings and ask for sauces on the side
- Lean meats, such as roast beef, chicken breast, lean ham, or turkey, or veggies
- One or two slices of lower-fat cheese (Swiss or mozzarella)
- Add low-fat dressing or mustard instead of mayo
- Ask for extra veggie toppings
- Choose whole-grain bread or take the top slice off the sub and eat it open-faced

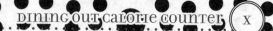

What to Remember When Dining Out at Asian Restaurants
Asian Options: Less Healthy Choices
- Fried egg rolls or spare ribs
- Battered or deep-fried dishes, such as sweet and sour pork or General Tso's chicken
- Deep-fried tofu
- Coconut milk, sweet and sour sauce, regular soy sauce
- Fried rice
- Salads with fried or crispy noodles
- Avoid anything "tempura"

Asian Options: Healthier Choices
- Egg drop, miso, wonton, or hot-and-sour soup
- Stir-fried, steamed, roasted, or broiled entrées, such as shrimp chow mein or chop suey
- Steamed or baked tofu
- Sauces, such as ponzu, rice-wine vinegar, wasabi, ginger, or low-sodium soy sauce
- Steamed brown rice
- Edamame, cucumber salad, stir-fried veggies

Insider Tip: Use the chopsticks—you'll eat more slowly and enjoy smaller bites!

What to Remember When Dining Out at Pasta Places
Pasta Places: Less Healthy Choices
- Thick-crust, deep-dish, or butter-crust pizza with extra cheese and meat toppings
- Garlic bread (say no to the endless bread bowl)
- Antipasto with meat
- Extra pesto sauces
- Pasta with cream or butter-based sauce
- Entrée with side of pasta
- Fried ("fritto") dishes

Insider Tip: Carbs may get a bad rap, but Italian food is actually one of the easiest types of cuisine to make healthy. Avoid fried, oily, and overly buttery items as well as thick-crust menu items. And as always, add extra veggies!

Pasta Places: Healthier Choices
- Thin-crust pizza with half the cheese and extra veggies
Insider Tip: Blot the oil when taking pizza to-go!
- Plain rolls or breadsticks
- Antipasto with vegetables
- Pasta with tomato sauce and veggies
- Entrée with side of veggies
- Grilled ("griglia") dishes
- Choose primavera dishes

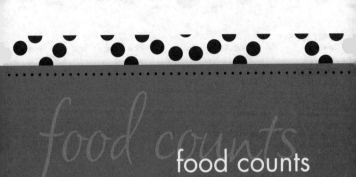

food counts

APPLEBEE'S

Item	Serving Size	Calories	Protein	Carb	Fiber	Sugar	Total Fat	Sat Fat	Sodium
APPETIZERS									
Appetizer sampler	as served	2440–2510	91–92	158–183	16	n/a	157–168	45–49	5740–6750
Boneless buffalo wings, classic	as served	1170	70	66	8	n/a	69	16	3790
Cheese quesadilla grande	as served	1270	43	84	4	n/a	84	36	3160
Cheeseburger sliders	as served	1240	51	81	3	n/a	80	25	2260
Chicken quesadilla grande	as served	1440	71	90	5	n/a	87	37	4030
Chicken wonton tacos	as served	610	40	58	4	n/a	24	4.5	2200
Chili cheese nachos	as served	1680	48	13	17	n/a	107	39	3850
Crunchy onion rings	as served	1230	14	161	12	n/a	59	11	2160
Dynamite shrimp	as served	730	22	40	n/a	n/a	54	10	1490
Mozzarella sticks	as served	940	45	84	6	n/a	46	20	2800
Pork wonton tacos	as served	940	55	71	4	n/a	47	14	2430
Potato skins	as served	1380	59	70	8	n/a	97	49	1860
Potato twisters	as served	840	25	64	7	n/a	24	20	3150
Queso blanco	as served	1360	36	115	13	n/a	84	28	2520
Queso blanco w/ chili	as served	1470	43	119	14	n/a	91	31	2800
Spinach & artichoke dip	as served	1470–1600	33–35	122–125	16	n/a	96–107	23–30	2440–2540
Steak quesadilla towers	as served	1200	58	76	4	n/a	71	33	3650
Veggie Patch pizza	as served	950	32	51	5	n/a	69	23	2310
ENTRÉES									
Asiago peppercorn steak	as served	390	43	26	5	n/a	14	6	1520
Bourbon Street steak	as served	700	54	31	4	n/a	41	10	2310
Grilled shrimp & Island rice	as served	380	29	59	6	n/a	4.5	1	2370
Sizzling Asian shrimp	as served	710	30	117	7	n/a	15	3	3830
Sizzling chicken w/ spicy queso blanco	as served	550	53	37	6	n/a	22	8	2500
Sizzling Skillet & cheese	as served	1070	67	54	7	n/a	65	22	3430

APPLEBEE'S continued

Item	Serving Size	Calories	Protein	Carb	Fiber	Sugar	Total Fat	Sat Fat	Sodium
Sizzling Skillet fajitas, chicken	as served	1150	72	103	10	n/a	50	22	4570
Sizzling Skillet fajitas, shrimp	as served	1040	47	104	10	n/a	49	22	4840
Sizzling Skillet fajitas, steak	as served	1180	72	105	10	n/a	53	24	5330
STEAKS									
House sirloin	7 oz	240	37	0	0	n/a	0	4	760
House sirloin	9 oz	310	48	0	0	n/a	13	5	970
New York strip	12 oz	590	60	0	0	n/a	39	18	550
Ribeye	12 oz	590	60	0	0	n/a	39	17	760
Chicken fried steak	as served	1290	53	123	13	n/a	65	15	4420
Shrimp 'N Parmesan sirloin	as served	540	66	5	0	n/a	28	14	2100
Steak & fried shrimp combo	as served	630	52	2	2	n/a	31	8	2030
Steak & grilled shrimp combo	as served	390	53	4	0	n/a	19	6	1740
Steak & honey BBQ chicken	as served	530	80	35	1	n/a	13	5	1840
Steak & riblets combo	as served	880–950	95	20–38	0–1	n/a	47	19	2650–3370
Steak topper: Grilled onions	as served	60	1	7	1	n/a	3	0.5	380
Steak topper: Sautéed garlic mushrooms	as served	130	1	2	0	n/a	14	7	200
Steak topper: Shrimp 'N Parmesan	as served	230	18	4	0	n/a	16	9	1120
RIBS									
Double-glazed baby back ribs	as served	1240–1460	61–70	87–129	7	n/a	73–75	23–24	2530–3650
Riblets basket	as served	1040–1110	62–63	71–89	5	n/a	56–57	18	2640–3360
Riblets platter	as served	1570–1700	98–100	10–130	7	n/a	87–88	29	4010–5650

APPLEBEE'S CONTINUED

Item	Serving Size	Calories	Protein	Carb	Fiber	Sugar	Total Fat	Sat Fat	Sodium
CHICKEN									
Chicken fried chicken	as served	1250	62	114	12	n/a	60	12	3450
Chicken Parmesan	as served	1330	81	114	12	n/a	61	20	3400
Chicken tenders basket	as served	1000	36	81	7	n/a	59	11	2140
Chicken tenders platter	as served	1300	49	104	10	n/a	77	14	2740
Crispy orange chicken	as served	2030	84	264	15	n/a	80	15	4480
Fiesta lime chicken	as served	1230	60	9	9	n/a	67	16	4390
Grilled chicken & portabello	as served	450	54	32	6	n/a	16	6	1810
Margherita chicken	as served	750	58	67	8	n/a	27	8	2320
Weight Watchers® garlic herb chicken	as served	370	49	37	7	n/a	6	1	1930
PASTAS									
Cheddar-Jack mac & cheese w/ chicken	as served	1250	58	70	4	n/a	83	38	3040
Chicken broccoli pasta Alfredo	as served	1420	69	109	9	n/a	81	40	2670
Florentine ravioli w/ chicken	as served	1410	86	70	6	n/a	90	42	3830
Provolone-stuffed meatballs w/ fettuccine	as served	1550	58	113	9	n/a	97	46	3910
Shrimp fettuccine Alfredo bowl	as served	1440	63	110	9	n/a	85	41	3320
Spicy shrimp diavolo	as served	500	32	79	12	n/a	10	3.5	1910
Three-cheese chicken penne	as served	1530	72	125	8	n/a	84	41	3130
BURGERS, SLIDERS, & SANDWICHES									
Bacon Cheddar cheeseburger	no sides	940	55	48	1	n/a	60	22	1610
Bacon cheese chicken grill	no sides	720	60	47	1	n/a	33	11	1810
BBQ pulled pork sliders	no sides	1020	55	89	3	n/a	48	15	2040
Blackened tilapia sandwich	no sides	710	35	52	2	n/a	41	8	1760

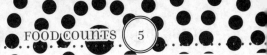

APPLEBEE'S CONTINUED

Item	Serving Size	Calories	Protein	Carb	Fiber	Sugar	Total Fat	Sat Fat	Sodium
California turkey club	no sides	1050	56	62	4	n/a	63	18	3600
Cheeseburger	no sides	850	48	47	1	n/a	52	19	1290
Chicken fajita rollup	no sides	1040	63	61	4	n/a	40	29	3280
Classic clubhouse grille	no sides	1130	56	77	3	n/a	65	21	3460
Cowboy burger	no sides	1120	58	74	3	n/a	67	23	2460
Fire Pit bacon burger	no sides	107	55	50	1	n/a	73	24	1900
French dip sliders	no sides	1310	56	82	3	n/a	85	27	2500
Green Garden turkey sandwich	no sides	780	37	58	8	n/a	45	8	2640
Hamburger	no sides	770	44	47	1	n/a	46	15	1170
Hand-battered fish sandwich	no sides	820	20	60	2	n/a	56	9	1160
Honey BBQ chicken sandwich	no sides	900	65	72	1	n/a	39	15	2380
Oriental chicken rollup	no sides	1060	31	110	6	n/a	54	11	2640
Philly burger	no sides	1090	60	70	5	n/a	63	25	2520
Quesadilla burger	no sides	1420	77	45	4	n/a	104	43	3740
Reuben	no sides	1130	54	49	7	n/a	80	28	3550
Slow simmered tender beef	no sides	940	33	96	5	n/a	48	12	2110
Southwest jalapeño burger	no sides	1110	52	65	1	n/a	70	24	2100
Spicy shrimp rollup	no sides	840	22	10	4	n/a	37	8	2580
Steakhouse burger w/ A.1. sauce	no sides	1190	50	63	3	n/a	82	24	2070
Veggie Burger	no sides	530	26	61	8	n/a	21	4	1390
Zesty ranch chicken sandwich	no sides	1140	43	74	4	n/a	75	22	2740

SOUPS & SIDES

Item	Serving Size	Calories	Protein	Carb	Fiber	Sugar	Total Fat	Sat Fat	Sodium
Baked potato	as served	380	5	8	2	n/a	29	19	520
Baked potato soup	1 bowl	420	17	27	2	n/a	30	14	1230
Broccoli Cheddar soup	1 bowl	360	13	18	2	n/a	26	16	1690
Clam chowder	1 bowl	350	13	22	1	n/a	24	14	1000
Chicken noodle soup	1 bowl	160	13	17	1	n/a	4	1	1120
Chicken tortilla soup	1 bowl	180	10	18	2	n/a	8	2.5	1570
Chili	1 bowl	540	38	24	4	n/a	32	15	1310
French onion soup	1 bowl	280	17	19	2	n/a	16	10	1380

APPLEBEE'S continued

Item	Serving Size	Calories	Protein	Carb	Fiber	Sugar	Total Fat	Sat Fat	Sodium
Fresh fruit	as served	70	1	17	3	n/a	0	0	0
Fried red potatoes	as served	150	4	22	3	n/a	5	1	640
Garlic mashed potatoes	as served	330	6	38	4	n/a	18	3.5	900
House salad	as served	230	13	12	2	n/a	15	7	390
Loaded baked potato	as served	45	10	28	2	n/a	35	21	680
Loaded mashed potatoes	as served	430	13	30	3	n/a	29	12	920
Seasonal vegetables	as served	40–60	1	8	2	n/a	0	n/a	340–400
Small Caesar salad	as served	90	5	10	3	n/a	3.5	1.5	125
Toasted garlic bread basket	as served	1190	16	75	3	n/a	93	28	1560
Tomato basil soup	1 bowl	250	5	27	3	n/a	14	7	1340

SALADS

Item	Serving Size	Calories	Protein	Carb	Fiber	Sugar	Total Fat	Sat Fat	Sodium
Apple walnut chicken salad	as served	1000	55	53	6	n/a	65	16	1670
Asian Crunch salad	as served	490	51	57	7	n/a	9	1	3170
California shrimp salad	as served	730	32	21	8	n/a	61	11	2080
Crispy shrimp Caesar salad	as served	1060	33	57	7	n/a	78	15	2270
Fried chicken salad	as served	1060	47	49	6	n/a	75	21	2130
Grilled chicken Caesar	as served	820	54	25	6	n/a	57	11	1640
Grilled shrimp 'n' spinach	as served	1050	50	68	13	n/a	72	11	2530
Grilled steak Caesar	as served	900	54	25	6	n/a	66	15	1860
Oriental chicken salad	as served	1310	34	88	11	n/a	93	15	1470
Oriental grilled chicken salad	as served	1240	53	87	9	n/a	77	12	2000
Pecan-crusted chicken salad	as served	1340	46	108	14	n/a	81	17	2600
Santa Fe chicken salad	as served	1300	60	58	11	n/a	94	25	3540
Weight Watchers® paradise chicken salad	as served	340	45	35	6	n/a	4.5	1	2060

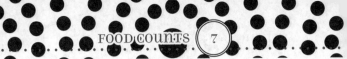

APPLEBEE'S continued

Item	Serving Size	Calories	Protein	Carb	Fiber	Sugar	Total Fat	Sat Fat	Sodium
DESSERTS									
Blue Ribbon brownie	as served	1290	16	172	6	n/a	63	31	740
Blue Ribbon brownie bite	as served	350	4	47	2	n/a	17	9	200
Chocolate chip cookie sundae	as served	1660	17	224	4	n/a	82	51	950
Chocolate mousse shooter	as served	450	3	44	2	n/a	31	20	280
Hot fudge sundae shooter	as served	340	3	45	0	n/a	18	14	150
Maple butter blondie	as served	990	13	116	5	n/a	52	28	870
Sizzling apple pie	as served	900	9	144	3	n/a	34	15	990
Strawberry cheesecake shooter	as served	380	5	41	1	n/a	23	16	270
Triple Chocolate Meltdown	as served	810	10	91	3	n/a	46	22	530

ARBY'S

Item	Serving Size	Calories	Protein	Carb	Fiber	Sugar	Total Fat	Sat Fat	Sodium
SANDWICHES									
All-American Roastburger®	each	390	19	40	2	10	16	5	1720
Arby's melt	each	320	18	38	2	6	11	3.5	900
Bacon & bleu Roastburger®	each	450	24	39	2	9	21	7	1750
Bacon Cheddar Roastburger®	each	430	26	39	2	8	18	8	1810
Chicken bacon & Swiss, boasted	each	470	32	43	3	10	19	6	1380
Chicken Cordon Bleu, boasted	each	490	35	40	3	8	20	5	1670
Classic Italian toasted sub	each	590	24	57	3	5	30	8	1870
French dip & Swiss toasted sub	each	500	29	59	2	2	17	7	2080
Ham & Swiss melt	each	300	18	37	2	6	8	3.5	1070
Jr. chicken sandwich	each	330	13	33	2	4	17	3	690
Jr. ham & Cheddar	each	200	13	26	2	5	5	1.5	890

ARBY'S continued

Item	Serving Size	Calories	Protein	Carb	Fiber	Sugar	Total Fat	Sat Fat	Sodium
Jr. roast beef	each	200	13	24	2	4	7	2.5	530
Pecan chicken salad sandwich	each	830	30	82	6	22	44	6	1390
Philly beef toasted sub	each	570	29	55	3	3	27	8	1490
Regular beef 'n Cheddar	each	430	23	42	2	10	19	6	1220
Regular roast beef	each	350	23	37	2	5	13	4.5	960
Reuben sandwich	each	690	36	65	4	7	32	9	2050
Roast beef & Swiss sandwich	each	780	39	78	5	17	37	11	1700
Roast beef gyro	each	420	20	32	2	3	23	6	1030
Roast beef patty melt	each	470	26	44	3	5	22	6	1790
Roast chicken club	each	500	31	38	2	8	23	7	1370
Roast chicken ranch sandwich	each	360	26	42	3	5	10	1.5	1030
Roast ham & Swiss sandwich	each	710	37	79	5	19	30	7	2030
Roast turkey & Swiss sandwich	each	710	41	78	5	18	28	7	1790
Roast turkey, ranch, & bacon sandwich	each	820	48	78	6	18	36	10	2270
Super roast beef	each	430	24	44	3	11	18	6	1070
Turkey bacon club toasted sub	each	570	33	56	3	4	24	6	1700
Ultimate BLT sandwich	each	850	34	78	6	18	46	10	1680

SIDES & SALADS

Item	Serving Size	Calories	Protein	Carb	Fiber	Sugar	Total Fat	Sat Fat	Sodium
Chopped farmhouse chicken salad, crispy	each	460	32	29	4	5	25	9	1090
Chopped farmhouse chicken salad, roasted	each	260	24	10	3	5	14	7	720
Chopped farmhouse salad, turkey, & ham	each	250	23	9	3	5	14	7	900
Chopped side salad	each	70	4	4	1	2	5	3	100
Crispy chicken tenders	regular	360	23	28	2	0	17	2.5	730
Curly fries	small	410	5	48	5	0	22	3	920
Curly fries	medium	540	7	64	6	0	29	4	1230
Curly fries	large	640	8	76	7	0	34	5	1460
Homestyle fries	small	350	4	49	4	0	15	2	720
Homestyle fries	medium	470	5	66	6	0	21	3	960

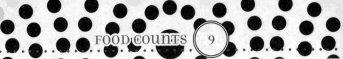

ARBY'S continued

Item	Serving Size	Calories	Protein	Carb	Fiber	Sugar	Total Fat	Sat Fat	Sodium
Homestyle fries	large	590	7	82	7	0	26	3.5	1200
Jalapeño Bites®	regular (5)	300	5	32	2	2	17	7	640
Jalapeño Bites®	large (8)	480	8	51	3	4	28	10	1030
Loaded Potato Bites®	regular (5)	340	10	29	2	1	20	6	760
Loaded Potato Bites®	large (8)	540	15	47	3	2	32	10	1210
Mozzarella sticks	regular (4)	430	20	36	2	3	23	9	1480
Mozzarella sticks	large (6)	650	30	54	2	4	35	13	2220
Onion petals	regular	330	4	38	2	7	18	2.5	280
Onion petals	large	600	7	70	4	12	33	5	510
Popcorn chicken	regular	360	26	27	2	0	24	3.5	280
Potato cakes	small	260	2	16	2	0	14	2	440
Potato cakes	medium	380	3	25	3	0	20	3	650
Potato cakes	large	510	4	33	5	0	27	4	870

SHAKES

Item	Serving Size	Calories	Protein	Carb	Fiber	Sugar	Total Fat	Sat Fat	Sodium
Chocolate swirl shake	regular	630	15	19	1	100	17	12	440
Jamocha swirl shake	regular	610	15	106	1	97	17	11	490
Vanilla swirl shake	regular	540	16	85	0	80	17	12	450

DESSERT ITEMS

Item	Serving Size	Calories	Protein	Carb	Fiber	Sugar	Total Fat	Sat Fat	Sodium
Apple turnover	1 turnover	270	4	32	1	11	15	7	290
Cherry turnover	1 turnover	270	4	31	1	10	15	7	300
Chocolate chunk cookies	2 each	420	4	54	2	34	21	10	55

KIDS' MEAL

Item	Serving Size	Calories	Protein	Carb	Fiber	Sugar	Total Fat	Sat Fat	Sodium
1% lowfat chocolate milk	as served	160	8	27	1	25	2.5	1.5	210
2% reduced fat milk	as served	130	8	13	0	12	5	3	125
Applesauce	as served	90	0	21	1	19	0	0	0
Capri Sun® fruit juice	as served	80	0	21	0	20	0	0	25
Curly fries	kids'	240	3	29	3	0	13	2	550
Homestyle fries	kids'	230	3	33	3	0	10	1.5	480
Jr. roast beef	each	200	13	24	2	4	7	2.5	530
Popcorn chicken	kids'	260	19	20	1	0	12	2	720
Potato cakes	2 cakes	260	2	16	2	0	14	2	440

ARTHUR TREACHER'S / NATHAN'S FAMOUS

Item	Serving Size	Calories	Protein	Carb	Fiber	Sugar	Total Fat	Sat Fat	Sodium
ENTRÉES									
Arthur Treacher's fish 'n chips	each	1515.8	34.1	156.3	9.9	40	95	15.1	2732.2
Arthur Treacher's fish sandwich	each	437.3	18.2	49.8	2.7	7.2	18.3	3.1	714.8
Arthur Treacher's seafood sampler	each	1964	47.3	195.5	15.8	46.8	122.7	19.9	2892.7
Arthur Treacher's shrimp 'n chips	each	1833.5	31.3	178.2	11.7	50.4	120.4	21.9	3394.9
Nathan's bacon cheeseburger	each	782.7	36.4	44.8	2.2	10.3	50.1	19.6	134.9
Nathan's cheese dog	each	390	12	30	1	5	25	8	1440
Nathan's chicken tender pita	each	823.1	21.9	66	5.4	14.6	52	7.7	1461.7
Nathan's chicken tender platter	each	1245	26	80.3	9.5	31	90	13.8	1352
Nathan's chicken tender sandwich	each	706.5	22.3	57.9	4.6	12.3	42.9	6.2	1165
Nathan's chicken tenders	each	526	21	24	3	7.5	39	5.5	900
Nathan's chicken wings	5 pieces	400	26.7	11.7	0	0	26.6	6.6	650
Nathan's chicken wings	10 pieces	800	53.3	23.3	0	0	53.3	13.3	1300
Nathan's chicken wings	20 pieces	1600	106.7	46.7	0	0	106.6	26.6	2600
Nathan's chili dog	each	400	16	33	2	5	23	6	1000
Nathan's corn dog on a stick	each	380	7	39	1	13	21	5	730
Nathan's double burger w/ cheese	each	1178.3	57.1	45	2.2	2.2	83.8	32.1	1298.8
Nathan's Famous hot dog	each	297	10.9	24	75	4	18.2	6.9	692
Nathan's grilled chicken Caesar wrap	each	700	38	60	1	2	34	11	1340
Nathan's grilled chicken platter	each	839.3	24.1	58.3	6.5	23.5	55.6	8.8	1133.7
Nathan's grilled chicken sandwich	each	554	27.4	39.9	2.6	3.3	31.9	5.1	1157.5
Nathan's hamburger w/ cheese	each	704.6	32.6	44.5	2.2	10.2	43.4	16.3	1070.5

ARTHUR TREACHER'S / NATHAN'S FAMOUS continued

Item	Serving Size	Calories	Protein	Carb	Fiber	Sugar	Total Fat	Sat Fat	Sodium
Nathan's hot dog nuggets	6 pieces	348.18	5	20	0	5	28	5.8	400.2
Nathan's Krispy Southwest chipotle wrap	each	750	68	62	1	3	39	13	1160
Nathan's Philly cheesesteak sandwich	each	849.2	43.9	70.2	2.4	1.2	44.6	20.5	1554.1
Nathan's Philly cheesesteak supreme	each	878.9	46.4	75.5	3.3	2.6	44.5	20.5	1625.1
Nathan's Philly chicken cheesesteak supreme	each	600.8	39.5	69.5	3.3	2.6	19.1	9	1719.2
Nathan's pretzel dog	each	390	12	49	1	7	16	6	970
Nathan's super cheeseburger	each	986.6	35.2	46.9	2.8	10.6	71.8	23	1348.6

SIDES & SNACKS

Item	Serving Size	Calories	Protein	Carb	Fiber	Sugar	Total Fat	Sat Fat	Sodium
Beer-battered onion rings	small	544.4	2.9	36.2	1.4	4.3	44.5	6.3	579.9
Beer-battered onion rings	large	786.3	4.2	52.3	2.1	6.3	64.3	9.1	837.6
Cheese fries	regular	563.9	4.7	41	3.7	4.7	42.1	6.7	785.3
Cheese fries	large	73.8	6.1	54.7	5.1	6.1	54.1	8.4	807
Cheese fries	super size	1199.2	9.9	162.8	7.9	9.9	89.4	14.2	1579.1
Corn on the cob	each	140	5	34	2	6	1.5	0	20
French fries	regular	463.9	3.7	35	3.7	3.7	34.1	4.7	55.3
French fries	large	633.8	5.1	48.7	5.1	5.1	46.1	6.4	77
French fries	super size	999.2	7.9	75.4	7.9	7.9	73.4	10.2	119.1
Mozzarella sticks	3 pieces	389.7	13.5	20.2	0.9	6.3	27.6	8	940.5
Pretzel	king size	180	6	38	1	1	1	0	940

DESSERTS

Item	Serving Size	Calories	Protein	Carb	Fiber	Sugar	Total Fat	Sat Fat	Sodium
Apple pie	each	314	3	33	0	9	19	3.8	310
Funnel cake	each	580	5	73	1	43	29	5	36

A&W

Item	Serving Size	Calories	Protein	Carb	Fiber	Sugar	Total Fat	Sat Fat	Sodium
SANDWICHES (INCLUDES BURGERS, CHICKEN, HOT DOGS, SHRIMP)									
Cheese dog	each	350	12	26	1	4	22	9	940
Cheeseburger	each	420	23	37	3	6	19	6	1040
Chicken strips	3	500	28	32	2	2	29	5	1050
Coney-chili cheese dog	each	380	14	28	2	5	23	9	1100
Coney-chili dog	each	340	14	26	2	5	20	9	900
Crispy chicken sandwich	each	550	30	52	5	6	25	4.5	1130
Crunchy shrimp	as served	340	13	34	2	1	19	5	820
Grilled chicken sandwich	each	400	35	31	4	7	15	3	820
Hamburger	each	380	21	33	4	7	30	10	880
Hot dog, plain	each	310	11	23	1	4	19	8	740
Original bacon cheeseburger	each	680	40	44	4	7	38	14	1330
Original bacon double cheeseburger	each	760	44	45	4	8	45	17	1570
Papa burger	each	690	40	44	4	8	39	14	1350
Papa single burger	each	470	23	38	4	7	25	8	1000
DIPPING SAUCES									
BBQ	as served	40	0	10	0	6	0	0	230
Cocktail	as served	25	0	6	0	5	0	0	250
Honey mustard	as served	100	0	12	0	6	6	1.5	170
Ketchup	as served	10	0	2	0	2	0	0	100
Marinara	as served	15	1	4	1	2	0	0	125
Ranch	as served	160	0	2	0	1	17	2.5	240
Sweet & sour	as served	45	0	12	0	7	0	0	120
Tartar	as served	100	0	4	0	3	9	1.5	250
SIDES									
Cheese curds	regular	570	27	62	7	4	27	7	990
Cheese curds	large	1140	54	27	2	3	40	21	1220
Cheese fries	as served	390	4	50	4	0	18	4.5	870
Chili	as served	190	12	54	4	6	80	42	640
Chili cheese fries	as served	410	8	52	5	1	17	5	990
Corn dog nuggets	small/kids'	180	5	20	1	6	8	2	520
Corn dog nuggets	regular	280	9	32	2	9	13	3	830
Extra burger patty	as served	170	15	22	12	0	6	2	170
French fries	small/kids'	200	2	28	3	0	8	2	290

A&W continued

Item	Serving Size	Calories	Protein	Carb	Fiber	Sugar	Total Fat	Sat Fat	Sodium
French fries	regular	310	3	45	4	0	12	3	460
French fries	large	430	5	61	6	1	17	4	640
Onion rings	regular	370	8	49	8	2	15	4	790
Onion rings	large	350	5	45	5	3	16	3.5	710

SWEETS & TREATS

Item	Serving Size	Calories	Protein	Carb	Fiber	Sugar	Total Fat	Sat Fat	Sodium
M&M'S Polar Swirl	as served	710	15	107	15	93	25	16	290
Oreo Polar Swirl	as served	690	14	107	14	79	24	11	570
Reese's Polar Swirl	as served	740	18	97	18	85	31	14	380

SHAKES

Item	Serving Size	Calories	Protein	Carb	Fiber	Sugar	Total Fat	Sat Fat	Sodium
Chocolate	small/kids'	700	11	100	0	60	29	18	200
Chocolate	medium	880	14	125	0	75	36	23	250
Strawberry	small/kids'	670	11	90	0	52	29	18	180
Strawberry	medium	840	14	113	0	65	36	23	230
Vanilla	small/kids'	720	12	97	0	57	31	19	210
Vanilla	medium	900	15	121	0	71	39	24	260
Vanilla cone	small/kids'	200	6	32	0	22	5	3	115
Vanilla cone	regular	260	7	41	0	29	7	4	145

FREEZES

Item	Serving Size	Calories	Protein	Carb	Fiber	Sugar	Total Fat	Sat Fat	Sodium
A&W root beer	small/kids'	370	7	68	0	62	8	5	170
A&W root beer	medium	480	9	89	1	81	10	6	230
A&W root beer	large	820	16	150	1	136	18	11	400
A&W root beer, diet	small/kids'	260	7	39	0	33	8	5	170
A&W root beer, diet	medium	340	9	53	1	45	10	6	230
A&W root beer, diet	large	600	16	92	1	78	18	11	400
Orange	small/kids'	450	7	108	24	79	8	5	170
Orange	medium	600	9	142	32	103	10	6	230
Orange	large	970	16	223	48	162	18	11	390

SUNDAES

Item	Serving Size	Calories	Protein	Carb	Fiber	Sugar	Total Fat	Sat Fat	Sodium
Caramel	each	340	8	57	0	13	9	4	230
Chocolate	each	320	8	53	0	15	8	4	180
Hot fudge	each	350	8	54	1	15	11	6	140
Strawberry	each	300	7	47	0	12	8	4	140

A&W continued

Item	Serving Size	Calories	Protein	Carb	Fiber	Sugar	Total Fat	Sat Fat	Sodium
FAMOUS FLOATS									
A&W root beer	small/kids'	330	2	70	0	57	5	3	100
A&W root beer	medium	350	2	77	0	64	5	3	105
A&W root beer	large	640	4	136	0	110	10	6	200
A&W root beer, diet	small/kids'	170	2	30	0	17	5	3	100
A&W root beer, diet	medium	170	2	30	0	17	5	3	105
A&W root beer, diet	large	350	4	60	0	34	10	6	200
Orange	small/kids'	320	4	74	8	63	4.5	3	115
Orange	medium	340	4	81	8	70	4.5	3	120
Orange	large	610	8	137	12	118	9	6	230
SMOOTHIES									
Pineapple banana	small/kids'	400	3	85	1	80	6	4.5	100
Pineapple banana	medium	480	3	104	1	98	6	4.5	104
Pineapple banana	large	750	6	160	2	151	10	7	200
Strawberry	small/kids'	360	3	70	0	59	6	4.5	85
Strawberry	medium	370	3	74	0	63	6	4.5	90
Strawberry	large	610	6	121	0	102	10	7	170
Strawberry banana	small/kids'	390	3	78	0	66	6	4.5	95
Strawberry banana	medium	420	3	86	0	74	6	4.5	100
Strawberry banana	large	680	6	137	0	118	10	7	190
BLENDRRR									
Chocolate fudge	small/kids'	490	4	68	1	46	30	25	100
Chocolate fudge	medium	560	4	92	3	56	32	27	125
Chocolate fudge	large	1010	8	152	3	97	5	49	220
Oreo cookies & cream	small/kids'	340	4	56	1	44	12	6	230
Oreo cookies & cream	medium	430	5	72	2	56	15	7	310
Oreo cookies & cream	large	190	8	109	2	84	21	10	450
Reese's peanut butter	small/kids'	700	7	103	3	66	41	30	180
Reese's peanut butter	medium	710	7	108	3	70	41	30	180
Reese's peanut butter	large	1360	14	203	5	131	79	57	360

A&W continued

Item	Serving Size	Calories	Protein	Carb	Fiber	Sugar	Total Fat	Sat Fat	Sodium
LIMEADES & SLUSHIES									
Blue raspberry slushie	small	280	0	67	0	63	0	0	35
Blue raspberry slushie	medium	380	0	91	0	85	0	0	45
Blue raspberry slushie	large	480	0	142	0	137	0	0	60
Cherry limeade	small	190	0	51	0	45	0	0	30
Cherry limeade	medium	300	0	79	0	70	0	0	45
Cherry limeade	large	340	0	90	0	80	0	0	55
Cherry slushie	small	330	0	83	0	63	0	0	25
Cherry slushie	medium	450	0	112	0	85	0	0	40
Cherry slushie	large	570	0	141	0	107	0	0	45
Lemon slushie	small	330	0	82	0	54	0	0	35
Lemon slushie	medium	440	0	110	0	74	0	0	45
Lemon slushie	large	560	0	139	0	94	0	0	60
Limeade	small	140	0	38	0	33	0	0	25
Limeade	medium	210	0	55	0	46	0	0	40
Limeade	large	250	0	66	0	56	0	0	45
Limeade slushie	small	280	0	69	0	54	0	0	35
Limeade slushie	medium	380	0	94	0	74	0	0	50
Limeade slushie	large	480	0	119	0	94	0	0	60
Strawberry limeade	small	230	0	58	0	49	0	0	35
Strawberry limeade	medium	290	0	75	0	62	0	0	45
Strawberry limeade	large	420	0	105	0	88	0	0	60
Watermelon slushie	small	270	0	73	0	77	0	0	50
Watermelon slushie	medium	360	0	99	0	104	0	0	65
Watermelon slushie	large	460	0	124	0	131	0	0	85
ROOT BEER									
A&W root beer, diet	small/kids'	0	0	0	0	0	0	0	40
A&W root beer, diet	medium	0	0	0	0	0	0	0	50
A&W root beer, diet	large	0	0	0	0	0	0	0	80
A&W root beer, regular	small/kids'	220	0	58	0	58	0	0	40
A&W root beer, regular	medium	270	0	72	0	72	0	0	50
A&W root beer, regular	large	440	0	116	0	116	0	0	80

AUNTIE ANNE'S

Item	Serving Size	Calories	Protein	Carb	Fiber	Sugar	Total Fat	Sat Fat	Sodium
PRETZELS & MORE									
Almond pretzel, soft pretzel, w/o butter	each	350	8	74	2	17	2	1	640
Cheese pretzel dog, w/o butter	each	340	12	33	1	5	17	7	640
Cinnamon sugar party pretzel	each	250	4	43	1	15	6	3.5	210
Cinnamon sugar pretzel nuggets, w/o butter	1 cup	460	9	99	2	3	2.5	0	300
Cinnamon sugar stix, w/o butter	6 sticks	380	8	84	2	29	1	0	400
Cinnamon sugar, soft pretzel, w/o butter	each	350	8	74	2	16	2	0	410
Garlic, soft pretzel, w/o butter	each	320	9	66	2	9	1	0	830
Jalapeño cheese pretzel dog, w/o butter	each	340	12	34	1	5	17	7	700
Jalapeño, soft pretzel, w/o butter	each	270	8	58	2	8	1	0	780
Original party pretzel	each	180	4	34	1	5	2	1.5	510
Original pretzel nuggets, w/o butter	1 cup	360	9	75	2	11	1.5	0	1280
Original stix, without butter	6 sticks	310	8	65	2	10	1	0	990
Original, soft pretzel, w/o butter	each	340	8	72	3	10	1	0	900
Pepperoni pretzel, w/o butter	each	440	15	65	2	10	12	5	850
Pretzel dog, w/o butter	each	320	11	33	1	5	16	6	740
Pretzel pocket, bacon, egg, cheese, w/o butter	each	550	23	71	2	12	20	8	790
Pretzel pocket, pepperoni & mozzarella, w/o butter	each	620	25	75	2	11	24	10	1120
Pretzel pocket, turkey & Cheddar, w/o butter	each	440	20	73	2	14	6	2.5	1050
Raisin pretzel, w/o butter	each	360	8	69	2	16	1	0	390
Sesame, soft pretzel, w/o butter	each	350	11	63	3	9	6	1	840
Sour cream & onion pretzel, w/o butter	each	330	9	68	2	12	0.5	0	1180

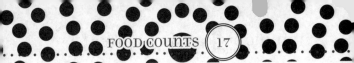

AUNTIE ANNE'S continued

Item	Serving Size	Calories	Protein	Carb	Fiber	Sugar	Total Fat	Sat Fat	Sodium
Whole wheat, soft pretzel, w/o butter	each	350	11	72	7	10	1.5	0	1100

DIPS

Item	Serving Size	Calories	Protein	Carb	Fiber	Sugar	Total Fat	Sat Fat	Sodium
Caramel	each	130	1	23	0	19	3	1.5	9
Cheese	each	100	3	2	0	0	8	3	470
Heated marinara sauce	each	20	1	5	2	4	0.5	0	330
Hot salsa cheese	each	90	2	4	0	3	7	3	450
Light cream cheese	each	80	3	1	0	0	6	4.5	120
Marinara sauce	each	45	1	7	2	4	1	0	240
Melted cheese	each	150	5	6	0	4	12	3	850
Sweet	each	130	0	32	0	32	0	0	0
Sweet mustard	each	60	2	10	0	9	2	1	0

BAJA FRESH

Item	Serving Size	Calories	Protein	Carb	Fiber	Sugar	Total Fat	Sat Fat	Sodium
BURRITO ULTIMO®									
Breaded fish	1 burrito	940	41	96	8	n/a	42	19	1950
Carnitas	1 burrito	920	46	86	9	n/a	44	21	2330
Chicken	1 burrito	880	54	84	9	n/a	36	18	2190
Mahi mahi	1 burrito	880	52	84	8	n/a	36	18	1890
Shrimp	1 burrito	860	48	85	8	n/a	36	18	2280
Steak	1 burrito	950	50	85	8	n/a	44	21	2310
BAJA BURRITO									
Breaded fish	1 burrito	850	40	78	7	n/a	44	16	1900
Carnitas	1 burrito	830	45	67	8	n/a	45	18	2280
Chicken	1 burrito	790	52	65	8	n/a	38	15	2140
Mahi mahi	1 burrito	780	51	66	7	n/a	38	15	1840
Shrimp	1 burrito	760	47	66	7	n/a	37	15	2230
Steak	1 burrito	850	49	67	7	n/a	46	18	2260
BURRITO MEXICANO									
Breaded fish	1 burrito	850	37	129	18	n/a	19	4	2040
Cabo style	1 burrito	980	50	81	11	n/a	52	20	1770
Caesar style	1 burrito	940	48	75	8	n/a	50	19	1930

BAJA FRESH continued

Item	Serving Size	Calories	Protein	Carb	Fiber	Sugar	Total Fat	Sat Fat	Sodium
Carnitas	1 burrito	830	42	119	19	n/a	20	6	2420
Chicken	1 burrito	790	50	117	20	n/a	13	3.5	2270
Diablo shrimp	1 burrito	1000	56	130	19	n/a	34	12	2930
Mahi mahi	1 burrito	790	49	117	18	n/a	13	3.5	1970
Nacho	1 burrito	1250	75	145	23	n/a	42	17	3200
Shrimp	1 burrito	770	44	117	18	n/a	13	3.5	2370
Steak	1 burrito	860	47	118	18	n/a	21	7	2400
BEAN AND CHEESE BURRITO									
Bare Burrito® w/ carnitas	1 burrito	680	37	99	20	n/a	14	4	2480
Bare Burrito® w/ steak	1 burrito	700	41	99	19	n/a	15	4.5	2450
Bare Burrito® w/ chicken	1 burrito	640	45	97	20	n/a	7	1	2330
Enchilado Style® to burrito add:	as served	630	23	45	7	n/a	40	19	1450
Breaded fish	1 burrito	1030	54	108	20	n/a	41	18	1990
Carnitas	1 burrito	1010	59	98	21	n/a	42	20	2370
Chicken	1 burrito	970	67	96	21	n/a	35	18	2230
Grilled veggies	1 burrito	800	32	94	16	n/a	33	17	1880
Mahi mahi	1 burrito	960	65	96	20	n/a	35	18	1930
No meat	1 burrito	840	39	96	20	n/a	33	17	1790
Shrimp	1 burrito	950	61	96	20	n/a	34	17	2320
Steak	1 burrito	1030	64	97	20	n/a	43	21	2350
Veggie & cheese Bare Burrito®	1 burrito	580	19	101	20	n/a	10	4	1950
TACOS									
Americano soft taco, breaded fish	1 taco	240	10	23	2	n/a	11	4.5	490
Americano soft taco, carnitas	1 taco	250	13	21	2	n/a	12	5	640
Americano soft taco, chicken	1 taco	230	16	20	2	n/a	10	4.5	590
Americano soft taco, mahi mahi	1 taco	240	17	20	2	n/a	10	4.5	490
Americano soft taco, shrimp	1 taco	230	15	21	2	n/a	10	4.5	640

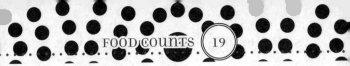

BAJA FRESH continued

Item	Serving Size	Calories	Protein	Carb	Fiber	Sugar	Total Fat	Sat Fat	Sodium
Americano soft taco, steak	1 taco	260	15	21	2	n/a	13	6	640
Baja fish taco, fried	1 taco	250	8	27	2	n/a	13	2	420
Carnitas Baja taco	1 taco	220	10	29	2	n/a	7	2	280
Chicken Baja taco	1 taco	210	12	28	2	n/a	5	1	230
Grilled mahi mahi	1 taco	230	12	26	4	n/a	9	1.5	300
Shrimp Baja taco	1 taco	200	11	28	2	n/a	5	1	280
Steak Baja taco	1 taco	230	11	28	2	n/a	8	2	260

QUESADILLAS

Item	Serving Size	Calories	Protein	Carb	Fiber	Sugar	Total Fat	Sat Fat	Sodium
Breaded fish	1 quesadilla	1400	62	96	8	n/a	86	38	2350
Charbroiled chicken	1 quesadilla	1330	75	84	9	n/a	80	37	2590
Charbroiled mahi mahi	1 quesadilla	1330	73	84	8	n/a	79	37	2290
Charbroiled shrimp	1 quesadilla	1310	69	84	8	n/a	79	37	2680
Charbroiled steak	1 quesadilla	1430	80	84	8	n/a	87	41	2600
Cheese	1 quesadilla	1200	47	84	8	n/a	78	37	2140
Savory pork carnitas	1 quesadilla	1370	67	86	9	n/a	87	40	2730
Veggie	1 quesadilla	1260	48	96	11	n/a	78	37	2310

NACHOS

Item	Serving Size	Calories	Protein	Carb	Fiber	Sugar	Total Fat	Sat Fat	Sodium
Breaded fish	as served	2090	78	176	31	n/a	116	41	2740
Charbroiled chicken	as served	2020	91	164	32	n/a	110	41	2980
Charbroiled Mahi mahi	as served	2020	90	164	31	n/a	110	41	2680
Charbroiled shrimp	as served	2000	85	164	31	n/a	110	41	3060
Charbroiled steak	as served	2120	96	163	31	n/a	118	44	2990
Cheese	as served	1890	63	163	31	n/a	108	40	2530
Savory pork carnitas	as served	2060	83	166	32	n/a	117	43	3120

TORTA

Item	Serving Size	Calories	Protein	Carb	Fiber	Sugar	Total Fat	Sat Fat	Sodium
W/ chips	as served	880	54	96	9	n/a	35	9	1580
W/o chips	as served	620	45	64	6	n/a	23	6	1330

BAJA FRESH continued

Item	Serving Size	Calories	Protein	Carb	Fiber	Sugar	Total Fat	Sat Fat	Sodium
FAJITAS									
Breaded fish w/ corn tortillas	as served	1060	51	130	22		37	9	2180
Breaded fish w/ flour tortillas	as served	1340	59	172	25		46	12	3020
Breaded fish w/ mixed tortillas	as served	1260	57	162	24		43	11	2740
Carnitas w/ corn tortillas	as served	920	50	108	23		34	11	2610
Carnitas w/ flour tortillas	as served	1190	58	150	26		43	14	3450
Carnitas w/ mixed tortillas	as served	1120	55	140	26		40	13	3170
Chicken taquitos w/ beans	as served	780	39	68	17		40	12	1810
Chicken taquitos w/ rice	as served	740	30	66	8		40	11	1770
Chicken w/ corn tortillas	as served	860	61	105	24		24	7	2400
Chicken w/ flour tortillas	as served	1140	69	147	27		33	10	3240
Chicken w/ mixed tortillas	as served	1070	67	137	26		30	9	2960
Mahi mahi w/ corn tortillas	as served	840	57	105	22		23	7	1960
Mahi mahi w/ flour tortillas	as served	1120	64	147	25		32	10	2800
Mahi mahi w/ mixed tortillas	as served	1050	62	138	24		29	9	2520
Shrimp w/ corn tortillas	as served	840	55	106	22		23	7	2570
Shrimp w/ flour tortillas	as served	1120	62	148	25		32	10	3410
Shrimp w/ mixed tortillas	as served	1045	60	138	24		29	9	3130
Steak w/ corn tortillas	as served	960	58	107	22		36	12	2600
Steak w/ flour tortillas	as served	1240	65	149	25		45	15	3440
Steak w/ mixed tortillas	as served	1170	63	139	24		42	14	3160

BAJA FRESH continued

Item	Serving Size	Calories	Protein	Carb	Fiber	Sugar	Total Fat	Sat Fat	Sodium
BAJA ENSALADA® (SALADS)									
Charbroiled chicken	as served	310	46	18	7		7	2	1210
Charbroiled shrimp	as served	230	28	18	6		6	2	1110
Charbroiled steak	as served	450	54	18	6		18	7	1240
Savory pork carnitas	as served	370	35	20	7		18	6	1410
TOSTADA SALAD									
Breaded fish	as served	1200	47	111	25		61	15	2140
Charbroiled chicken	as served	1140	60	98	27		55	14	2370
Charbroiled fish	as served	1130	59	99	25		55	14	2070
Charbroiled shrimp	as served	1120	55	99	25		55	14	2460
Charbroiled steak	as served	1230	65	98	25		63	17	2380
Mango chipotle chicken salad	as served	930	42	67	10		2.5	9	1960
No meat	as served	1010	32	98	25		53	13	1930
Savory pork carnitas	as served	1180	52	100	26		62	17	2520
DRESSINGS, SOUPS, & SIDES									
Black beans	side	360	23	61	26		2.5	1	1120
Breaded fish	side	390	30	25	0		16	2.5	410
Carnitas	side	300	35	4	2		16	6	1010
Chicken	side	230	48	0	2		3.5	0.5	760
Chicken tortilla soup w/charbroiled chicken	as served	320	17	29	4		14	4	2760
Chicken tortilla soup w/o charbroiled chicken	as served	270	8	29	4		14	4	2600
Chips & Salsa Baja™	as served	810	13	98	14		37	4	1140
Corn tortilla chips	1.5 oz	210	3	29	3		9	1	55
Corn tortilla chips	5 oz	740	10	90	9		34	3.5	170
Fat-free salsa verde	as served	15	0	3	1		0	0	370
Guacamole	8 oz	310	6	14	6		35	3	710
Mahi mahi	side	210	44	1	0		3	1	240
Olive oil vinaigrette	as served	290	0	2	0		31	4.5	290
Pico de gallo	8 oz	50	2	12	3		0.5	0	890
Pinto beans	side	320	19	56	21		1	0	840
Ranch dressing	as served	260	2	4	0		26	6	470
Rice	side	280	5	55	4		4	0.5	980

BAJA FRESH continued

Item	Serving Size	Calories	Protein	Carb	Fiber	Sugar	Total Fat	Sat Fat	Sodium
Rice & beans plate	as served	420	18	72	18		5	1.5	1320
Salsa Baja™	8 oz	70	2	7	4		2.5	0	970
Salsa roja	8 oz	70	3	13	4		1	0	1080
Salsa verde	8 oz	50	2	11	3		0	0	1170
Shrimp	side	150	31	1	0		2	0.5	740
Steak	side	330	48	0	0		14	6	670
Tostada shell	each	490	7	44	4		28	3.5	600
Veggie mix (grilled peppers, chilies, & onions)	as served	110	3	24	6		0	0	330

BASKIN-ROBBINS

Item	Serving Size	Calories	Protein	Carb	Fiber	Sugar	Total Fat	Sat Fat	Sodium
ICE CREAM, SORBET, & FROZEN YOGURT									
Butter almond crunch reduced-fat ice cream	2.5 oz	140	4	19	3	4	7	3	90
Butter pecan, old-fashioned ice cream	2.5 oz	170	3	15	1	14	11	6	60
Chocolate chip cookie dough ice cream	2.5 oz	180	3	22	0	19	9	6	80
Fat-free vanilla frozen yogurt	2.5 oz	90	4	20	0	19	0	0	65
Lemon blueberry frozen yogurt	2.5 oz	120	3	21	0	19	3.5	2.5	45
Lemon sorbet	2.5 oz	80	0	21	0	20	0	0	10
Pink grapefruit sorbet	2.5 oz	80	0	21	0	20	0	0	10
Premium churned light aloha brownie ice cream	2.5 oz	150	3	26	1	21	5	3	95
Premium churned light cappuccino chip ice cream	2.5 oz	140	3	20	1	18	5	2.5	70
Premium churned light dulce de leche ice cream	2.5 oz	140	3	24	0	22	4.5	3	90
Premium churned reduced-fat, no sugar added, Cabana Berry Banana ice cream	2.5 oz	90	3	17	2	4	3.5	2	45

BASKIN-ROBBINS continued

Item	Serving Size	Calories	Protein	Carb	Fiber	Sugar	Total Fat	Sat Fat	Sodium
Premium churned feduced-fat, no sugar added, Caramel Turtle Truffle ice cream	2.5 oz	120	3	24	2	4	5	3.5	75
Real fruit strawberry sorbet	2.5 oz	80	0	21	0	21	0	0	5
Rocky Road ice cream	2.5 oz	180	3	22	0	20	10	5	75
Vanilla pomegranate parfait frozen yogurt	2.5 oz	150	3	23	0	19	5	3.5	55
SUNDAES									
Two-scoop	as served	530	8	61	0	51	29	19	200
Banana Royale	as served	620	9	87	5	73	28	19	200
Brownie	as served	920	12	119	2	97	47	22	460
Chocolate chip cookie dough	as served	990	13	138	2	107	43	28	540
Classic banana split	as served	1010	12	173	8	125	34	20	240
Made with Snickers	as served	1000	16	138	3	113	46	25	710
Reese's peanut butter cup	as served	1220	27	109	6	92	80	32	700
Strawberry soft serve	regular	450	12	59	1	57	18	11	310
31° BELOW™ SHAKES									
Chocolate chip cookie dough	medium	940	20	143	1	114	34	20	660
Chocolate Oreo	medium	1290	22	187	3	154	55	29	1080
Fudge brownie	medium	1390	26	199	2	164	58	28	990
Jamoca Oreo	medium	860	19	128	2	94	33	19	710
Oreo	medium	1000	21	143	3	110	41	21	920
Reese's peanut butter cup	medium	1220	33	134	5	121	67	28	870

BLIMPIE

Item	Serving Size	Calories	Protein	Carb	Fiber	Sugar	Total Fat	Sat Fat	Sodium
SUBS & BURGERS									
Blimpie Best®	6"	450	24	49	3	10	17	6	1330
Blimpie burger	each	460	21	42	2	6	24	10	1280
Blimpie dog	each	510	17	45	1	4	29	12	1420
B.L.T.	6"	430	15	43	2	6	22	5	960
Chicken Caesar wrap	each	560	30	56	4	5	24	8	1480
Chicken Cheddar bacon ranch	6"	600	36	48	3	8	29	10	1570
Chicken teriyaki	6"	450	33	52	2	13	12	5	1280
Ciabatta, Buffalo chicken	each	540	31	49	3	5	23	7	1970
Ciabatta, French dip	each	430	31	49	2	2	11	4.5	1820
Ciabatta, grilled chicken Caesar	each	580	34	62	3	4	20	5	1480
Ciabatta, Mediterranean	each	450	26	65	3	6	8	3	1720
Ciabatta, roast beef, turkey, Cheddar	each	520	25	51	3	6	24	8	1780
Ciabatta, Sicilian	each	590	29	66	3	9	22	6	2170
Ciabatta, spicy chicken & pepperoni	each	710	33	65	3	4	34	11	2070
Ciabatta, Tuscan	each	570	28	65	3	6	20	6	2030
Ciabatta, ultimate club	each	520	27	47	2	5	24	7	1600
Club	6"	410	23	49	3	9	13	4	1050
Cuban	6"	410	29	43	1	6	11	4.5	1630
French dip	6"	410	30	46	1	3	11	5	1650
Ham & American cheese kids' sub	3"	260	14	32	2	6	8	4.5	900
Ham & Swiss	6"	420	23	49	3	10	14	4.5	1020
Ham, salami, & provolone	6"	470	24	49	3	9	20	7	1270
Hot pastrami	6"	430	30	42	1	5	16	7	1350
Meatball	6"	580	27	50	4	6	31	13	1960
Philly steak & onion	6"	600	25	46	1	7	35	11	1410
Reuben	6"	530	34	52	3	7	20	6	1740
Roast beef & provolone	6"	430	28	46	3	7	14	5	980
Southwestern wrap	each	530	23	61	4	10	22	6	1770
Special vegetarian (Doritos sub)	6"	590	16	66	4	10	30	9	1170
Tuna	6"	470	24	43	2	5	21	3	770
Tuna kids' sub	3"	280	14	30	2	4	11	1.5	460

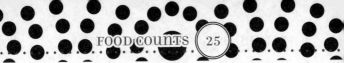

BLIMPIE continued

Item	Serving Size	Calories	Protein	Carb	Fiber	Sugar	Total Fat	Sat Fat	Sodium
Turkey & avocado	6"	360	21	51	4	8	7	1	1340
Turkey & bacon, Super Stacked™	6"	367	43	49	2	9	29	10	2690
Turkey & cranberry	6"	350	20	58	3	14	4	0.5	1220
Turkey & provolone	6"	410	24	49	3	8	13	4	1310
Turkey kids' sub	3"	190	10	31	2	5	2.5	0	600
Veggie & cheese	6"	460	19	50	3	9	21	9	1420
Veggie supreme	6"	550	26	50	3	9	27	13	1500
VegiMax™	6"	520	28	56	5	8	20	6	1270

SALADS

Item	Serving Size	Calories	Protein	Carb	Fiber	Sugar	Total Fat	Sat Fat	Sodium
Antipasto	as served	250	20	12	4	6	14	6	1630
Buffalo chicken	as served	220	25	10	4	5	9	5	840
Chicken Caesar	as served	190	25	6	3	3	8	4	460
Cole slaw, side	side	160	1	20	2	17	9	1.5	240
Garden	as served	30	2	6	3	3	0	0	15
Macaroni salad, side	side	330	5	28	2	8	22	5	790
Northwest potato salad, side	side	260	3	22	3	3	17	4	390
Potato salad, side	side	230	3	28	3	8	12	2.5	490
Tuna salad	as served	270	18	6	3	3	19	2.5	370
Ultimate club	as served	260	23	10	3	5	14	7	1070

SOUPS

Item	Serving Size	Calories	Protein	Carb	Fiber	Sugar	Total Fat	Sat Fat	Sodium
Bean w/ ham	1 serving	140	8	23	11	2	1	0	1070
Beef steak and noodle	1 serving	120	8	14	0	4	4	1.5	780
Beef stew	1 serving	170	17	18	2	2	4	3.5	890
Captain's corn chowder	1 serving	210	6	29	4	7	7	2.5	890
Chicken & dumpling	1 serving	170	11	19	3	4	7	3	970
Chicken gumbo	1 serving	90	6	13	2	4	2	0	1280
Chicken noodle	1 serving	130	7	18	2	5	4	1	1040
Chicken w/ white & wild rice	1 serving	250	14	15	4	4	10	2.5	1030
Cream of broccoli w/ cheese	1 serving	250	7	13	<1	2	19	11	1040
Cream of potato	1 serving	190	5	24	3	3	9	2.5	860

BLIMPIE continued

Item	Serving Size	Calories	Protein	Carb	Fiber	Sugar	Total Fat	Sat Fat	Sodium
French onion	1 serving	80	2	11	1	6	4	0.5	1020
Garden vegetable	1 serving	80	5	14	3	5	1	0	620
Grande chili w/ bean & beef	1 serving	310	20	31	9	9	9	4	1440
Harvest vegetable	1 serving	100	4	19	3	4	1	0	920
Italian style wedding	1 serving	130	7	17	0	0	4	1.5	900
Minestrone	1 serving	90	4	14	4	4	3	0	1150
New England clam chowder	1 serving	170	7	28	2	5	3	2	1060
Pasta fagioli w/ sausage	1 serving	150	7	22	4	2	5	1.5	910
Split pea w/ ham	1 serving	130	8	21	6	1	2	0	1090
Tomato basil w/ raviolini	1 serving	110	4	22	0	5	1	0	720
Vegetable beef	1 serving	80	4	13	2	3	2	0.5	1010
Yankee pot roast	1 serving	80	5	12	2	2	2	0.5	750

BREAKFAST ITEMS

Item	Serving Size	Calories	Protein	Carb	Fiber	Sugar	Total Fat	Sat Fat	Sodium
Bagel	each	290	11	58	3	12	1	0	700
Bagel, cream cheese	each	390	13	59	3	12	11	6	780
Biscuit, bacon, egg, & cheese	each	520	22	38	1	4	30	18	1940
Biscuit, egg & cheese	each	380	13	37	1	4	20	15	1380
Biscuit, ham, egg, & cheese	each	420	19	39	1	5	21	15	1660
Biscuit, sausage, egg, & cheese	each	530	19	37	1	4	34	20	1690
Biscuit w/ sausage gravy	each	460	12	43	2	4	27	14	132
Bluffin, bacon, egg, & cheese	each	270	14	27	2	2	12	5	890
Bluffin, egg & cheese	each	240	12	27	2	2	10	5	770
Bluffin, ham, egg, & cheese	each	280	17	29	2	4	10	5	1050
Bluffin, plain	each	130	5	25	2	2	1	0	240
Bluffin, sausage, egg, & cheese	each	390	18	27	2	2	24	10	1080
Burrito, bacon, egg, & cheese	each	580	26	57	5	2	28	12	2320

BLIMPIE continued

Item	Serving Size	Calories	Protein	Carb	Fiber	Sugar	Total Fat	Sat Fat	Sodium
Burrito, egg & cheese	each	50	21	57	5	2	23	10	2010
Burrito, ham, egg, & cheese	each	580	32	60	5	5	24	10	2560
Burrito, sausage, egg, & cheese	each	800	33	57	5	2	50	20	2620
Burrito, turkey, egg, & cheese	each	560	29	59	5	3	23	10	2530
Cinnamon roll	each	450	9	60	2	17	20	9	730
Egg & cheese on a roll	each	200	10	22	1	2	9	4	650
Grilled breakfast sandwich, bacon	each	480	25	44	1	4	23	10	1620
Grilled breakfast sandwich, ham	each	480	30	47	1	7	6	9	1860
Grilled breakfast sandwich, sausage	each	710	32	44	1	4	45	18	1920
Grilled breakfast sandwich, turkey	each	460	28	46	1	5	18	8	1830
DESSERTS									
Brownie	each	230	3	28	1	21	10	4	115
Chocolate chunk cookie	each	200	2	25	0	16	10	4.5	150
Oatmeal raisin cookie	each	180	2	27	<1	16	7	3	150
Peanut butter cookie	each	210	3	21	<1	13	13	5	170
Sugar cookie	each	320	3	42	0	23	16	6	240
White chocolate macadamia nut cookie	each	200	2	25	0	16	11	4.5	110

BOB EVANS

Item	Serving Size	Calories	Protein	Carb	Fiber	Sugar	Total Fat	Sat Fat	Sodium
APPETIZERS									
Breaded garlic mushrooms	as served	461	11	63	3	2	18	3	1585
County Fair cheese bites	as served	942	41	47	5	4	66	32	1757
Fried green tomatoes	as served	554	6	3	6	10	22	3	2278
Loaded potato bites	as served	1008	16	93	6	7	63	1	2180
Wildfire chicken quesadilla	as served	765	62	55	6	19	34	17	1512
BREAKFAST ITEMS									
Biscuit sandwich	each	584	22	33	1	3	39	17	1475
Blueberry crepe	each	306	5	40	2	25	14	6	292
Blueberry pancake, no topping	each	335	5	60	0	15	8	4	784
Blueberry-banana mini fruit & yogurt parfait	each	166	4	36	3	32	1	0	60
Blueberry-stuffed French toast	each	730	15	90	5	60	19	9	990
Border Scramble® biscuit bowl	each	1028	53	75	5	8	57	25	3055
Border Scramble® omelet	each	635	39	14	2	7	46	18	1519
Buttermilk hotcake, no topping	each	329	5	58	0	14	8	4	783
Country biscuit breakfast	each	594	21	41	1	3	39	18	1524
Farmer's Market omelet	each	631	37	14	1	6	45	21	2129
French toast	each	164	4	18	1	9	3	1	283
Fresh fruit plate with low-fat strawberry yogurt	each	353	7	84	8	70	2	0	73
Garden Harvest omelet	each	542	30	14	2	6	38	17	1762
Grits	1 bowl	265	4	4	2	1	11	5	252
Ham & Cheddar omelet	each	515	40	4	0	2	36	13	1808
Hardcooked egg	each	57	6	1	0	0	4	1	52
Meat Lovers BoBurrito	each	805	44	40	3	7	52	19	1883
Mini fruit & yogurt parfait	each	177	4	39	3	34	1	0	61
Multigrain hotcake, no topping	each	341	8	62	4	16	7	4	878
Mush	each	171	2	25	5	10	7	1	1012
Oatmeal	1 bowl	168	6	31	4	1	3	0	9

BOB EVANS continued

Item	Serving Size	Calories	Protein	Carb	Fiber	Sugar	Total Fat	Sat Fat	Sodium
Plain crepe	each	255	5	27	1	14	14	6	285
Pot roast hash	each	749	43	32	3	6	49	16	1307
Roasted caramel apple crepe	each	361	5	52	2	26	14	6	328
Roasted caramel-apple-stuffed French toast	each	839	15	116	5	61	20	9	1063
Sausage & Cheddar omelet	each	552	35	4	0	2	43	16	1253
Sausage biscuit bowl	each	998	32	76	4	4	61	28	3166
Sausage breakfast patty	each	140	8	0	0	0	11	4	323
Sausage gravy	1 bowl	294	8	23	0	2	19	12	1375
Sausage link	each	133	5	0	0	0	12	3	184
Scrambled Bob Evans Egg Lites®	each	28	6	1	0	1	0	0	119
Scrambled egg whites	each	25	6	1	0	0	0	0	90
Smoked ham	each	99	16	3	0	1	3	1	1293
Spinach, bacon & tomato biscuit bowl	each	1013	36	79	4	7	60	29	3510
Stacked & stuffed blueberry cream hotcakes	each	1031	15	170	3	75	33	18	1835
Stacked & stuffed cinnamon cream hotcakes	each	1053	14	160	1	67	40	22	1895
Stacked & stuffed strawberry banana cream hotcakes	each	1151	16	202	9	98	33	18	1821
Strawberry & banana crepes	each	314	6	43	3	26	14	6	285
Strawberry banana & yogurt parfait	each	151	4	33	3	28	1	0	55
Strawberry blueberry mini fruit & yogurt parfait	each	151	4	33	3	28	1	0	55
Strawberry-stuffed French toast	each	685	15	80	5	49	19	9	977
Stuffed French toast, no topping	each	627	14	65	3	37	19	9	977
Sunshine Skillet®	each	565	26	34	3	1	35	13	1767
Sweet cinnamon hotcake, no topping	each	374	5	64	0	19	11	5	784
Sweet cream waffle, no topping	each	378	9	61	2	17	10	5	795

BOB EVANS continued

Item	Serving Size	Calories	Protein	Carb	Fiber	Sugar	Total Fat	Sat Fat	Sodium
Three cheese omelet	each	528	2	5	0	2	40	18	1451
Turkey & spinach omelet	each	618	9	9	1	5	40	17	2435
Turkey sausage	each	72	9	1	0	0	4	1	404
Turkey sausage breakfast	each	362	27	48	5	18	18	2	1009
Western BoBurrito	each	738	45	42	3	7	44	15	2081
Western omelet	each	529	41	8	1	4	36	13	1809

SALAD DRESSINGS

Item	Serving Size	Calories	Protein	Carb	Fiber	Sugar	Total Fat	Sat Fat	Sodium
Blue cheese	2.8 oz	411	3	5	0	3	44	8	630
Buttermilk ranch	2.8 oz	291	3	3	0	3	29	5	582
Caesar	2.8 oz	432	2	2	0	1	47	7	655
Colonial	2.8 oz	433	0	22	0	22	38	6	361
French	2.8 oz	410	0	18	0	15	38	6	461
Honey mustard	2.8 oz	358	0	15	0	13	33	5	461
Hot bacon	2.8 oz	198	0	33	0	31	6	2	353
Lite ranch	2.8 oz	192	2	4	0	2	18	3	704
Raspberry reduced-fat	2.8 oz	199	0	27	0	26	10	2	169
Sweet Italian	2.8 oz	253	0	12	0	10	23	4	741
Swiss bacon	2.8 oz	423	3	3	0	3	48	8	741
Thousand Island	2.8 oz	397	0	13	0	11	37	5	661
Vinegar & oil	2.8 oz	54	0		0	0	6	1	0
Wildfire ranch	2.8 oz	225	1	16	0	3	17	3	573

SALADS

Item	Serving Size	Calories	Protein	Carb	Fiber	Sugar	Total Fat	Sat Fat	Sodium
Cobb	regular	517	51	10	3	4	31	7	1673
Cobb	savor size	362	36	7	2	3	22	12	1146
Country spinach	regular	428	44	12	5	4	25	8	1297
Country spinach	savor size	384	35	10	4	4	24	7	1082
Cranberry pecan chicken	regular	639	46	33	5	24	36	13	1511
Cranberry pecan chicken	savor size	545	31	32	4	23	33	13	1244
Garden	regular	58	2	9	1	2	1	0	132
Heritage chef	regular	398	34	11	3	6	25	12	1324
Heritage chef	savor size	294	25	7	2	4	18	9	926
Specialty garden	regular	124	6	10	1	2	7	3	334
Wildfire fried chicken	regular	711	32	70	7	18	34	9	1332
Wildfire fried chicken	savor size	543	23	54	5	13	27	8	995

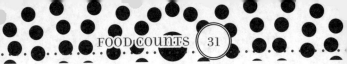

BOB EVANS continued

Item	Serving Size	Calories	Protein	Carb	Fiber	Sugar	Total Fat	Sat Fat	Sodium
Wildfire grilled chicken	regular	389	2	37	6	1	16	5	963
Wildfire grilled chicken	savor size	340	24	35	5	13	13	5	769
SANDWICHES									
Bacon cheeseburger	as served	719	25	35	2	5	38	17	1355
Cheeseburger	as served	648	24	35	2	5	31	13	1247
Chicken Caesar wrap	as served	605	31	55	5	6	29	8	1576
Chicken salad	as served	565	19	5	5	10	31	5	1139
Chicken salad wrap	as served	605	21	66	9	14	29	5	1348
Fried chicken club	as served	637	40	47	3	4	31	11	1567
Fried chicken	as served	489	35	47	3	4	18	4	1109
Grilled cheese	as served	350	9	22	2	4	15	6	729
Grilled chicken club	as served	512	41	34	2	4	23	10	1435
Grilled chicken	as served	370	36	33	2	4	10	3	986
Hamburger	as served	542	18	34	2	4	22	8	776
Knife & Fork meatloaf	as served	808	24	51	4	14	35	16	2647
Knife & Fork turkey	as served	702	26	47	3	6	37	13	3034
Pot roast	as served	642	35	52	2	11	32	12	1342
Turkey bacon melt	as served	588	33	49	2	7	28	11	2093
Turkey club wrap	as served	695	37	58	5	8	34	13	2246
LUNCH & DINNER									
Chicken & broccoli Alfredo	regular	871	53	62	6	9	46	17	2183
Chicken & broccoli Alfredo	savor size	471	30	35	6	6	24	9	1157
Chicken Parmesan w/ meat sauce	regular	1134	64	94	6	14	55	19	3100
Chicken Parmesan w/ meat sauce	savor size	818	52	56	4	9	42	15	2442
Chicken salad plate	as served	774	22	71	12	57	48	7	1099
Chicken-N-Noodles deep-dish dinner	as served	699	30	66	3	6	29	15	2233
Country fried steak w/ gravy	each	549	19	38	0	0	36	13	1507
Country fried steak, w/o gravy	each	496	18	31	0	0	33	11	1217
Fried haddock	each	363	24	27	2	2	18	4	608

BOB EVANS continued

Item	Serving Size	Calories	Protein	Carb	Fiber	Sugar	Total Fat	Sat Fat	Sodium
Garlic butter grilled chicken breast	each	180	31	1	0	0	6	2	738
Garlic butter salmon	each	256	41	1	0	0	9	2	174
Meatloaf	each	403	15	22	1	11	18	7	1583
Open-faced roast beef	each	472	33	21	1	9	24	8	790
Pot roast stroganoff	regular	813	42	65	2	14	43	15	1782
Pot roast stroganoff	savor size	425	2	33	1	7	23	9	905
Potato-crusted flounder	each	177	19	9	0	1	7	3	486
Salmon	each	243	40	0	0	0	8	2	101
Sirloin steak	each	421	33	3	0	0	29	9	638
Slow-roasted chicken pot pie	as served	862	31	63	4	12	56	22	2623
Slow-roasted Chicken-N-Noodles	as served	229	17	30	2	4	5	1	719
Slow-roasted turkey	each	136	18	3	0	2	5	1	985
Spaghetti w/ meat sauce	regular	778	32	81	5	14	36	12	2002
Spaghetti w/ meat sauce	savor size	462	2	43	3	8	23	8	1343
Turkey & dressing	as served	688	42	54	3	21	33	10	3096
Turkey bacon & tomato pasta	regular	1132	76	66	3	15	62	26	4740
Turkey bacon & tomato pasta	savor size	580	39	33	2	8	32	13	2410

SIDES

Item	Serving Size	Calories	Protein	Carb	Fiber	Sugar	Total Fat	Sat Fat	Sodium
Applesauce	side	69	0	18	2	13	0	0	11
Baked potato	side	193	8	50	6	6	0	0	0
Bread & celery dressing	side	299	6	29	2	2	19	6	790
Broccoli florets	side	44	5	8	5	3	1	0	41
Coleslaw	side	208	1	19	1	17	14	2	243
Corn	side	166	2	17	2	2	12	5	253
Cottage cheese	side	92	11	4	1	3	4	2	310
Cranberry relish	side	68	0	16	1	15	0	0	7
French fries	side	319	4	46	1	0	13	3	92
Fresh fruit cup	side	148	1	38	4	32	1	0	8
Garden vegetables	side	148	3	1	4	4	12	5	306
Glazed carrots	side	101	1	14	3	9	5	2	99

BOB EVANS continued

Item	Serving Size	Calories	Protein	Carb	Fiber	Sugar	Total Fat	Sat Fat	Sodium
Green beans	side	47	3	6	2	1	2	1	515
Grilled mushrooms	side	87	4	10	5	0	5	1	865
Hash browns	side	324	6	53	3	3	8	1	1091
Home fries	side	164	3	24	3	0	6	1	680
Loaded baked potato	side	395	19	53	6	7	16	9	472
Loaded hash browns	side	526	18	56	4	4	24	10	1564
Macaroni & cheese	side	321	14	29	2	4	17	8	1045
Mashed potatoes	side	192	2	16	1	1	7	4	428
Onion petals	side	288	3	35	2	3	14	2	464
Sweet potato fries	side	465	3	49	6	15	29	5	468

SOUPS

Item	Serving Size	Calories	Protein	Carb	Fiber	Sugar	Total Fat	Sat Fat	Sodium
Bean soup	1	204	14	28	8	1	4	1	1016
Cheddar baked potato soup	1	332	14	26	1	5	19	11	1531
Sausage chili	1	397	23	27	10	3	25	9	1017
Vegetable beef soup	1	162	10	23	4	5	3	1	949

DESSERTS

Item	Serving Size	Calories	Protein	Carb	Fiber	Sugar	Total Fat	Sat Fat	Sodium
Apple crumb pie à la mode	as served	621	7	87	3	51	28	14	396
Blackberry cobbler	as served	553	4	82	1	41	24	10	530
Blackberry cobbler à la mode	as served	665	6	96	1	52	29	14	566
Coconut cream pie	as served	514	7	59	3	40	29	20	451
French silk pie	as served	655	6	59	1	43	44	26	318
Lemon meringue pie	as served	432	2	77	1	56	13	6	379
Lemon Supreme pie	as served	642	5	71	2	50	38	24	363
NSA apple pie	as served	486	3	52	3	8	27	12	380
NSA apple pie à la mode	as served	597	5	65	3	18	33	16	415
Peanut butter brownie bites	as served	1026	12	137	6	96	50	13	689
Peanut butter brownie sundae	as served	764	10	104	3	76	35	14	429
Pecan pie	as served	704	7	87	1	71	36	13	375
Pumpkin pie	as served	490	6	65	2	42	24	10	304
Pumpkin supreme pie	as served	615	7	61	2	40	38	22	402
Vanilla ice cream	as served	111	2	13	0	10	6	4	36

BOSTON MARKET

Item	Serving Size	Calories	Protein	Carb	Fiber	Sugar	Total Fat	Sat Fat	Sodium
ENTRÉES & SANDWICHES									
Chicken, dark meat, without skin, rotisserie garlic	1/4 chicken	190	22	1	0	1	10	3	440
Chicken, with skin, rotisserie garlic	1/2 chicken	590	70	4	0	4	33	10	1010
Chicken & queso sandwich	each	550	38	62	3	5	21	7	1590
Chicken Carver sandwich, w/ cheese & sauce	each	640	38	61	4	13	29	7	980
Chicken pot pie	as served	750	26	57	2	4	46	14	1530
Country chicken, crispy baked	as served	420	26	31	5	1	22	5	880
Lean pork ham, honey-glazed	as served	210	24	10	0	10	8	3	1460
Marinated grilled chicken sandwich	each	670	42	45	2	5	36	6	810
Meatloaf Carver sandwich, w/ cheese	each	730	39	85	5	18	29	12	1590
Meatloaf, double sauce, Angus	as served	310	22	16	1	3	19	8	650
Turkey, breast, w/o skin, low-fat, rotisserie	as served	170	36	3	0	3	1	0	850
Turkey Carver® sandwich, w/ cheese & sauce	each	630	40	64	4	14	26	7	1350
SIDES									
Chicken gravy	as served	15	0	2	0	0	0.5	0	180
Cornbread	1 piece	200	3	33	1	13	6	1.5	390
Creamed spinach	as served	260	9	11	2	2	20	13	740
Macaroni & cheese	as served	280	13	33	1	8	11	7	1100
Mashed potatoes w/ gravy, homestyle	as served	230	4	32	3	4	9	5	780
Potato salad, homestyle	as served	200	3	22	2	5	12	2	440
Rice pilaf w/ vegetables	as served	140	2	24	1	2	4	0.5	520
Sesame broccoli	as served	80	3	13	2	10	2.5	0	390

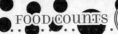

BOSTON MARKET continued

Item	Serving Size	Calories	Protein	Carb	Fiber	Sugar	Total Fat	Sat Fat	Sodium
Squash, butternut	as served	150	2	25	6	12	6	4	560
Steamed vegetables	as served	30	2	6	2	2	0	0	135
Stuffing, savory	as served	190	4	27	2	5	8	1.5	620
Tomato bisque soup	as served	380	6	25	4	11	29	13	1660
Tortilla soup w/ toppings	as served	170	8	18	2	2	8	2.5	1060
DESSERTS									
Apple pie	1 slice	550	4	66	3	16	31	13	690
Brownie	1 order	580	9	88	6	65	23	5	350
Chocolate cake	1 slice	650	4	86	2	68	32	8	320
Chocolate chip cookie	1 order	390	4	51	2	28	19	10	340
Chocolate chip fudge brownie	each	320	5	49	3	36	13	3	220
Cornbread	each	200	3	34	1	13	5	2	300
Hot apples w/ cinnamon	1 order	250	0	56	3	49	4.5	0.5	45
Pecan pie	1 slice	640	7	74	2	46	36	11	340
Pumpkin pie	1 slice	430	6	57	2	35	22	10	380
SALADS									
Asian grilled chicken	full	570	40	33	5	15	31	5	1280
Asian grilled chicken	half	290	20	17	3	8	16	2.5	640
Caesar	half	360	23	21	2	4	22	4.5	960
Caesar w/ chicken	full	650	45	26	3	8	42	10	1680
Caesar w/o chicken	full	500	14	25	3	7	39	9	1190
Mediterranean	full	670	40	27	3	11	45	10	1380
Mediterranean	half	340	20	14	1	6	22	5	690
Southwest Santa Fe	full	690	41	41	5	11	42	9	1560
Southwest Santa Fe	half	350	20	20	2	5	21	4.5	780

BRUEGGER'S BAGELS

Item	Serving Size	Calories	Protein	Carb	Fiber	Sugar	Total Fat	Sat Fat	Sodium
BAGELS, BREADS, & WRAPS									
Asiago Parmesan bagel	each	330	14	61	4	7	4	1	730
Bagel bowl	each	720	30	136	8	22	9	3	152
Baked apple bagel	each	320	10	67	5	18	2	0	510
Blueberry bagel	each	310	11	62	3	14	2	0	500
Chocolate chip bagel	each	330	10	65	3	18	3.5	2	470
Ciabatta	each	250	9	48	2	2	2.5	0	730
Cinnamon raisin bagel	each	310	11	65	4	10	2	0	480
Cinnamon sugar bagel	each	320	14	63	4	13	2	0	420
Cranberry orange bagel	each	310	10	64	4	16	2	0	480
Egg bagel	each	310	11	63	4	10	2.5	0	530
Everything bagel	each	310	12	62	4	7	2.5	0	710
Focaccia bagel	each	390	15	61	4	9	10	3.5	700
Fortified multigrain bagel	each	340	12	66	6	10	2.5	0	500
Garlic bagel	each	300	12	61	4	7	2	0	520
Hearty white, slice	2 slices	260	10	54	2	2	1	0	620
Honey grain bagel	each	310	11	61	4	10	2.5	0	490
Honey wheat, slice	2 slices	280	12	54	2	6	3	0	520
Jalapeño bagel	each	310	12	62	4	7	2	0	530
Onion bagel	each	300	12	61	4	8	2	0	530
Plain bagel	each	300	12	60	4	7	2	0	530
Poppy bagel	each	310	12	61	4	7	2.5	0	610
Pumpernickel bagel	each	300	11	62	4	10	2	0	560
Rosemary olive oil bagel	each	330	11	59	4	8	6	0.5	510
Rye bagel	each	330	11	59	5	8	2	0	560
Salt bagel	each	300	12	61	4	7	2	0	1540
Sesame bagel	each	310	12	60	4	7	3	0	610
Sourdough bagel	each	290	11	56	4	7	2	0	540
Square Asiago Parmesan bagel	each	360	15	68	4	11	4.5	1.5	760
Square everything bagel	each	350	12	64	4	8	2	0	740
Square plain bagel	each	330	12	67	4	11	2.5	0	640
Square sesame bagel	each	370	14	70	4	11	3.5	0	690
Sundried tomato bagel	each	280	10	57	4	10	2	0	550
Trail mix bagel	each	310	11	60	5	14	3.5	0	340
White wrap	each	180	6	32	3	1	1.5	1	420
Whole wheat bagel	each	300	13	56	5	10	3.5	0	670

BRUEGGER'S BAGELS continued

Item	Serving Size	Calories	Protein	Carb	Fiber	Sugar	Total Fat	Sat Fat	Sodium
SWEETS									
Banana nut muffin	each	450	5	50	2	24	26	4	379
Blueberry muffin	each	430	5	53	1	30	22	3.5	310
Cappuccino muffin	each	490	6	60	1	34	26	5	340
Chocolate chip cookie	each	390	5	52	2	32	17	8	150
Chocolate chunk brownie	each	310	4	38	2	26	18	9	25
Double chocolate cookie	each	390	5	51	3	33	19	9	160
Everything cookie	each	380	5	49	2	29	18	9	260
Marshmallow chew	each	280	2	55	0	29	6	3	330
Seven layer bar	each	650	10	58	5	42	43	23	280
Toffee almond bar	each	400	4	53	1	34	19	8	340
BEVERAGES									
Brueggaccino	16 oz	460	8	43	0	43	28	18	150
Brueggaccino	24 oz	690	12	65	0	65	42	27	225
Café au lait	12 oz	150	8	11	0	11	8	4.5	8
Café au lait	16 oz	200	11	15	0	15	10.6	6	11
Café au lait	20 oz	249	13	18	0	18	13.3	7.5	14
Café latte	12 oz	170	9	13	0	13	9	5	8
Café latte	16 oz	226	12	17	0	17	12	6.7	11
Café latte	20 oz	283	15	22	0	22	15	8.3	14
Café mocha	12 oz	210	9	23	0	21	9	5	8
Café mocha	16 oz	279	12	31	0	28	12	6.7	11
Café mocha	20 oz	349	15	38	0	35	15	8.3	14
Cappuccino	12 oz	130	7	11	0	11	7	4	8
Cappuccino	16 oz	173	9	15	0	15	9.3	5.3	11
Cappuccino	20 oz	216	12	18	0	18	11.7	6.7	14
Espresso	2 oz	5	0	1	0	1	0	0	10
Espresso	3 oz	8	0	2	0	2	0	0	15
Espresso	4 oz	10	0	2	0	2	0	0	20
Flavored, French roast, house blend decaf, iced coffees	12 oz	4	n/a	n/a	n/a	n/a	n/a	n/a	8
Flavored, French roast, house blend decaf, iced coffees	16 oz	5	n/a	n/a	n/a	n/a	n/a	n/a	11

BRUEGGER'S BAGELS continued

Item	Serving Size	Calories	Protein	Carb	Fiber	Sugar	Total Fat	Sat Fat	Sodium
Flavored, French roast, house blend decaf, iced coffees	20 oz	6	n/a	n/a	n/a	n/a	n/a	n/a	14
Hot chocolate	8 oz	140	2	31	1	26	1.5	1.5	190
Oregon chai tea	12 oz	117	3	29	0	27	n/a	n/a	12
SYRUPS									
Almond flavored	1 oz	90	0	23	0	23	0	0	0
Caramel flavored	1 oz	100	0	24	0	24	0	0	0
Chocolate flavored	1 oz	88	<1	20	<1	15	0.7	0.5	12
Hazelnut flavored	1 oz	90	0	22	0	21	0	0	7
Vanilla flavored	1 oz	100	0	25	0	25	0	0	0
CREAM CHEESES									
Bacon scallion	1.5 oz	140	3	5	0	2	12	7	150
Cucumber dill	1.5 oz	150	3	3	<1	1	14	7	130
Garden veggie	1.5 oz	130	3	5	1	2	11	6	140
Honey walnut	1.5 oz	150	3	8	<1	3	12	6	125
Jalapeño	1.5 oz	140	3	4	0	2	13	8	150
Light garden veggie	1.5 oz	90	6	3	0	2	6	4	105
Light garlic herb	1.5 oz	100	6	4	0	2	6	3.5	125
Light plain	1.5 oz	100	6	4	<1	3	6	3	130
Olive pimiento	1.5 oz	140	3	3	0	1	13	6	130
Onion & chive	1.5 oz	140	3	3	0	2	13	8	105
Plain	1.5 oz	130	3	6	<1	2	11	7	125
Pumpkin	1.5 oz	120	3	4	0	3	11	7	135
Smoked salmon	1.5 oz	150	3	3	<1	2	13	6	150
Strawberry	1.5 oz	140	3	4	0	2	13	7	100
Vermont maple	1.5 oz	120	3	4	0	3	11	7	135
SALADS									
Caesar, w/ dressing	as served	270	9	22	2	5	17	4.5	900
Caesar, w/o dressing	as served	160	7	14	2	3	8	2.5	220
Caesar w/ chicken, w/ dressing	as served	380	28	23	2	5	20	6	1420
Mandarin Medley, w/ balsamic dressing	as served	340	8	36	4	27	17	5	660
Mandarin Medley, w/o dressing	as served	220	8	29	4	21	8	4.5	300

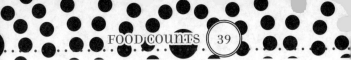

BRUEGGER'S BAGELS continued

Item	Serving Size	Calories	Protein	Carb	Fiber	Sugar	Total Fat	Sat Fat	Sodium
Mandarin Medley w/ chicken, w/ dressing	as served	450	26	37	4	27	21	6	1180
Sesame Salad, w/ Asian Sesame dressing	as served	380	23	29	2	18	26	2.5	270
Sesame Salad, w/o dressing	as served	120	4	12	2	3	4.5	0	75
Sesame Salad w/ chicken, w/ dressing	as served	490	42	30	2	18	29	3.5	790
BREAKFAST SANDWICHES									
Breakfast bagel w/ egg, cheese	as served	470	23	63	4	8	14	5	840
Breakfast bagel w/ egg, cheese, & bacon	as served	480	27	64	4	9	21	8	1210
Breakfast bagel w/ egg, cheese, & ham	as served	490	29	65	4	10	13	4	1350
Breakfast bagel w/ egg, cheese, & sausage	as served	630	31	64	4	8	35	14	1300
Classic wrap w/ bacon	as served	730	40	39	3	6	44	17	1710
Classic wrap w/ ham	as served	570	36	38	3	5	27	11	1640
Classic wrap w/ sausage	as served	690	34	37	3	3	41	17	1280
Rio Grande w/ bacon	as served	640	32	41	3	7	38	10	1570
Rio Grande w/ ham	as served	480	27	41	3	6	21	4.5	1500
Rio Grande w/ sausage	as served	600	26	39	3	4	35	10	1140
Smoked salmon, plain bagel	as served	460	26	66	4	10	10	4.5	1520
Spinach, Cheddar & sausage omelet, plain bagel	as served	550	32	66	4	10	17	7	1590
Spinach & Cheddar omelet, bacon, plain bagel	as served	570	29	64	4	9	22	8	1210
Spinach & Cheddar omelet, ham, plain bagel	as served	670	31	64	4	8	31	13	1230

BRUEGGER'S BAGELS continued

Item	Serving Size	Calories	Protein	Carb	Fiber	Sugar	Total Fat	Sat Fat	Sodium
Spinach & Cheddar omelet, plain bagel	as served	500	24	64	4	8	16	6	990
Western, plain bagel	as served	760	27	66	4	10	56	12	1580
DELI SANDWICHES									
BLT, plain bagel	each	530	19	64	4	10	23	5	1000
BLT, hearty white	each	720	23	62	0	8	42	10	1550
Chicken breast, hearty white	each	610	35	94	0	41	4	1.5	1520
Chicken breast, plain bagel	each	550	37	81	4	27	6	1.5	1330
Garden veggie, plain bagel	each	360	12	72	5	13	2	0	550
Garden veggie, wheat	each	360	13	67	4	13	3	0	540
Ham, honey wheat	each	540	38	64	2	12	16	6	2430
Ham, plain bagel	each	430	25	64	4	11	8	3	1490
Roast beef, hearty white	each	560	53	59	0	5	18	7	2050
Roast beef, plain bagel	each	450	33	63	4	9	11	3.5	1250
Tuna salad, hearty white	each	810	31	58	1	8	46	6	1390
Tuna salad, plain bagel	each	570	22	63	4	10	25	3	920
Turkey, hearty white	each	560	41	60	2	10	15	7	2060
Turkey, plain bagel	each	440	26	64	4	9	8	3.5	1300
HOT PANINI									
Four cheese & tomato, hearty white	each	700	42	56	0	4	34	18	1420
Ham & Swiss, honey wheat	each	600	40	72	2	24	17	7	1870
Primo pesto chicken, hearty white	each	700	49	56	2	3	32	10	1870
Tuna & Cheddar melt, honey wheat	each	970	43	57	3	11	61	13	1520
Turkey Toscana, hearty white	each	650	40	58	1	4	28	10	1840
SIGNATURE & CLASSIC SANDWICHES									
Herby turkey, sesame bagel	each	530	26	73	4	11	14	4.5	1190
Leonardo da Veggie, plain softwich	each	560	25	76	4	17	15	8	1170

BRUEGGER'S BAGELS continued

Item	Serving Size	Calories	Protein	Carb	Fiber	Sugar	Total Fat	Sat Fat	Sodium
Roma roast beef, hearty white	each	770	46	62	3	6	44	12	1740
Tarragon chicken salad, hearty white	each	750	61	75	2	16	37	5	1380
Thai peanut chicken, plain bagel	each	580	28	91	7	17	11	3.5	1190
Turkey chipotle club, honey wheat	each	800	31	57	3	8	51	7	1840

SIGNATURE SOUPS

Item	Serving Size	Calories	Protein	Carb	Fiber	Sugar	Total Fat	Sat Fat	Sodium
Beef chili	8 oz	190	10	18	6	3	8	3	880
Butternut squash	8 oz	240	4	21	1	2	17	9	650
Chicken spaetzle	8 oz	140	8	15	1	3	5	2.5	1200
Chicken wild rice	8 oz	280	8	12	1	2	22	10	840
Fire-roasted tomato	8 oz	130	2	17	2	10	6	3	920
Four cheese broccoli	8 oz	260	9	12	1	2	20	10	1240
New England clam chowder	8 oz	230	23	16	<1	12	14	4.5	600
Spinach & lentil	8 oz	110	7	16	7	2	3.5	1	570
White chicken chili	8 oz	240	14	26	7	2	9	0	630

BUFFALO WILD WINGS

Item	Serving Size	Calories	Protein	Carb	Fiber	Sugar	Total Fat	Sat Fat	Sodium
APPETIZERS									
Ballpark sampler	as served	137	22	103	5	20	77	18	2515
Cheeseburger Slammers™	as served	1559	66	98	7	10	92	34	1451
Chicken quesadilla	as served	800	51	70	5	6	35	18	1810
Chili con queso dip	as served	920	28	100	8	8	48	14	2240
Chips & salsa	as served	500	4	46	2	0	30	14	1180
Crispy Southwest Dippers®	as served	630	24	78	8	10	25	10	1974
Mini corn dogs	as served	713	13	49	2	16	24	5	1270
Mozzarella sticks	as served	560	30	52	0	2	22	15	1800
Naked tenders	6 each	260	10	34	2	10	12	1	3420
Popcorn shrimp	3/4 lb	880	34	88	4	6	44	6	2900
Pulled Pork Slammers™	as served	1167	61	105	4	17	51	13	1867

BUFFALO WILD WINGS continued

Item	Serving Size	Calories	Protein	Carb	Fiber	Sugar	Total Fat	Sat Fat	Sodium
Queso chili fries	as served	862	26	92	10	10	40	15	2654
Roasted garlic mushrooms	as served	360	6	44	2	4	18	3	1240
The Sampler	as served	1520	76	128	8	20	76	20	3120
Ultimate nachos	as served	960	24	108	8	8	52	14	2680
Ultimate nachos w/ chicken	as served	1120	52	108	8	8	52	14	3200

SIDES

Item	Serving Size	Calories	Protein	Carb	Fiber	Sugar	Total Fat	Sat Fat	Sodium
Buffalo Chips™	basket	514	9	93	9	5	9	2	70
Buffalo Chips™	regular	257	5	47	5	2	5	1	35
Buffalo Chips™ w/ cheese	basket	734	23	95	9	5	27	14	430
Buffalo Chips™ w/ cheese	regular	367	12	48	5	2	14	7	215
Coleslaw	side	170	0	6	0	6	15	0	39
French fries	basket	560	8	84	8	4	20	6	1320
French fries	regular	280	4	42	4	2	10	3	660
Onion rings	basket	1100	10	130	10	20	55	10	2200
Onion rings	regular	460	4	52	4	8	26	5	960
Potato wedges	basket	560	9	79	9	5	28	7	2147
Potato wedges	regular	280	5	40	5	2	14	4	1073
Potato wedges w/ cheese	basket	780	23	81	9	5	46	19	2507
Potato wedges w/ cheese	regular	390	12	41	5	2	23	10	1253
Side salad	side	210	6	14	4	4	15	5	385

TENDERS, POPCORN SHRIMP, & WINGS

Item	Serving Size	Calories	Protein	Carb	Fiber	Sugar	Total Fat	Sat Fat	Sodium
Boneless wings	each	88	5	3	0	0	6	2	178
Breaded tenders	each	170	5	15	1	5	11	3	573
Naked tenders	each	43	2	6	0	2	2	0	570
Popcorn shrimp	1/2 lb	587	23	59	3	4	29	4	1933
Wings	each	72	6	0	0	0	5	1	66

BUFFALO WILD WINGS continued

Item	Serving Size	Calories	Protein	Carb	Fiber	Sugar	Total Fat	Sat Fat	Sodium
RIBS & COMBO MEALS									
Boneless wings & traditional wings	as served	1480	66	68	6	2	98	20	7940
Chicken tenders & popcorn shrimp	as served	1120	24	110	10	30	62	12	3220
Popcorn shrimp & fish	as served	820	50	70	4	6	36	6	2520
Ribs & boneless wings	as served	1960	102	88	6	16	126	40	4380
Ribs & chicken tenders	as served	1860	88	112	8	30	118	38	2980
Ribs & more ribs	as served	2380	144	88	6	28	158	58	5320
Ribs & popcorn shrimp	as served	1480	80	84	4	20	92	32	2980
Ribs & traditional wings	as served	1860	108	74	6	16	124	40	3800
SALADS									
Chicken Caesar	as served	490	5	10	5	4	27	6	790
Chicken tender	as served	990	26	74	11	24	68	17	2580
Garden	as served	420	12	28	7	8	30	10	770
Grilled blackened chicken	as served	660	55	23	7	9	39	11	840
Grilled chicken	as served	640	55	20	6	8	38	11	790
Honey BBQ™ chicken	as served	733	19	87	8	43	38	11	3850
BURGERS W/O FRIES									
Bacon Cheddar	as served	860	46	44	3	4	57	24	1170
Big Jack Daddy™	as served	900	50	53	3	9	56	23	1630
Black & bleu	as served	770	37	44	3	4	51	20	860
Cheeseburger	as served	780	42	44	3	4	51	22	870
Chili queso	as served	880	49	49	3	5	57	26	1270
Honey BBQ™	as served	890	46	51	3	10	57	24	1340
WRAPS & BUFFALITOS® W/O CHIPS									
Buffalo ranch chicken wrap	as served	1020	28	97	16	16	59	18	2120
Chicken Caesar wrap	as served	560	39	68	4	4	15	6	1770
Chicken tender wrap	as served	1040	37	125	25	25	46	17	2800

BUFFALO WILD WINGS continued

Item	Serving Size	Calories	Protein	Carb	Fiber	Sugar	Total Fat	Sat Fat	Sodium
Grilled Chicken Buffalitos®	as served	380	40	44	4	4	9	6	1240
Naked tenders wrap	as served	600	54	68	4	4	14	9	1980
Southwest chicken queso wrap	as served	490	39	73	6	6	7	4	2660
SATISFYING SANDWICHES W/O FRIES									
Buffalo ranch chicken	as served	800	32	60	3	5	49	13	1460
Crispy fish	as served	550	8	22	3	1	22	6	760
Gardenburger	as served	250	40	63	3	7	5	2	1060
Grilled chicken	as served	470	51	50	3	10	7	3	750
Honey BBQ bacon chicken	as served	530	50	42	3	4	18	9	890
Jerk chicken	as served	530	51	56	3	16	10	3	1140
Pulled pork	as served	570	30	61	2	15	25	7	3160
WILD FLATBREADS™									
Buffalo chicken	as served	908	53	56	4	1	49	17	2298
Create Own	as served	783	52	61	4	8	32	14	1908
Honey BBQ™ chicken	as served	813	52	71	4	14	32	14	1848
Parmesan Garlic™	as served	863	54	55	4	2	44	16	2188
DESSERTS									
Chocolate fudge cake	as served	820	11	127	3	108	33	13	95
Deep-dish apple pie	as served	590	7	105	4	66	18	9	260
New York cheesecake	as served	460	6	47	1	39	28	16	20
WILD-CHILD(REN) W/O FRIES									
Boneless wings	4 pieces	288	24	0	0	0	20	5	24
Chicken tenders	3 pieces	510	14	44	4	15	32	8	1720
French fries	regular	280	4	42	4	2	10	3	660
Kids' cheeseburger Slammer™	as served	400	21	20	1	3	26	10	400
Kids' ice cream	as served	210	3	33	1	30	8	5	95
Macaroni & cheese	as served	380	16	49	3	9	13	5	1240
Mini corn dogs	5 pieces	357	7	25	1	5	12	3	735
Naked tenders	3 pieces	130	5	17	1	5	6	1	1710
Traditional wings	4 pieces	384	31	1	0	0	28	7	352

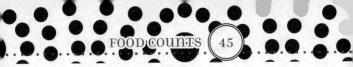

BUFFALO WILD WINGS continued

Item	Serving Size	Calories	Protein	Carb	Fiber	Sugar	Total Fat	Sat Fat	Sodium
SAUCES & DRESSINGS									
Asian Zing	1 oz	90	0	22	0	2	0	0	580
Blazin	1 oz	60	0	2	0	0	5	0	1280
Blue cheese	1 oz	280	2	2	0	2	30	6	480
Caribbean jerk	1 oz	80	0	12	0	12	3	0	500
Desert Heat	1/2 tsp	8	0	1	0	1	0	0	380
Honey BBQ	1 oz	70	0	18	0	14	0	0	400
Honey mustard	1 oz	80	0	6	0	6	6	0	320
Hot	1 oz	50	0	2	0	0	4	0	1200
Hot BBQ	1 oz	40	0	6	0	4	2	0	740
Mango habanera	1 oz	80	0	20	0	14	0	0	460
Medium	1 oz	40	0	2	0	0	4	0	1160
Mild	1 oz	50	0	2	0	0	5	0	1040
Parmesan garlic	1 oz	120	2	2	0	2	12	2	740
Pepper infusion	1 oz	90	0	2	1	1	9		780
Ranch dressing	1 oz	320	0	2	0	2	30	4	440
Southwestern ranch	1 oz	320	0	2	0	2	34	5	740
Spicy garlic	1 oz	50	0	4	0	0	4	0	1220
Sweet BBQ	1 oz	40	0	8	0	8	0	0	460
Teriyaki	1 oz	70	0	14	0	12	0	0	1100
Wild	1 oz	50	0	4	0	0	4	0	1160

BURGER KING

Item	Serving Size	Calories	Protein	Carb	Fiber	Sugar	Total Fat	Sat Fat	Sodium
BREAKFASTS									
Bacon, egg, cheese, w/ biscuit, sandwich	each	520	20	38	1	4	46	16	1360
BK® breakfast bowl	each	540	24	17	2	2	42	13	1020
Cheesy bacon BK® wrapper	each	380	13	28	2	2	24	7	1020
Egg, cheese, & sausage, w/ croissant, sandwich	each	460	19	27	1	5	31	11	1000
Egg, w/ biscuit, sandwich	each	390	11	37	1	4	22	5	1020
Egg & cheese, w/ croissant, sandwich	each	340	14	26	1	5	19	8	840

BURGER KING continued

Item	Serving Size	Calories	Protein	Carb	Fiber	Sugar	Total Fat	Sat Fat	Sodium
Pancake platter, w/ sausage & syrup	as served	670	14	78	1	36	34	9	1010
Pancakes w/ syrup	3 pancakes	500	7	77	1	36	19	4.5	700
Sausage, w/ biscuit, sandwich	each	510	13	35	1	3	35	15	1090
Sausage & cheese, w/ croissant, sandwich	each	380	14	26	1	3	24	10	780
BURGERS & SANDWICHES									
American original chicken sandwich	each	730	29	49	3	5	47	12	1830
BK® big fish sandwich	each	710	24	67	4	4	38	5	1370
BK® broiler chicken sandwich	each	550	30	52	3	5	25	5	1110
BK® double stacker	each	560	30	29	1	7	36	15	1040
BK® quad stacker	each	920	58	31	1	8	63	28	1730
BK® triple stacker	each	740	43	30	1	7	50	22	1390
BK® veggie burger	each	410	22	44	7	8	16	2.5	1030
Cheeseburger	each	286	15	24	3	5	14.8	6.8	602
Chicken Tenders® sandwich	each	450	14	37	2	4	27	7	1100
Double Stacker cheeseburger w/ bacon	each	610	38	32	2	5	37	15	1380
Double Whopper® sandwich	each	900	47	51	3	11	57	19	1050
Double Whopper® w/ cheese	each	990	52	53	3	11	65	24	1480
Hamburger	each	275	14	27	2	5	12	5.1	455
Hamburger, double	each	480	31	30	2	5	26	8	550
Italian original chicken sandwich	each	520	32	50	3	5	22	7	1670
Original chicken club sandwich	each	690	29	48	3	5	43	9	1590
Original chicken sandwich	each	630	24	46	3	4	39	7	1390
Spicy Chick'n Crisp® sandwich	each	460	13	34	2	4	30	5	810
Tendercrisp® chicken sandwich	each	1460	22	124	5	13	102	17	2720
Tendergrill® chicken sandwich	each	1130	27	96	4	11	74	12.5	2180

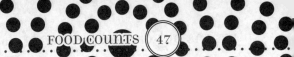

BURGER KING continued

Item	Serving Size	Calories	Protein	Carb	Fiber	Sugar	Total Fat	Sat Fat	Sodium
Triple Whopper® sandwich	each	1140	67	51	3	11	75	27	1110
Triple Whopper® w/ cheese	each	1230	71	53	3	11	82	32	1550
Whopper Jr®. sandwich	each	340	14	28	2	6	19	5	510
Whopper Jr.® w/ cheese	each	380	16	29	2	6	23	8	730
Whopper® sandwich	each	670	29	51	3	11	40	11	980
Whopper® sandwich, w/ cheese	each	760	33	53	3	11	47	16	1410
Whopper® chicken sandwich	each	216	12	19	2	3	11	2.2	433
SIDES									
Chicken fries	6 pieces	250	14	16	1	1	15	2.5	820
Chicken fries	9 pieces	80	21	24	2	1	2	4	1220
Chicken fries	12 pieces	500	28	32	3	1	29	5	1630
Chicken Tenders®	4 pieces	180	9	13	0	0	11	2	310
Chicken Tenders®	5 pieces	230	11	16	0	0	13	2.5	380
Chicken Tenders®	6 pieces	270	14	19	0	0	16	3	460
Chicken Tenders®	8 pieces	360	18	25	0	0	21	4	610
French fries	small	340	4	44	4	0	17	3.5	530
French fries	medium	440	5	56	5	0	22	4.5	670
French fries	large	540	6	69	6	0	27	6	830
French toast sticks	3 pieces	349	6	41	1	10	18	2	280
French toast sticks	5 pieces	380	5	49	2	13	18	3	430
Hash browns	small	250	2	24	3	0	16	3.5	410
Hash browns	medium	500	4	48	7	0	33	7	810
Hash browns	large	670	5	65	9	0	44	9	1080
Mozzarella sticks	4 pieces	280	11	24	2	2	15	5	650
Onion rings	small	310	4	36	3	4	17	3	490
Onion rings	medium	400	6	47	4	5	21	3.5	630
Onion rings	large	490	7	57	5	7	26	4.5	770
SHAKES									
Chocolate	12 oz	340	7	60	1	51	9	7	270
Chocolate	16 oz	440	9	78	1	67	11	8	360
Chocolate	20 oz	650	12	119	2	103	16	12	530
Chocolate	30 oz	960	17	176	2	153	23	17	780

BURGER KING continued

Item	Serving Size	Calories	Protein	Carb	Fiber	Sugar	Total Fat	Sat Fat	Sodium
Strawberry	12 oz	330	6	58	0	51	8	6	230
Strawberry	16 oz	430	8	77	0	66	11	8	290
Strawberry	20 oz	630	11	116	0	102	15	11	400
Strawberry	30 oz	930	6	172	0	151	21	16	590
Vanilla	12 oz	290	7	46	0	38	9	7	230
Vanilla	16 oz	370	9	60	0	50	12	9	310
Vanilla	20 oz	520	12	84	0	69	16	12	420
Vanilla	30 oz	760	18	124	0	102	24	18	630

CALIFORNIA PIZZA KITCHEN (CPK)

Item	Serving Size	Calories	Protein	Carb	Fiber	Sugar	Total Fat	Sat Fat	Sodium
SMALL CRAVINGS									
Asparagus & arugula	as served	173	4	8	2	n/a	n/a	2	442
Crispy artichoke hearts	as served	321	8	17	3	n/a	n/a	4	550
Korean BBQ steak tacos	as served	454	21	55	9	n/a	n/a	3	645
Mediterranean plate	as served	398	8	36	3	n/a	n/a	4	827
Spicy chicken tinga quesadilla	as served	455	18	34	3	n/a	n/a	9	953
The Wedge salad	as served	280	5	5	1	n/a	n/a	6	470
Tuscan panzanella salad	as served	337	6	28	8	n/a	n/a	3	557
White corn guacomole & chips	as served	362	6	48	7	n/a	n/a	3	759
APPETIZERS									
Avocado club egg rolls	as served	1172	45	58	4	n/a	n/a	19	2667
Garlic cheese focaccia	as served	951	30	119	6	n/a	n/a	11	2790
Lettuce wraps w/ chicken	as served	911	36	122	8	n/a	n/a	2	2877
Lettuce wraps w/ chicken & shrimp	as served	1054	65	123	8	n/a	n/a	2	1519
Lettuce wraps w/ shrimp	as served	895	41	123	8	n/a	n/a	1	1564

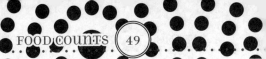

CALIFORNIA PIZZA KITCHEN (CPK) continued

Item	Serving Size	Calories	Protein	Carb	Fiber	Sugar	Total Fat	Sat Fat	Sodium
Sesame ginger chicken dumplings	as served	326	20	50	0	n/a	n/a	0	1185
Singapore shrimp rolls	as served	633	15	105	5	n/a	n/a	2	3693
Spinach artichoke dip	as served	873	20	103	9	n/a	n/a	15	1242
Tortilla spring rolls	any 2 rolls	636–888	26–32	62–86	8–10	n/a	n/a	10–14	1814–2370
Tortilla spring rolls	any 3 rolls	978–1356	39–48	93–129	12–15	n/a	n/a	18–21	2721–3555
Tuscan hummus	as served	861	21	124	7	n/a	n/a	4	1562

SOUPS

Item	Serving Size	Calories	Protein	Carb	Fiber	Sugar	Total Fat	Sat Fat	Sodium
Asparagus	1 bowl	213	8	32	4	n/a	n/a	1	1862
Asparagus	1 cup	106	4	16	2	n/a	n/a	1	929
Dakota smashed peas & barley	1 bowl	368	25	70	26	n/a	n/a	0	2100
Dakota smashed peas & barley	1 cup	106	4	16	2	n/a	n/a	1	929
Sedona tortilla	1 bowl	541	7	54	7	n/a	n/a	18	1831
Sedona tortilla	1 cup	184	12	35	13	n/a	n/a	0	1050
Tuscan white bean minestrone	1 bowl	262	10	35	5	n/a	n/a	3	672
Tuscan white bean minestrone	1 cup	157	5	21	3	n/a	n/a	2	383

SALADS

Item	Serving Size	Calories	Protein	Carb	Fiber	Sugar	Total Fat	Sat Fat	Sodium
Chinese chicken	full	707	30	95	9	n/a	n/a	0	2460
Chinese chicken	half	376	18	49	5	n/a	n/a	0	1254
Classic Caesar	full	553	16	29	8	n/a	n/a	14	1030
Classic Caesar	half	277	8	15	4	n/a	n/a	7	515
CPK Cobb w/ ranch	full	1015	51	22	10	n/a	n/a	19	1508
CPK Cobb w/ ranch	half	512	26	12	5	n/a	n/a	10	757
Field greens	full	998	18	68	15	n/a	n/a	12	805
Field greens	half	499	9	34	7	n/a	n/a	6	403
Grilled vegetable	full	810	34	58	19	n/a	n/a	8	2104
Grilled vegetable	half	440	13	50	6	n/a	n/a	4	1056
Miso shrimp	full	1177	53	109	17	n/a	n/a	53	2661
Miso shrimp	half	588	26	54	9	n/a	n/a	26	1330
Moroccan chicken	full	825	25	60	14	n/a	n/a	25	617
Moroccan chicken	half	412	12	30	7	n/a	n/a	12	309

CALIFORNIA PIZZA KITCHEN (CPK) continued

Item	Serving Size	Calories	Protein	Carb	Fiber	Sugar	Total Fat	Sat Fat	Sodium
Original BBQ chicken	full	1133	46	95	13	n/a	n/a	16	1460
Original BBQ chicken	half	576	23	50	6	n/a	n/a	8	785
Original chopped	full	952	50	31	10	n/a	n/a	17	2134
Original chopped	half	476	25	19	7	n/a	n/a	8	1097
Thai Crunch	full	1155	53	106	16	n/a	n/a	7	1309
Thai Crunch	half	578	27	53	8	n/a	n/a	4	654
Waldorf chicken	full	1485	53	95	16	n/a	n/a	16	1864
Waldorf Chicken	half	743	26	48	8	n/a	n/a	8	932

PIZZAS

Item	Serving Size	Calories	Protein	Carb	Fiber	Sugar	Total Fat	Sat Fat	Sodium
BBQ chicken w/ bacon	as served	1316	72	136	6	n/a	n/a	25	3288
BLT	as served	1364	55	122	8	n/a	n/a	25	2869
Buffalo chicken	as served	1247	61	124	8	n/a	n/a	23	3377
California club	as served	1560	71	129	13	n/a	n/a	26	3542
Carne Asada	as served	1323	62	125	7	n/a	n/a	27	3496
Cheeseburger	as served	1444	59	132	8	n/a	n/a	26	2901
Chipotle chicken	as served	1198	59	127	7	n/a	n/a	19	2773
Five-cheese & tomato	as served	1114	51	139	12	n/a	n/a	25	2539
Goat cheese w/ peppers	as served	1177	47	81	9	n/a	n/a	23	2638
Hawaiian	as served	1074	49	134	8	n/a	n/a	16	2565
Hawaiian BBQ chicken	as served	1159	60	141	7	n/a	n/a	19	2569
Italian tomato & basil	as served	1033	46	125	7	n/a	n/a	17	1218
Jamaican jerk chicken	as served	1356	74	137	9	n/a	n/a	24	4236
Mushroom pepperoni sausage	as served	1426	67	127	8	n/a	n/a	31	3336
Original BBQ chicken	as served	1136	60	136	6	n/a	n/a	19	2568
Pear & Gorgonzola	as served	1195	44	128	8	n/a	n/a	24	2175
Pepperoni	as served	1140	47	122	7	n/a	n/a	22	2637
Roasted garlic chicken	as served	1125	58	122	7	n/a	n/a	20	2111
Thai chicken	as served	1301	61	139	9	n/a	n/a	17	3002
The Greek	as served	1424	61	118	6	n/a	n/a	22	2979
The Meat Cravers	as served	1530	77	127	7	n/a	n/a	33	4134
The Works	as served	1430	63	131	9	n/a	n/a	29	3335
Tostada	as served	1438	51	158	18	n/a	n/a	27	2626
Traditional cheese	as served	998	42	131	9	n/a	n/a	16	2161

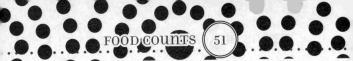

CALIFORNIA PIZZA KITCHEN (CPK) continued

Item	Serving Size	Calories	Protein	Carb	Fiber	Sugar	Total Fat	Sat Fat	Sodium
Vegetarian w/ eggplant	as served	1166	51	127	7	n/a	n/a	19	2808
White pizza	as served	1103	49	118	6	n/a	n/a	21	2455
Wild mushroom	as served	1244	44	135	6	n/a	n/a	23	2473
THIN-CRUST PIZZAS									
Four Seasons	as served	953	50	87	10	n/a	n/a	18	3134
Margherita	as served	1105	54	106	7	n/a	n/a	20	3188
Pepperoni Supremo	as served	1016	48	105	7	n/a	n/a	21	3048
Pesto chicken	as served	1329	59	110	9	n/a	n/a	21	2737
Roasted artichoke & spinach	as served	855	43	81	9	n/a	n/a	18	2302
Sicilian	as served	1225	66	101	6	n/a	n/a	29	3107
Tricolore salad pizza	as served	1000	37	125	7	n/a	n/a	15	1911
PIZZA CRUSTS									
Honey-wheat whole grain	as served	602	19	106	10	n/a	n/a	2	945
Thin crust	as served	439	15	91	3	n/a	n/a	0	958
Traditional	as served	614	15	111	4	n/a	n/a	2	1115
PASTAS									
Asparagus & spinach spaghettini	as served	1115	32	119	10	n/a	n/a	10	2078
Baby clam linguini	as served	956	28	91	5	n/a	n/a	29	1274
Broccoli sun-dried tomato fusilli	as served	1287	37	121	10	n/a	n/a	14	2368
Chicken tequila fettucine	as served	1225	34	95	6	n/a	n/a	42	1247
Four cheese ravioli	as served	947	28	49	2	n/a	n/a	41	1554
Garlic cream fettuccine	as served	1300	28	89	4	n/a	n/a	51	1706
Jambalaya	as served	1188	62	106	8	n/a	n/a	15	2206
Kung pao spaghetti	as served	1165	33	135	11	n/a	n/a	7	1230
Pesto chram penne	as served	1347	27	111	6	n/a	n/a	49	1765
Portobello mushroom ravioli	as served	718	21	81	5	n/a	n/a	10	1550
Spaghetti bolognese	as served	890	33	117	5	n/a	n/a	8	1931
Thai linguini	as served	1521	32	158	10	n/a	n/a	20	2780

CALIFORNIA PIZZA KITCHEN (CPK) continued

Item	Serving Size	Calories	Protein	Carb	Fiber	Sugar	Total Fat	Sat Fat	Sodium
Tomato basil spaghettini	as served	1038	21	118	5	n/a	n/a	12	1991
SPECIALTIES									
Baja fish tacos	as served	976	36	95	8	n/a	n/a	10	1796
Chicken Marsala	as served	1412	89	113	6	n/a	n/a	15	3038
Chicken Milanese	as served	579	36	16	3	n/a	n/a	10	995
Chicken piccata	as served	1539	82	99	5	n/a	n/a	30	3617
Ginger salmon	as served	979	51	74	6	n/a	n/a	8	2299
Pan-sautéed salmon	as served	1309	66	71	5	n/a	n/a	30	1721
Steak tacos	as served	985	34	74	8	n/a	n/a	15	2006
Wild-caught mahi mahi	as served	1212	67	77	8	n/a	n/a	12	2419
FOCACCIA SANDWICHES									
California club chicken	as served	937	36	92	7	n/a	n/a	8	2069
California club turkey	as served	976	42	93	7	n/a	n/a	8	2932
Cranberry walnut chicken	as served	857	23	93	5	n/a	n/a	6	1727
Grilled chicken Caesar	as served	937	36	92	7	n/a	n/a	8	2069
Grilled dijon chicken	as served	737	50	93	5	n/a	n/a	3	2017
Grilled vegetable sandwich	as served	830	22	96	7	n/a	n/a	9	2531
Italian deli	as served	1127	38	91	5	n/a	n/a	19	2979
Turkey stack	as served	749	37	94	5	n/a	n/a	3	2815
SIDES									
Caesar salad	as served	208	4	8	2	n/a	n/a	5	422
Szechuan slaw	as served	342	3	29	4	n/a	n/a	3	1328
DESSERTS									
Apple crisp	as served	510	3	100	5	n/a	n/a	6	26
Butter cake	as served	1084	8	95	3	n/a	n/a	45	530
Chocolate soufflé cake	as served	676	7	50	4	n/a	n/a	31	43
Hot caramel sundae	as served	966	13	77	2	n/a	n/a	36	172
Hot fudge brownie sundae	as served	1065	10	108	4	n/a	n/a	30	299

CALIFORNIA PIZZA KITCHEN (CPK) continued

Item	Serving Size	Calories	Protein	Carb	Fiber	Sugar	Total Fat	Sat Fat	Sodium
Hot fudge sundae	as served	975	10	67	2	n/a	n/a	39	125
Key lime pie	as served	839	9	92	1	n/a	n/a	27	280
Red velvet cake	as served	743	7	91	1	n/a	n/a	17	355
Tiramisu	as served	530	5	53	0	n/a	n/a	19	125
White chocolate strawberry cheesecake	as served	1101	13	96	0	n/a	n/a	47	600

CAPTAIN D'S SEAFOOD KITCHEN

Item	Serving Size	Calories	Protein	Carb	Fiber	Sugar	Total Fat	Sat Fat	Sodium
FISH, SHRIMP, & OTHER SELECTIONS									
Batter-dipped fish	1 piece	182	9	8	1	0	12	6	454
Bite size shrimp	1 order	460	13	51	2	6	21	9	840
Catfish	1 piece	105	7	6	0	0	6	2	233
Chicken tender	1 piece	170	9	11	0	0	10	4	430
Clams	1/2 lb	770	22	64	6	2	47	8	1450
Coconut shrimp	3 shrimp	321	11	27	1	3	19	10	638
Country style fish	1 piece	195	14	14	1	0	10	5	584
Crab cake	1 piece	174	7	12	1	2	11	5	467
Fried flounder	1 piece	213	14	12	0	0	13	6	473
Oysters	1 order	320	10	31	1	0	18	8	710
Premium shrimp	3 pieces	154	8	0	0	0	6	3	323
Scampi shrimp	4 shrimp	28	4	0	0	0	0	0	120
Seasoned tilapia dinner	1 piece	130	24	1	0	0	3	2	520
Shrimp skewers	6 shrimp	100	22	0	0	0	0	0	780
Stuffed crab shell	1 crab shell	100	5	9	0	1	5	2	22
Wild Alaskan salmon	1 piece	140	33	1	0	1	1	0	410
SANDWICHES									
Classic fish sandwich	each	714	27	63	4	4	38	14	1453
Chicken ranch sandwich	each	680	27	69	2	4	33	11	1488
Great little fish sandwich	each	642	17	56	2	5	38	15	1456
Wild Alaskan salmon sandwich	each	490	42	48	2	5	15	2	955

CAPTAIN D'S SEAFOOD KITCHEN continued

Item	Serving Size	Calories	Protein	Carb	Fiber	Sugar	Total Fat	Sat Fat	Sodium
SALADS									
Bite size shrimp	each	267	10	33	4	8	10	4	437
Fried chicken salmon	each	207	11	18	3	5	10	4	447
Side	1 order	232	1	3	2	3	0	0	9
Wild Alaskan salmon	each	177	35	8	3	6	1	0	427
SIDES									
Baked potato, plain	each	255	6	54	6	3	0	0	25
Breadstick	each	150	3	21	1	3	6	2	150
Broccoli	1 order	100	2	5	2	1	1	0	30
Cole slaw	1 order	109	1	13	2	10	12	2	310
Corn on the cob	1 each	163	5	37	4	5	2	0	10
Cracklins	1 oz	28	1	11	0	0	12	6	557
French fries	1 order	99	3	38	4	0	15	7	450
Fried okra	1 order	113	3	23	2	2	14	6	410
Green beans	1 order	113	1	10	3	2	2	0	400
Hush puppies	1 order (2)	50	2	18	1	2	13	6	330
Macaroni & cheese	1 order	113	6	17	0	2	7	2	570
Roasted red potatoes	1 order	124	3	25	3	1	7	4	1200
Seasoned rice	1 order	113	4	35	1	1	1	0	670
SAUCES									
Blue cheese dressing	1 pkt	43	2	2	0	2	24	4	440
Cocktail	3/4 oz	21	0	6	0	4	0	0	250
Fat Free Italian dressing	1 pkt	28	0	2	0	1	0	0	440
Ginger Teriyaki	5 fl oz	68	2	13	0	9	0	0	1300
Honey mustard dressing	1 pkt	28	0	5	0	3	16	2	125
Ranch dressing	1 pkt	29	0	1	0	1	12	2	210
Scampi butter	2 fl oz	57	2	5	0	1	10	6	360
Sweet chili	2 fl oz	68	0	25	0	23	0	0	960
Tartar	3/4 oz	21	0	1	0	1	10	2	75
DESSERTS									
Cheesecake	1 slice	113	6	35	1	24	27	14	300
Cheesecake w/ strawberries	1 slice	142	6	45	1	27	26	9	220
Chocolate cake	1 slice	85	3	49	2	35	11	2	270
Pecan pie	1 slice	113	5	56	0	26	26	4	270
Pineapple cream cheese pie	1 slice	106	6	43	0	33	14	6	300

CARL'S JR.

Item	Serving Size	Calories	Protein	Carb	Fiber	Sugar	Total Fat	Sat Fat	Sodium
BREAKFAST									
Bacon & egg burrito	each	550	29	37	1	2	32	10	990
Breakfast burger	each	780	38	64	3	13	41	15	1460
French toast dips, w/o syrup	5 pieces	460	9	60	3	16	21	4	570
Hash brown nuggets	1 order	350	3	32	3	0	23	4	440
Loaded breakfast burrito	each	780	36	51	3	3	49	16	1480
Sourdough breakfast sandwich	each	470	26	37	1	2	25	9	1090
Steak & egg burrito	each	650	41	43	1	4	36	14	1750
Sunrise croissant	each	590	20	27	1	4	44	17	810
BURGERS & SANDWICHES									
Bacon Swiss Crispy Chicken® sandwich	each	750	36	62	4	9	40	9	1990
Big hamburger	each	470	24	55	3	14	17	8	1010
Carl's Catch Fish Sandwich®	each	680	20	70	4	9	37	6	1260
Charbroiled BBQ chicken sandwich	each	380	30	51	3	13	7	1.5	1070
Charbroiled Chicken Club™ sandwich	each	560	36	46	3	10	27	7	1330
Charbroiled Santa Fe Chicken™ sandwich	each	630	32	46	3	10	35	8	1460
Chicken Stars	4 pieces	170	8	12	1	0	10	2	360
Chicken Stars	6 pieces	260	12	18	2	0	16	3.5	540
Chicken Stars	9 pieces	390	18	26	3	0	23	5	810
Famous Star® w/ cheese	each	660	27	53	3	11	39	13	1240
Fish & chips	each	710	22	69	7	0	38	6	1410
Hand-Breaded Chicken Tenders™	kids'	220	19	10	1	0	12	2.5	770
Hand-Breaded Chicken Tenders™	3 pieces	340	28	14	1	1	19	3.5	1160
Hand-Breaded Chicken Tenders™	5 pieces	560	47	24	2	1	31	6	1930
Jalapeño burger	each	720	27	51	6	9	47	14	1350
Kids' cheeseburger	each	290	12	25	1	5	15	7	790
Kids' hamburger	each	230	9	24	1	5	10	3.5	510
Single Teriyaki Burger™	each	610	28	60	3	19	29	11	1020

CARL'S JR. continued

Item	Serving Size	Calories	Protein	Carb	Fiber	Sugar	Total Fat	Sat Fat	Sodium
Spicy chicken sandwich	each	420	12	37	3	3	26	5	1260
Super Star w/ cheese	each	920	47	55	3	12	58	24	1580
The Big Carl	each	910	47	52	2	11	58	23	1350
The Guacamole Bacon Six Dollar Burger®	each	1040	49	51	4	10	72	24	2240
The Jalapeno Six Dollar Burger®	each	930	45	51	6	9	63	21	2200
The Low Carb Six Dollar Burger®	each	570	38	9	1	5	43	19	1460
The Original Six Dollar Burger®	each	900	45	59	3	18	54	21	2000
The Portobello Mushroom Six Dollar Burger®	each	870	47	52	4	9	53	19	1730
The Western Bacon Six Dollar Burger®	each	1000	52	77	4	15	53	22	2370
Western Bacon Cheeseburger™	each	710	32	70	4	14	33	13	1430
Western Bacon Cheeseburger™, Double	each	960	52	71	4	14	52	23	1770

SIDES

Item	Serving Size	Calories	Protein	Carb	Fiber	Sugar	Total Fat	Sat Fat	Sodium
Chili cheese fries	1 serving	950	28	88	8	1	56	19	2350
CrissCut fries	1 serving	450	5	42	4	0	29	5	900
Fish & chips	1 serving	730	22	72	6	0	39	7	1630
Fried zucchini	1 serving	330	6	36	2	7	18	3	610
Natural-cut fries	kids	240	3	29	2	0	11	2	580
Natural-cut fries	small	310	4	42	4	0	15	3	830
Natural-cut fries	medium	430	5	60	5	0	22	4.5	1180
Natural-cut fries	large	470	6	65	5	0	24	5	1290
Onion rings	1 serving	530	8	61	3	6	28	4.5	590

SALADS

Item	Serving Size	Calories	Protein	Carb	Fiber	Sugar	Total Fat	Sat Fat	Sodium
Cranberry, apple, walnut grilled chicken	each	300	26	25	4	15	11	3.5	840
Original grilled chicken	each	200	24	13	3	6	6	3	610
Side	each	50	3	5	2	2	2.5	1.5	75
Southwest grilled chicken salad	each	440	35	24	5	4	23	8	1100

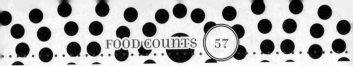

CARL'S JR. continued

Item	Serving Size	Calories	Protein	Carb	Fiber	Sugar	Total Fat	Sat Fat	Sodium
SALAD DRESSINGS									
Blue cheese	each	320	2	1	0	1	34	7	410
Chipotle Caesar	each	270	2	5	1	3	27	4.5	860
House	each	220	1	3	0	2	22	3.5	440
Low-fat balsamic vinaigrette	each	35	0	5	0	3	1.5	0	480
Raspberry vinaigrette	each	160	0	12	0	11	12	2	150
DESSERTS									
Chocolate Cake	each	300	3	48	1	36	12	3	350
Chocolate Chip Cookie	each	370	3	48	2	27	19	10	350
Strawberry Swirl Cheesecake	1 slice	290	6	30	0	21	16	9	230
SHAKES & MALTS									
Chocolate Hand-Scooped Ice Cream malt™	each	780	15	100	1	82	34	24	370
Chocolate Hand-Scooped Ice Cream shake™	each	710	14	86	1	71	33	23	300
Oreo cookie Hand-Scooped Ice Cream malt™	each	790	17	95	1	76	38	25	440
Oreo cookie Hand-Scooped Ice Cream shake™	each	730	15	81	1	64	38	25	360
Strawberry Hand-Scooped Ice Cream malt™	each	770	15	99	0	86	34	24	320
Strawberry Hand-Scooped Ice Cream shake™	each	700	14	85	0	75	33	23	250
Vanilla Hand-Scooped Ice Cream malt™	each	780	15	101	0	87	34	24	320
Vanilla Hand-Scooped Ice Cream shake™	each	710	14	86	0	76	33	23	240

CHEVYS FRESH MEX

Item	Serving Size	Calories	Protein	Carb	Fiber	Sugar	Total Fat	Sat Fat	Sodium
APPETIZERS & QUESADILLAS									
Carnitas quesadilla	as served	1650	59	112	4	11	107	48	3100
Chile con queso	as served	1510	53	131	8	5	85	41	2190
Crab & shrimp quesadilla	as served	1790	77	86	3	7	126	63	3440
Crispy chicken flautas	as served	970	39	82	6	34	56	17	1710
'Dilla-Duo-Dinner	as served	765–963	38–52	58–70	4–8	4–9	43–51	19–20	1224–2255
Farmers' Market quesadilla	as served	1590	63	105	6	11	104	52	3080
Fresh Mex® Sampler	as served	2560	144	179	25	19	139	53	4130
Grilled steak quesadilla	as served	1380	69	78	3	2	88	41	223
Guac-My-Way	as served	730	10	62	24	4	53	7	1030
Nachos Grande	as served	1890	69	163	22	9	105	41	2280
Original chicken quesadilla	as served	1260	57	77	4	4	80	39	229
Original fajita nachos	as served	1540–1654	92–89	81–89	21	4–9	91–108	44–50	2160–2234
Red chile pork taquitos	as served	610	28	44	6	5	37	12	870
San Antonio chicken quesadilla	as served	1170	73	72	4	15	65	34	2140
Shrimp & sweet corn cake tamalito	as served	690	26	55	6	15	42	20	3050
Spicy wings	as served	1520	108	37	3	14	99	22	3760
SOUPS & SALADS									
BBQ chicken salad	as served	1140	60	72	11	27	69	21	2170
Grilled chicken Caesar	as served	860	33	32	7	5	69	8	960
Grilled fajita salad	as served	1448–1582	48–64	65–69	10	31–33	107–127	27–34	1449–1941
Homemade tortilla soup	1 bowl	390	26	35	7	9	17	3.5	1200
Kickin' chicken corn chowder	1 serving	280	8	28	3	5	16	9	1020
Sante Fe chopped	as served	670	52	30	9	11	39	16	1820
Tostada salad	as served	1547–1682	63–80	100–105	18	8–11	94–115	37–45	2213–2536

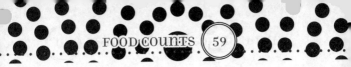

CHEVYS FRESH MEX continued

Item	Serving Size	Calories	Protein	Carb	Fiber	Sugar	Total Fat	Sat Fat	Sodium
SIZZLING FAJITAS									
Carnitas	as served	1291	49	103	19	22	77	28	2823
Fresh salmon	as served	1127	71	96	19	16	51	16	2684
Juicy achiote shrimp	as served	1200	56	102	19	18	64	27	3268
Mix & Match	as served	1235–1438	47–73	115–120	22–23	20–23	55–88	22–34	2483–2826
Mixed grill	as served	1533	83	103	19	21	87	35	3327
Original famous chicken	as served	932	67	95	18	17	32	11	2225
Sizzling steak	as served	1030	63	94	18	16	46	17	2083
Veggie fajitas & chile relleno	as served	1080	38	119	23	29	53	24	2710
À LA CARTE ITEMS									
Beans a la Charra	each	210	13	32	11	1	4	2	790
Carnitas crispy taco	each	270	16	27	3	3	12	4	230
Carnitas enchilada	each	300	12	15	2	2	21	8	470
Carnitas soft taco	each	360	11	27	2	3	23	7	680
Cheddar cheese enchilada	each	390	22	17	2	2	27	14	590
Chile relleno	each	260	16	7	3	4	30	14	320
Crispy chicken flautas	each	430	19	36	3	12	23	8	830
Crispy picadillo beef taco	each	240	10	18	3	2	15	4	260
Crispy salsa chicken taco	each	230	10	17	2	2	13	3	320
El Machino tortilla	each	140	3	22	1	0	4	2	300
Fresh Mex® rice	as served	180	3	29	1	1	5	1	600
Guacamole	as served	130	2	7	5	1	12	2	320
Homemade black beans	as served	190	12	32	11	2	2	0.5	750
Mini chimichanga	each	600	24	47	4	2	35	14	1170
Picadillo beef enchilada	each	260	15	18	2	3	14	6	370
Refried beans	as served	280	11	28	9	2	14	5	670
Salsa chicken enchilada	each	230	15	17	2	3	11	5	430
Salsa chicken tamale	each	330	14	49	9	3	10	4	400
Slow-roasted pork tamale	each	370	17	54	10	5	10	4	450
Soft picadillo beef taco	each	290	12	27	2	2	15	5	560
Soft salsa chicken taco	each	280	12	26	2	2	14	4	620
Sour cream	as served	180	3	4	0	0	18	11	45
Sweet corn tamalito	as served	190	3	29	2	9	7	3	170

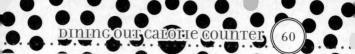

CHEVYS FRESH MEX continued

Item	Serving Size	Calories	Protein	Carb	Fiber	Sugar	Total Fat	Sat Fat	Sodium
FRESH MEX SPECIALTIES									
Chile verde	as served	1030	43	113	6	11	44	15	2510
Crispy chicken flautas	as served	1510	55	156	20	40	76	24	3220
Red chile pork taquitos	as served	1350	54	136	22	15	69	23	2750
SIGNATURE ENCHILADAS									
Chicken mole enchiladas	as served	950	43	84	9	13	51	19	1690
Chipotle chicken enchiladas	as served	1070	39	87	8	13	64	30	2000
Fresh Mex® artichoke/mushroom	as served	1120	24	94	9	14	75	36	1810
Shrimp & crab enchilada	as served	1360	41	87	7	11	97	49	2070
MESQUITE GRILLED TACOS									
Grilled chicken tacos	as served	1050	56	125	16	11	35	9	2590
Grilled fresh fish tacos	as served	1060	50	125	16	11	39	10	2910
Grilled steak tacos	as served	1110	53	124	16	11	44	13	2490
Grilled tacos combo	as served	1080	54	125	16	11	40	11	2540
FRESH MEX BURRITOS									
Cheeseburger	as served	1550	70	139	11	10	79	29	2290
Fajita burrito steak	as served	1320–1420	56–69	151–153	22	16–19	51–67	21–28	3400–3540
Grande chimi beef	as served	1720–1730	77–85	152–153	26–29	17–20	88–90	40–44	4280–4590
Smothered	as served	1490–1540	67–69	157–159	22	20–21	68–73	30–31	3860–3800
Smothered chile verde	as served	1360	52	134	11	16	71	29	3130
Veggie	as served	1440	49	177	26	23	62	26	3780
DESSERTS									
Chevys flan	each	740	16	116	0	115	23	12	150
Chiquita sundae	each	560–590	8	68–72	2	37–40	28–31	12–13	450–460
Deep-fried ice cream	each	1100	15	131	3	78	60	25	750
Ooey Gooey Chewy Sundae	each	1020	12	145	4	105	48	23	650
Sopapillas	each	550	7	78	2	37	24	1	560

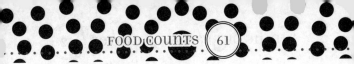

CHEVYS FRESH MEX continued

Item	Serving Size	Calories	Protein	Carb	Fiber	Sugar	Total Fat	Sat Fat	Sodium
KIDS' MENU									
Bean & cheese burrito	as served	1020	26	131	12	26	45	15	1580
Cheese quesadilla	as served	1020	28	125	8	25	47	20	1450
Flour flautas	as served	1100–1240	35–45	120–125	9–12	25–29	53–71	18–29	1610–1980
Fresh Mex® chicken bites	as served	810	28	97	7	25	36	9	1380
Kiddie cheeseburger	as served	1060	43	112	7	29	5	19	1120
Taco	as served	750–840	20–28	96–106	7–8	26–27	33–35	10–12	810–1080
SIZZLING LUNCH FAJITAS									
Juicy achiote shrimp	as served	923	35	88	15	13	48	21	2620
Original famous chicken	as served	820	51	90	17	14	29	10	2032
Sizzling steak	as served	885	48	89	17	14	39	14	1937
Slow-roasted carnitas	as served	956	34	93	17	17	51	19	2260
LUNCH DUOS									
Baby greens	side	80	2	13	3	2	3	1	100
Caesar salad	side	360	4	16	4	2	32	3	350
Chicken quesadilla	as served	490	27	35	0	1	27	13	970
Grilled Steak quesadilla	as served	550	33	35	0	0	31	14	930
Sante Fe chopped salad	as served	370	26	15	5	4	23	9	910
LUNCH BOWLS									
Chicken mole enchilada	as served	860	41	70	8	8	47	18	1610
Chili verde	as served	510	33	39	3	9	25	6	1430
Grilled fresh salmon	as served	540	12	45	5	6	26	7	1300
Red chile pork taquitos	as served	770	36	55	7	5	48	16	1610
Smothered chile verde burrito	as served	1130	49	109	8	11	57	23	2840

CHEVYS FRESH MEX continued

Item	Serving Size	Calories	Protein	Carb	Fiber	Sugar	Total Fat	Sat Fat	Sodium
MISC. DIPS / TOPPINGS									
Guacamole	1 tbsp	20	0	1	1	0	2	0	45
Pico de gallo	1 tbsp	5	0	1	0	0	0	0	40
Sour cream	1 tbsp	30	0	1	0	0	3	2	10
Sweet corn tamalito	1 tbsp	30	0	5	0	2	1	0	30

CHICK-FIL-A

Item	Serving Size	Calories	Protein	Carb	Fiber	Sugar	Total Fat	Sat Fat	Sodium
DESSERTS									
Cheesecake	1 slice	340	6	30	2	25	21	12	270
Fudge nut brownie	each	330	4	45	2	29	15	3.5	210
Ice cream, Icedream®	small	230	5	39	0	39	6	3.5	100
Lemon pie	1 slice	320	7	51	3	39	10	3.5	220
SANDWICHES & WRAPS									
Charbroiled cicken wrap	each	390	31	53	3	6	7	3	1120
Chargrilled chicken breast fillet	each	100	20	1	0	1	1.5	0	690
Chicken Caesar wrap	each	460	38	51	3	5	11	6	1540
Chicken deluxe sandwich	each	420	28	39	2	5	16	3.5	1300
Chicken salad sandwich on whole wheat	each	350	20	32	5	6	15	3	880
Chicken sandwich	each	410	28	38	1	5	16	3.5	1300
Spicy chicken wrap	each	390	31	51	3	5	7	3.5	1150
SIDES & SALADS									
Chargrilled chicken Caesar salad	each	240	31	6	2	3	10	6	1170
Chicken nuggets	8 pieces	260	26	12	1	3	12	2.5	1090
Chick-n-Strips, breaded & fried	4 pieces	250	25	12	0	2	11	2.5	570
Chick-n-Strips salad	each	340	30	19	3	5	16	5	680
Garden salad w/ chargrilled chicken	each	180	23	8	3	4	6	3	730
Hearty chicken breast soup	1 cup	100	9	13	1	2	1.5	0	940
Salad	each	80	5	6	2	3	5	2.5	110
Waffle fries	small	280	3	37	5	0	14	5	105

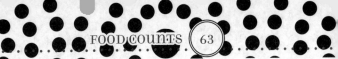

CHILI'S

Item	Serving Size	Calories	Protein	Carb	Fiber	Sugar	Total Fat	Sat Fat	Sodium
ENTRÉES									
Chicken platter	as served	563	38	83	4	5	9	3	3284
Chicken salad w/ dressing	as served	272	29	27	6	20	5	1	1475
Chili's classic sirloin w/o sides	as served	400	49	7	0	n/a	19	9	1490
Classic bacon burger	as served	1520	64	115	9	0	88	26	3630
Crispy chicken tacos w/ corn tortillas	as served	1670	64	182	13	n/a	76	21	4110
Crispy shrimp tacos w/ corn tortillas	as served	1610	60	186	22	n/a	70	19	4420
Flame-grilled rib eye w/o sides	as served	900	50	18	2	n/a	68	32	1980
Grilled BBQ chicken salad w/ dressing	as served	1060	76	50	12	4	63	19	2190
Grilled salmon w/ garlic & herbs	as served	320	44	1	1	n/a	16	5	600
Memphis dry rub ribs, 1/2 rack	as served	860	42	80	8	n/a	42	8	3390
Original ribs, 1/2 rack	as served	860	43	73	8	n/a	43	15	2970
Pasta w/ veggies & chicken	as served	786	53	106	6	6	15	5	1195
Pulled pork tacos w/ corn tortillas	as served	800	52	99	12	n/a	22	8	2870
Shiner Bock BBQ ribs, 1/2 rack	as served	930	44	90	8	n/a	43	15	2890
Smoked chicken tacos w/ corn tortillas	as served	700	45	98	12	n/a	15	6	3060
SIDES & SALADS									
Asian salad w/ grilled chicken	as served	540	33	40	5	n/a	29	8	2110
Asian salad w/ salmon	small	650	42	40	9	n/a	32	8	2310
Asian salad w/ steak	as served	610	39	41	7	n/a	33	8	2760
Black beans	as served	100	6	17	5	n/a	1	0	620
Boneless Buffalo wings w/ blue cheese	1 order	1060	38	44	2	2	81	14	3330
Buffalo chicken salad	as served	1110	46	49	6	n/a	79	17	4150

CHILI'S continued

Item	Serving Size	Calories	Protein	Carb	Fiber	Sugar	Total Fat	Sat Fat	Sodium
Caribbean salad w/ grilled chicken	as served	620	36	66	9	n/a	25	4	530
Caribbean salad w/ grilled shrimp	as served	620	20	66	7	n/a	31	6	1000
Chicken Caesar salad	as served	710	42	25	8	n/a	58	6	1010
Cinnamon apples	as served	200	0	35	7	n/a	8	2	95
Guiltless Grill Asian salad	as served	410	40	22	8	n/a	21	3	890
Guiltless Grill Caribbean salad	as served	550	35	54	9	n/a	22	3	630
Homestyle fries	as served	380	4	55	6	n/a	16	3	1210
Loaded beef nachos	1/8 order	144	8	5	1	0	10.3	4.8	418
Loaded mashed potatoes	as served	380	12	28	3	n/a	25	9	1140
Mashed potatoes w/ black pepper gravy	as served	280	4	31	3	n/a	15	4	1300
Ranch only as served w/ whips	as served	460	3	5	0	n/a	48	9	910
Rice	as served	240	4	41	1	n/a	6	1	410
Salsa only as served w/ chips	as served	30	1	6	2	n/a	0	0	1120
Salsa ranch only as served w/ chips	as served	250	2	5	1	n/a	24	5	1010
Seasonal veggies	as served	80	3	7	3	n/a	6	3	490
Sour cream	as served	60	1	2	0	n/a	6	4	55
Spicy cole slaw	as served	180	2	9	3	n/a	15	3	810
Sweet corn on the cob w/ butter	as served	200	5	32	3	n/a	7	1	420

DRESSINGS

Item	Serving Size	Calories	Protein	Carb	Fiber	Sugar	Total Fat	Sat Fat	Sodium
Ancho chili ranch	as served	170	1	3	0	n/a	17	4	390
Asian vinaigrette	as served	150	1	5	0	n/a	15	2	690
Avocado ranch	as served	110	1	2	1	n/a	11	2	230
Blue cheese	as served	240	1	1	0	n/a	25	5	310
Caribbean Guiltless Grill	as served	190	0	5	0	n/a	19	3	430
Citrus balsamic vinaigrette	as served	250	0	6	0	n/a	25	4	220
Honey lime	as served	200	0	13	0	n/a	17	3	250

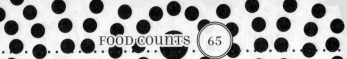

CHILI'S continued

Item	Serving Size	Calories	Protein	Carb	Fiber	Sugar	Total Fat	Sat Fat	Sodium
Honey mustard	as served	180	0	1	0	n/a	21	3	380
Honey mustard, non-fat	as served	70	0	10	0	n/a	0	0	510
Jalapeño ranch	as served	140	1	2	0	n/a	15	3	360
Low-fat ranch	as served	45	1	4	0	n/a	3	0	440
Ranch	as served	170	1	2	0	n/a	18	4	340

APPETIZERS

Item	Serving Size	Calories	Protein	Carb	Fiber	Sugar	Total Fat	Sat Fat	Sodium
Boneless Buffalo wing w/ blue cheese	as served	1060	38	44	2	n/a	81	14	3330
Bottomless tostada chips w/ salsa	as served	480	4	26	5	n/a	39	5	2050
Classic nachos, beef	12 piece	1600	98	66	9	n/a	106	50	3590
Classic nachos, beef	8 piece	1090	66	46	6	n/a	73	34	2450
Classic nachos, chicken	12 piece	1530	108	62	10	n/a	98	46	2630
Classic nachos, chicken	8 piece	1050	72	43	7	n/a	67	32	1810
Crispy onion string & jalapeño stack w/ jalapeño ranch	as served	1020	8	49	6	n/a	86	13	1780
Fire-grilled corn guacamole w/ chips	as served	1390	16	150	27	n/a	84	15	2320
Fried cheese w/ marinara sauce	as served	730	36	60	2	n/a	39	17	2270
Hot spinach & artichoke dip w/ chips	as served	1130	31	41	3	n/a	90	39	2460
Skillet queso w/ chips	as served	920	30	46	9	n/a	73	30	4040
Southwestern eggrolls w/ avocado ranch	as served	910	27	72	7	n/a	57	14	1980
Texas cheese fries, 1/2 order w/ chili & jalapeño ranch	as served	1510	70	65	7	n/a	109	49	3970
Texas cheese fries, 1/2 order w/ jalapeño ranch	as served	1410	64	60	6	n/a	103	48	3630
Texas cheese fries, w/ chili & jalapeño ranch	as served	2070	94	105	12	n/a	144	64	5950
Texas cheese fries, w/ jalapeño ranch	as served	1920	84	98	11	n/a	134	61	5450

CHILI'S continued

Item	Serving Size	Calories	Protein	Carb	Fiber	Sugar	Total Fat	Sat Fat	Sodium
Triple Dipper™ Big Mouth Bites® w/ jalapeño ranch	as served	790	31	49	1	n/a	51	14	1780
Triple Dipper™ Boneless Buffalo Wings w/ blue cheese	as served	750	24	27	1	n/a	60	11	1990
Triple Dipper™ Chicken Crispers® w/o dressing	as served	320	28	19	1	n/a	14	4	1040
Triple Dipper™ crispy onion string & jalapeño stack	as served	410	3	16	2	n/a	37	6	790
Triple Dipper™ fried cheese w/ marinara sauce	as served	430	21	36	1	n/a	23	10	1380
Triple Dipper™ hot spinach & artichoke dip w/ chips	as served	570	16	20	2	n/a	45	20	1230
Triple Dipper™ Southwestern eggrolls w/ avocado ranch	as served	640	18	48	5	n/a	42	10	1400
Triple Dipper™ Wings Over Buffalo® w/ blue cheese	as served	800	34	4	1	n/a	69	15	1860
Wings Over Buffalo® w/ blue cheese	as served	1320	67	4	1	n/a	110	25	2240
SOUPS									
Broccoli cheese soup	1 bowl	240	10	17	2	n/a	15	7	1270
Broccoli cheese soup	1 cup	120	5	8	1	n/a	8	4	640
Chicken & green chili	1 bowl	250	16	33	3	n/a	6	1	1060
Chicken & green chili	1 cup	120	8	17	1	n/a	3	0	530
Chicken enchilada	1 bowl	430	28	22	2	n/a	26	10	1350
Chicken enchilada	1 cup	220	14	11	1	n/a	13	5	670
Chili's Terlingua chili w/ toppings	1 bowl	460	24	24	4	n/a	30	12	2190
Chili's Terlingua chili w/ toppings	1 cup	230	12	12	2	n/a	15	6	1090
Loaded baked potato soup	1 bowl	400	15	21	1	n/a	30	18	1150

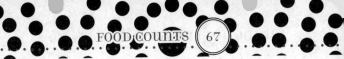

CHILI'S continued

Item	Serving Size	Calories	Protein	Carb	Fiber	Sugar	Total Fat	Sat Fat	Sodium
Loaded baked potato soup	1 cup	200	8	11	1	n/a	15	9	570
Sweet corn soup	1 bowl	450	4	31	1	n/a	36	20	960
Sweet corn soup	1 cup	230	2	16	1	n/a	18	10	480

SANDWICHES

Item	Serving Size	Calories	Protein	Carb	Fiber	Sugar	Total Fat	Sat Fat	Sodium
BBQ pulled pork sandwich	as served	1250	41	149	11	n/a	54	14	3320
Buffalo chicken ranch sandwich	as served	1520	51	138	8	n/a	82	15	3790
GG grilled chicken sandwich w/ veggies	as served	610	44	78	8	n/a	12	5	1310
GG Sante Fe chicken wrap w/ veggies	as served	610	34	75	9	n/a	22	4	1740
Grilled chicken sandwich	as served	1240	56	114	9	n/a	62	14	2510
Sante Fe chicken wrap w/ Ancho Chili ranch	as served	1270	41	121	12	n/a	70	16	2580
Smoked turkey combo, w/o soup or salad	as served	830	26	83	7	n/a	43	11	2180
Smoked turkey sandwich	as served	1240	44	110	8	n/a	66	17	3060
Steakhouse sandwich	as served	1080	38	115	11	n/a	51	20	3780

TACOS

Item	Serving Size	Calories	Protein	Carb	Fiber	Sugar	Total Fat	Sat Fat	Sodium
Chicken club tacos	as served	1280	59	130	11	n/a	57	17	4120
Crispy chicken tacos	as served	1650	64	181	13	n/a	76	21	4080
Crispy shrimp tacos	as served	1600	59	186	22	n/a	69	19	4380

BURGERS

Item	Serving Size	Calories	Protein	Carb	Fiber	Sugar	Total Fat	Sat Fat	Sodium
Big Mouth® Bites w/ jalapeño ranch	as served	1930	65	145	7	n/a	117	31	4400
Classic bacon burger	as served	1520	64	115	9	n/a	88	26	3630
Ground peppercorn burger w/ blue cheese	as served	1520	55	120	12	n/a	88	21	3330
Jalapeño smokehouse burger w/ jalapeño ranch	as served	2140	94	125	10	n/a	139	44	6710
Mushroom-Swiss burger	as served	1500	61	116	10	n/a	85	25	3750

CHILI'S continued

Item	Serving Size	Calories	Protein	Carb	Fiber	Sugar	Total Fat	Sat Fat	Sodium
Oldtimer®	as served	1260	53	118	10	n/a	62	16	3140
Shiner Bock BBQ burger	as served	1510	59	138	9	n/a	78	22	3570
Southern smokehouse burger w/ Ancho Chili BBQ	as served	2090	93	139	10	n/a	127	42	6310
KIDS' MENU W/O SIDES									
Pepper Pals® cheese pizza	as served	570	23	67	3	n/a	24	9	1120
Pepper Pals® cheese quesadilla	as served	460	20	42	2	n/a	24	12	1000
Pepper Pals® chocolate shake	as served	490	6	67	0	n/a	24	14	140
Pepper Pals® corn dog	as served	280	5	25	2	n/a	17	4	650
Pepper Pals® Crispy Chicken Crispers	as served	380	26	19	2	n/a	22	4	630
Pepper Pals® grilled cheese sandwich	as served	520	10	28	0	n/a	41	12	860
Pepper Pals® grilled chicken platter	as served	150	31	1	1	n/a	3	1	140
Pepper Pals® grilled chicken sandwich	as served	180	19	17	1	n/a	4	0	180
Pepper Pals® Little Crispy Chicken Crispers	as served	320	28	19	1	n/a	14	4	1040
Pepper Pals® Little Mouth Burger	as served	310	22	17	1	n/a	17	5	570
Pepper Pals® Little Mouth Cheeseburger	as served	380	25	18	1	n/a	23	9	890
Pepper Pals® macaroni & cheese	as served	500	16	69	3	n/a	18	6	930
Pepper Pals® side celery sticks w/ ranch	as served	50	2	5	0	n/a	3	0	460
Pepper Pals® side cinnamon apples	as served	200	0	35	7	n/a	8	2	95
Pepper Pals® side corn cob w/o butter	as served	150	5	32	3	n/a	2	0	5
Pepper Pals® side homestyle fries	as served	250	3	36	4	n/a	10	2	790

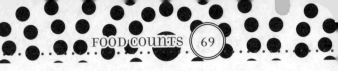

CHILI'S continued

Item	Serving Size	Calories	Protein	Carb	Fiber	Sugar	Total Fat	Sat Fat	Sodium
Pepper Pals® side kernel corn	as served	130	4	23	6	n/a	2	0	0
Pepper Pals® side mandarin oranges	as served	70	0	17	0	n/a	0	0	10
Pepper Pals® side mashed potatoes w/o gravy	as served	120	2	14	1	n/a	7	2	430
Pepper Pals® side pineapple	as served	35	0	9	1	n/a	0	0	0
Pepper Pals® side rice	as served	240	4	41	1	n/a	6	1	410
Pepper Pals® side salad w/ low-fat ranch	as served	100	4	9	1	n/a	6	2	540
Pepper Pals® side steamed broccoli	as served	30	3	6	3	n/a	0	0	30
DESSERTS									
Brownie sundae	each	1290	14	195	8	n/a	61	30	930
Cheesecake	each	710	12	68	0	n/a	42	26	460
Chocolate Chip Paradise Pie	each	1290	16	163	5	n/a	68	33	680
Frosty chocolate shake	each	740	8	100	0	n/a	35	21	210
Molten chocolate cake	each	1070	11	143	5	n/a	51	28	820
Sweet Shot key lime pie	each	240	4	30	0	n/a	12	8	75
Sweet Shot red velvet cake	each	250	3	39	1	n/a	9	5	200
Sweet Shot warm cinnamon roll	each	280	3	38	1	n/a	13	8	95
Sweet Shot warm double chocolate fudge brownie	each	420	1	51	1	n/a	24	14	25
White chocolate molten cake	each	1250	14	150	0	n/a	65	24	450

CHIPOTLE MEXICAN GRILL

Item	Serving Size	Calories	Protein	Carb	Fiber	Sugar	Total Fat	Sat Fat	Sodium
SHELLS									
Chips	4 oz	570	8	73	8	n/a	27	3.5	420
Crispy taco shell	each	60	<1	9	1	n/a	2	0.5	10
Flour tortilla (burrito)	each	290	7	44	2	n/a	9	3	670
Flour tortilla (taco)	each	90	2	13	<1	n/a	2.5	1	200
MEAT									
Barbacoa	4 oz	170	24	2	0	n/a	7	2.5	510
Carnitas	4 oz	190	27	1	0	n/a	8	2.5	540
Chicken	4 oz	190	32	1	0	n/a	6.5	2	370
Steak	4 oz	190	30	2	0	n/a	6.5	2	320
TOPPINGS									
Black beans	4 oz	120	7	23	11	n/a	1	0	250
Cheese	1 oz	100	8	0	0	n/a	8.5	5	180
Cilantro-lime rice	3 oz	130	2	23	0	n/a	3	0.5	150
Corn salsa	3.5 oz	80	3	15	3	n/a	1.5	0	410
Green tomatillo salsa	2 fl oz	15	1	3	1	n/a	0	0	230
Guacamole	3.5 oz	150	2	8	6	n/a	13	2	190
Fajita vegetables	2.5 oz	20	1	4	1	n/a	0.5	0	170
Pinto beans	4 oz	120	7	22	10	n/a	1	0	330
Red tomatillo salsa	2 fl oz	40	2	8	4	n/a	1	0	510
Romaine lettuce (salad)	2.5 oz	10	1	2	1	n/a	0	0	5
Romaine lettuce (tacos)	1 oz	5	0	1	1	n/a	0	0	0
Sour cream	2 oz	120	2	2	0	n/a	10	7	30
Tomato salsa	3.5 oz	20	1	4	<1	n/a	0	0	470
Vinaigrette	2 fl oz	260	0	12	1	n/a	24.5	4	700

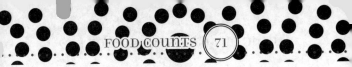

CHURCH'S CHICKEN

Item	Serving Size	Calories	Protein	Carb	Fiber	Sugar	Total Fat	Sat Fat	Sodium
MAIN COURSE									
Boneless wings w/ BBQ sauce	6 pieces	550	33	60	2	23	21	4	2420
Boneless wings w/ Buffalo sauce	6 pieces	460	33	36	1	1	21	4	2620
Chicken fried steak	1 pieces	470	21	36	1	4	28	7	1620
Chicken sandwich w/ cheese	each	503	19	48	3	5	26	7	1461
Double chicken N cheese sandwich	each	738	32	63	4	5	39	12	250
Nuggets	5 pieces	162	9	13	1	0	7	2	759
Original breast	1 piece	200	22	3	1	0	11	3	450
Original chicken sandwich	each	458	16	48	3	5	22	4	1241
Original leg	1 piece	110	10	3	0	0	6	2	280
Original thigh	1 piece	330	21	8	1	0	23	6	680
Original wing	1 piece	300	27	7	3	0	19	5	540
Shrimp & fries basket	3 basket	750	21	86	6	3	36	6	1980
Spicy breast	1 piece	320	21	12	2	0	20	5	760
Spicy chicken sandwich	each	456	15	47	3	5	21	4	1292
Spicy leg	1 piece	180	12	8	1	0	11	3	470
Spicy Tender Strips™	1 piece	135	11	7	4	0	7	2	480
Spicy thigh	1 piece	480	22	20	2	0	35	9	1035
Spicy wing	4 piece	430	29	17	2	0	27	7	1020
Steak fingers	3 pieces	494	20	23	2	2	36	12	1036
Tender Strips™	1 piece	120	12	6	0	0	6	2	440
SIDES & DESSERTS									
Apple pie	1 pie	260	2	39	1	15	11	4	250
Cajun rice	regular	130	1	16	0	0	7	3	260
Cajun rice	large	350	3	43	0	0	19	8	693
Cajun rice	family	520	4	64	0	0	28	12	1040
Churro, caramel	1 piece	140	2	18	1	4	7	2	120
Cole slaw	regular	150	1	15	2	7	10	2	170
Cole slaw	large	400	3	40	5	19	27	5	453
Cole slaw	family	600	4	60	8	28	40	8	680
Corn on the cob	1 piece	140	4	24	9	2	3	0	15
French fries	value	215	2	28	3	1	10	2	235

CHURCH'S CHICKEN continued

Item	Serving Size	Calories	Protein	Carb	Fiber	Sugar	Total Fat	Sat Fat	Sodium
French fries	regular	290	3	38	4	1	14	3	320
French fries	large	595	6	78	8	2	29	6	656
French fries	family	890	9	117	12	3	43	9	982
Honey-butter biscuit	each	190	2	22	1	3	10	2	430
Jalapeño Cheese Bombers®	value	180	6	22	2	4	8	5	730
Jalapeño Cheese Bombers®	regular	240	8	29	3	5	10	6	970
Jalapeño Cheese Bombers®	large	480	16	58	6	10	20	12	1940
Jalapeño Cheese Bombers®	family	720	24	87	9	15	30	18	2910
Jalapeño Pepper	1 pepper	5	0	1	1	1	0	0	195
Macaroni & cheese	regular	221	7	24	2	2	10	5	799
Macaroni & cheese	large	585	8	63	5	5	27	14	2115
Macaroni & cheese	family	884	27	95	7	7	41	20	3196
Mashed potatoes & gravy	regular	70	2	12	1	2	2	0	480
Mashed potatoes & gravy	large	190	5	32	3	5	5	0	1280
Mashed potatoes & gravy	family	280	8	48	4	8	8	0	1920
Okra	regular	350	3	36	5	3	22	7	590
Okra	large	718	6	74	10	6	45	15	1210
Okra	family	1075	9	111	15	9	68	21	1811
Strawberry short cake	1 piece	505	4	95	6	71	14	5	788

CONDIMENTS

Item	Serving Size	Calories	Protein	Carb	Fiber	Sugar	Total Fat	Sat Fat	Sodium
BBQ sauce	1 pkg	24	0	6	0	2	0	0	96
Creamy Jalapeño sauce	1 pkg	80	0	1	0	0	9	4	112
Honey mustard sauce	1 pkg	88	0	3	0	1	9	4	104
Hot sauce	1 pkg	18	0	0	0	0	0	0	210
Ketchup	1 pkg	14	0	4	0	3	0	0	148
Purple pepper sauce	1 pkg	45	0	12	0	6	0	0	26
Ranch sauce	1 pkg	104	0	1	0	0	10	2	256
Sweet & sour sauce	1 pkg	24	0	6	0	2	0	0	96

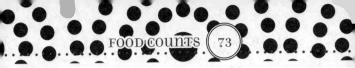

COLD STONE CREAMERY

Item	Serving Size	Calories	Protein	Carb	Fiber	Sugar	Total Fat	Sat Fat	Sodium
ICE CREAM									
Amaretto	Like It	330	5	33	0	29	20	12	80
Banana	Like It	310	5	33	0	28	18	12	70
Black cherry	Like It	330	5	36	0	32	19	12	75
Blueberry	Like It	320	5	33	0	31	2	13	55
Butter pecan	Like It	320	5	32	0	28	19	12	105
Cake batter	Like It	340	5	41	0	32	19	12	180
Caramel apple	Like It	320	4	44	0	38	16	10	110
Cheesecake	Like It	320	4	36	0	32	19	13	85
Chocolate	Like It	320	6	33	1	30	20	13	95
Chocolate cake batter	Like It	340	5	42	1	33	19	11	210
Chocolate-dipped strawberry	Like It	310	5	32	2	29	19	12	65
Chocolate peanut butter	Like It	410	10	36	3	31	28	13	200
Cinnamon	Like It	330	5	34	<1	29	20	12	80
Cinnamon bun	Like It	350	4	47	1	37	18	12	190
Coconut	Like It	330	5	33	0	28	20	12	80
Coffee	Like It	330	5	34	0	29	20	12	80
Cookie batter	Like It	360	4	43	0	37	20	12	270
Cotton candy	Like It	330	5	34	0	28	19	12	75
Dark chocolate	Like It	340	7	32	3	29	20	12	95
French toast	Like It	330	5	35	0	30	19	12	150
French vanilla	Like It	340	5	37	0	33	19	14	80
Fudge brownie batter	Like It	350	5	43	2	37	19	12	125
Ghirardelli chocolate	Like It	330	7	37	4	27	20	12	75
Irish cream	Like It	330	5	33	0	29	20	13	80
Key lime	Like It	340	5	39	0	36	20	13	50
Macadamia nut	Like It	330	5	34	0	29	20	12	75
Mango	Like It	310	5	33	0	28	18	12	70
Marshmallow	Like It	330	5	41	0	35	17	12	50
Mint	Like It	330	5	36	0	31	19	12	75
Mocha	Like It	320	6	33	1	29	20	12	95
Oatmeal cookie batter	Like It	340	5	36	0	28	19	12	110
Orange dreamsicle	Like It	320	5	35	0	28	19	12	75
Oreo crème	Like It	440	4	41	0	38	31	14	80
Peach	Like It	310	4	44	0	39	15	10	45
Peanut butter	Like It	370	7	33	<1	28	24	13	130

COLD STONE CREAMERY continued

Item	Serving Size	Calories	Protein	Carb	Fiber	Sugar	Total Fat	Sat Fat	Sodium
Pecan praline	Like It	330	5	37	0	31	19	12	90
Pistachio	Like It	330	5	34	0	29	20	12	85
Pumpkin	Like It	290	4	33	1	28	15	10	105
Pumpkin cheesecake	Like It	300	4	35	1	31	16	11	100
Raspberry	Like It	330	5	36	0	31	19	12	75
Sinless cake batter	Like It	210	7	43	1	15	1	0.5	160
Sinless Sans Fat™	Like It	170	8	35	1	11	0	0	250
Strawberry	Like It	320	5	35	0	30	18	12	75
Strawberry cheesecake	Like It	320	5	39	0	32	21	12	50
Sweet cream	Like It	330	5	33	0	29	20	13	80
Vanilla bean	Like It	330	5	32	0	28	19	12	75
White chocolate	Like It	320	5	33	0	28	19	12	75

SHAKES & SMOOTHIES
SINLESS SMOOTHIES

Item	Serving Size	Calories	Protein	Carb	Fiber	Sugar	Total Fat	Sat Fat	Sodium
2 to Mango™	Like It	220	0	55	1	43	0	0	25
Berry Trinity™	Like It	110	2	28	6	15	1	0	25
Citrus Sunsation™	Like It	190	0	48	1	42	0	0	40
Man-Go Bananas™	Like It	240	1	59	2	42	0	0	20
On the YoGo™	Like It	210	1	24	2	40	1	0	20
Strawberry Bananza™	Like It	140	2	37	4	24	1	0	30

SINLESS SHAKES

Item	Serving Size	Calories	Protein	Carb	Fiber	Sugar	Total Fat	Sat Fat	Sodium
Sinless Cake 'n Shake	16 fl oz	670	24	140	1	57	7	2	780
Sinless milk & cookies	16 fl oz	510	23	109	1	37	4.5	1	400
Sinless Oh Fudge	16 fl oz	490	23	110	0	44	2	2	360
Sinless very vanilla	16 fl oz	500	22	113	0	41	1	0.5	330

LIFESTYLE SHAKES

Item	Serving Size	Calories	Protein	Carb	Fiber	Sugar	Total Fat	Sat Fat	Sodium
Banana banana	Like It	340	3	78	5	46	3.5	2.5	150
Banana strawberry	Like It	280	3	64	4	40	4	2	150
Blueberry banana	Like It	250	2	57	3	36	3	2	150
Blueberry pineapple	Like It	230	1	49	2	34	3	2	150
Mango pineapple	Like It	390	1	90	1	67	3	2	150
Mango strawberry	Like It	380	2	89	2	65	3.5	2	150
Pineapple coconut orange	Like It	370	2	64	3	47	12	11	170
Raspberry banana	Like It	290	2	65	6	38	3	2	150
Strawberry raspberry	Like It	250	2	55	4	35	3.5	2	150

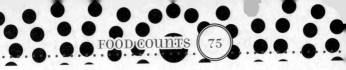

COLD STONE CREAMERY continued

Item	Serving Size	Calories	Protein	Carb	Fiber	Sugar	Total Fat	Sat Fat	Sodium
ORIGINAL SHAKES									
Cake 'n Shake™	Like It	1140	18	140	<1	106	60	36	700
Cherry Cheeseshake™	Like It	1090	16	135	<1	92	54	34	260
Cream de Menthe™	Like It	1160	17	124	4	109	67	42	240
Lotta Caramel Latte™	Like It	1320	19	175	0	134	62	39	430
Milk and Cookies™	Like It	1090	18	117	<1	97	63	38	370
Oh Fudge!™	Like It	1250	22	141	4	127	70	45	460
PB&C™	Like It	1280	27	119	5	104	82	45	470
Savory Strawberry™	Like It	1000	16	116	2	98	55	35	240
Very Vanilla™	Like It	1180	16	149	0	121	57	40	370
SORBETS & FROZEN YOGURTS									
Countrytime pink lemonade sorbet	5 oz*	240	0	59	0	59	0	0	25
Lemon sorbet	5 oz*	150	0	40	0	34	0	0	15
Raspberry sorbet	5 oz*	160	0	42	0	36	0	0	15
Tart & tangy berry yogurt	5 oz*	150	3	36	0	27	0	0	65
Tart & tangy yogurt	5 oz*	140	3	33	0	24	0	0	70
Watermelon sorbet	5 oz*	160	0	41	0	35	0	0	15
MIX-INS									
CANDY MIX-INS									
Almond Joy candy	1 piece	170	1	21	2	16	9	6	50
Butterfinger candy	1/2 bar	140	2	22	<1	15	6	3	35
Chocolate chips	1 oz	130	1	16	1	14	7	4.5	0
Chocolate shavings	0.5 oz	90	<1	9	2	8	5	3	0
Ghirardelli caramel square	1 each	70	1	9	0	8	4	2.5	20
Gumballs	1 oz	90	0	23	<1	24	0	0	0
Gummi bears	1 oz	120	0	30	0	13	0	0	15
Heath toffee bar	1 bar	110	<1	12	0	12	7	3.5	75
Kit Kat wafer bar	1/2 bar	110	1	13	0	10	5	3.5	15
M&M'S, peanut	1 oz	150	3	18	<1	14	8	3.5	30
M&M'S, plain	1 oz	170	2	25	<1	22	7	4.5	20
Nestlé Crunch bar	1/2 bar	130	2	16	<1	14	7	4	35
Reese's peanut butter cups	1 piece	190	4	19	1	17	11	4	110
Reese's pieces candy	1 oz	180	4	21	1	19	9	6	70

COLD STONE CREAMERY continued

Item	Serving Size	Calories	Protein	Carb	Fiber	Sugar	Total Fat	Sat Fat	Sodium
Snickers candy bar	1/2 bar	170	3	2	<1	7	9	3	95
Twix candy	1 piece	150	1	20	0	14	7	2.5	60
White chocolate chips	1 oz	160	2	18	0	18	9	8	45
Whoppers candy	1 oz	120	1	19	0	15	4	3.5	85
York peppermint patties	2 pieces	120	<1	24	<1	18	2	1.5	10

FRUIT MIX-INS

Item	Serving Size	Calories	Protein	Carb	Fiber	Sugar	Total Fat	Sat Fat	Sodium
Apple pie filling	0.75 oz	60	0	16	<1	14	0	0	25
Bananas	1/2 piece	50	<1	14	2	9	0	0	0
Black cherries	0.75 oz	80	0	18	0	17	0	0	10
Blackberries	0.75 oz	10	0	2	<1	2	0	0	0
Blueberries	0.75 oz	10	0	2	0	2	0	0	0
Cherry pie filling	0.75 oz	50	0	13	0	0	0	0	10
Maraschino cherries	1 piece	5	0	1	0	1	0	0	0
Peach pie filling	1 oz	60	0	16	<1	14	0	0	25
Pineapple chunks	0.75 oz	15	0	4	0	4	0	0	0
Raisins	1 oz	70	<1	20	<1	16	0	0	0
Raspberries	0.75 oz	25	0	5	1	2	0	0	0
Strawberries	0.75 oz	20	0	7	<1	4	0	0	0

OTHER MIX-INS

Item	Serving Size	Calories	Protein	Carb	Fiber	Sugar	Total Fat	Sat Fat	Sodium
Brownies	1 piece	170	2	32	1	22	3.5	1	180
Coconut	0.5 oz	80	0	7	<1	6	5	4.5	40
Cookie dough	1 piece	180	1	26	0	26	8	2.5	150
Graham cracker pie crust	1 oz	130	1	17	1	7	6	2.5	135
Granola	1 oz	120	2	23	2	0	2	0	30
Marshmallows	1 oz	100	<1	24	0	24	0	0	10
Nilla wafers	3 cookies	70	<1	11	0	6	2.5	0	50
Oreo cookies	2 cookies	120	1	18	<1	10	5	1.5	140
Oreo pie crust	1 oz	180	0	19	0	10	8	1.5	190
Peanut butter	0.75 oz	150	6	5	1	2	13	2.5	125
Toasted coconut	0.5 oz	90	<1	7	<1	6	7	6	5
Yellow cake	1 piece	80	2	13	0	8	0.5	0.5	140

NUT MIX-INS

Item	Serving Size	Calories	Protein	Carb	Fiber	Sugar	Total Fat	Sat Fat	Sodium
Cashews	1 oz	170	5	9	1	2	14	2.5	90
Macadamia nuts	1 oz	180	2	3	2	<1	19	3	65
Peanuts	1 oz	210	10	5	3	0	18	3	110

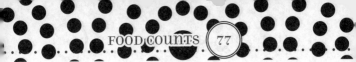
COLD STONE CREAMERY continued

Item	Serving Size	Calories	Protein	Carb	Fiber	Sugar	Total Fat	Sat Fat	Sodium
Pecan pralines	1 oz	210	2	5	2	1	21	1.5	230
Pecans	1 oz	140	2	3	2	<1	15	1.5	80
Pistachio nuts	1 oz	200	7	10	4	<1	16	2	0
Roasted almonds	1 oz	150	5	4	3	1	14	1	85
Sliced almonds	1 oz	210	7	6	4	0	20	2	0
Walnuts	1 oz	130	3	3	1		13	1	0

TOPPINGS

Item	Serving Size	Calories	Protein	Carb	Fiber	Sugar	Total Fat	Sat Fat	Sodium
Butterscotch fat-free	1 oz	8	<1	19	0	15	0	0	85
Caramel	1 oz	90	<1	21	0	13	1	0.5	50
Caramel fat-free	1 oz	80	<1	19	0	14	0	0	85
Chocolate sprinkles	1 oz	25	0	6	0	6	0	0	0
Cinnamon	1/8 tsp	0	0	0	0	0	0	0	0
Fudge	1 oz	90	1	18	0	16	2	2	80
Fudge fat-free	1 oz	80	<1	20	0	16	0	0	15
Honey	1 oz	90	0	25	0	25	0	0	0
Marshmallow crème	1 oz	100	0	24	0	20	0	0	20
Rainbow sprinkles	1 oz	25	0	6	0	6	0	0	0
Reddi-wip original	1 dollop	45	<1	5	0	2	2.5	1	15
Rich's On Top	1 dollop	50	0	4	0	0	3.5	3.5	0

CONES & BOWLS

Item	Serving Size	Calories	Protein	Carb	Fiber	Sugar	Total Fat	Sat Fat	Sodium
Dipped waffle cone	each	310	3	46	2	31	15	7	70
Sugar cone	each	50	<1	11	0	3	0	0	20
Waffle cone or bowl	each	160	2	29	0	14	4	1	70

CORNER BAKERY CAFÉ

Item	Serving Size	Calories	Protein	Carb	Fiber	Sugar	Total Fat	Sat Fat	Sodium

BREAKFAST ENTRÉES, SANDWICHES, & SIDES, ALL MADE W/ WHOLE EGGS AS APPLICABLE

Item	Serving Size	Calories	Protein	Carb	Fiber	Sugar	Total Fat	Sat Fat	Sodium
All-American Scrambler w/ bacon	as served	350	21	3	0	2	27	9	780
Anaheim panini	each	640	25	51	5	4	37	13	1200
Anaheim Scrambler	as served	570	29	9	4	4	45	17	1060
Bacon	3 slices	110	2	0	0	0	11	3.5	390
Baked French toast, incl. vanilla syrup	as served	850	13	138	5	73	28	13	380

CORNER BAKERY CAFÉ continued

Item	Serving Size	Calories	Protein	Carb	Fiber	Sugar	Total Fat	Sat Fat	Sodium
Baked French toast w/ bacon & fresh fruit	as served	980	15	145	6	79	39	17	770
Baked French toast w/bacon & scrambled eggs	as served	1200	33	141	5	75	55	22	1150
Breakfast potatoes	as served	140	2	21	2	1	5	0.5	290
Farmer's Scrambler	as served	420	28	13	2	4	28	11	670
Fresh berry & yogurt parfait	each	390	11	65	6	36	12	2	170
Ham & Swiss panini	each	530	34	48	2	3	22	9	1530
Harvest toast	as served	160	6	31	3	4	1	0	280
Oatmeal w/ all toppings	as served	330	12	49	4	23	9	1	240
Oatmeal w/o all toppings	as served	140	10	21	1	11	1.5	0.5	230
Seasonal fruit medley	as served	70	1	17	2	14	0	0	0
Smoked bacon & Cheddar panini	each	590	25	46	2	2	33	13	1310
Sweet crisp	as served	150	3	25	1	8	4	1	115
Swiss oatmeal	as served	360	11	78	5	63	3	1	130
The Commuter croissant	each	690	26	43	3	9	45	22	1140
Vanilla Syrup, incl. w/ French toast	included	220	0	56	0	30	0	0	30
BAGELS									
8-grain	each	330	11	72	4	8	2	0	500
Blueberry	each	340	11	73	3	10	2	0	650
Cinnamon raisin	each	330	10	72	3	12	2	0	540
Everything	each	330	11	69	3	6	2.5	0.5	800
Plain	each	330	11	70	3	6	2	0	660
Sesame seed	each	340	11	69	3	6	3.5	1	650
SPREADS									
Hand-crafted cream cheese	as served	130	2	2	0	2	13	8	200
Hand-crafted green onion cream cheese	as served	130	2	2	0	2	12	7	190
Hand-crafted strawberry cream cheese	as served	110	2	3	0	3	10	6	150
Hand-crafted veggie cream cheese	as served	110	2	2	0	2	11	6	160

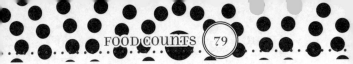

CORNER BAKERY CAFÉ continued

Item	Serving Size	Calories	Protein	Carb	Fiber	Sugar	Total Fat	Sat Fat	Sodium
Peanut butter	as served	240	9	2	2	4	21	4	190

MUFFINS & SWEET BREADS

Item	Serving Size	Calories	Protein	Carb	Fiber	Sugar	Total Fat	Sat Fat	Sodium
Banana muffin	each	530	7	67	1	36	26	5	500
Blueberry muffin	each	510	6	70	1	36	22	7	390
Chocolate muffin	each	530	8	60	2	36	28	7	630
Cinnamon crumb muffin	each	660	7	90	2	50	30	10	460
Cinnamon roll	each	660	9	95	2	47	24	7	480
Croissant	each	340	8	39	2	6	16	10	37
Pumpkin muffin	each	460	6	69	2	48	18	3	430

SALADS, SERVED W/ DRESSING

Item	Serving Size	Calories	Protein	Carb	Fiber	Sugar	Total Fat	Sat Fat	Sodium
Asian wonton	entrée size	480	35	56	8	25	15	1	1890
Caesar	entrée size	710	15	22	6	6	63	12	1330
Caesar salad w/ roasted chicken	entrée size	800	31	24	6	5	65	13	1660
Chopped	entrée size	800	34	31	11	14	59	18	2070
Harvest	entrée size	770	22	72	11	37	45	12	1460
Harvest salad w/ roasted chicken	entrée size	860	37	74	11	37	47	13	1790
Mixed green	entrée size	420	5	26	4	5	33	4	910
Santa Fe ranch	entrée size	760	33	54	9	11	45	11	1400
The Greek	entrée size	530	16	39	7	24	35	14	2790

SALAD DRESSINGS

Item	Serving Size	Calories	Protein	Carb	Fiber	Sugar	Total Fat	Sat Fat	Sodium
Asian	entrée size	130	2	30	0	16	10	1	1280
Balsamic Vinaigrette	entrée size	130	0	10	0	8	8	1	330
Caesar	entrée size	460	2	3	0	2	48	8	790
Caesar	side size	80	0	1	0	0	8	1	130
House	entrée size	280	0	8	0	2	27	4	680
House	side size	70	0	2	0	1	7	1	170
Light ranch	entrée size	160	2	2	0	2	16	3	440
White Balsamic Vinaigrette	entrée size	210	0	15	0	12	15	3	570

TRIO, COMBO, & SIDE SALADS

Item	Serving Size	Calories	Protein	Carb	Fiber	Sugar	Total Fat	Sat Fat	Sodium
Asian edamame salad	side size	140	6	11	4	6	8	0.5	720
Caesar salad	side size	230	5	8	2	2	20	3.5	420
D.C. chicken salad	side size	360	16	22	3	14	21	2.5	750

CORNER BAKERY CAFÉ continued

Item	Serving Size	Calories	Protein	Carb	Fiber	Sugar	Total Fat	Sat Fat	Sodium
Egg salad	side size	340	16	5	0	2	27	6	780
Greek vegetable salad	side size	90	3	9	2	5	4.5	1.5	890
Mixed greens w/ dressing	side size	120	2	9	2	3	8	1	240
Mixed greens w/ dressing, garnish	garnish only	30	0	1	0	0	2.5	0	70
Pasta Caprese salad	side size	210	9	18	2	2	10	5	250
Seasonal fruit medley	side size	100	2	25	3	21	0	0	15
Tuna salad	side size	400	29	3	<1	1	29	4.5	770

SOUPS

Item	Serving Size	Calories	Protein	Carb	Fiber	Sugar	Total Fat	Sat Fat	Sodium
Big Al's chili w/ Cheddar cheese	1 bowl	590	39	44	11	7	27	12	1790
Big Al's chili w/ Cheddar cheese	1 cup	380	25	29	8	4	17	7	1180
Cheddar broccoli	1 bowl	550	19	28	2	7	41	24	1900
Cheddar broccoli	1 cup	370	12	19	1	4	28	16	1270
Country bread boule	1 cup	1040	35	213	9	4	3	0	2990
Loaded baked potato w/ Cheddar cheese & green onion	1 bowl	630	21	36	2	6	43	26	1570
Loaded baked potato w/ Cheddar cheese & green onion	1 cup	410	13	24	1	4	27	17	1030
Mom's chicken noodle	1 bowl	210	11	28	2	4	6	2	1620
Mom's chicken noodle	1 cup	140	8	19	1	3	4	1.5	1080
Roasted poblano corn chowder	1 bowl	420	7	43	5	8	25	10	1130
Roasted poblano corn chowder	1 cup	280	4	29	3	6	16	7	750
Roasted tomato basil w/ croutons	1 cup	200	8	31	3	15	7	0	1500
Roasted tomato basil w/ croutons	1 bowl	320	12	49	4	22	11	0	2290
Three lentil vegetable	1 bowl	210	11	36	13	4	4	0	1390
Three lentil vegetable	1 cup	140	8	24	9	4	2.5	0	930
Zesty chicken tortilla w/ strips	1 bowl	360	11	41	9	9	16	1	1980
Zesty chicken tortilla w/ strips	1 cup	230	7	26	6	6	11	1	1310

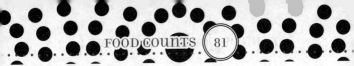

CORNER BAKERY CAFÉ continued

Item	Serving Size	Calories	Protein	Carb	Fiber	Sugar	Total Fat	Sat Fat	Sodium
PASTAS									
Chicken carbonara	combo	620	28	56	4	3	30	16	850
Chicken carbonara	entrée	1140	53	93	6	7	60	31	1690
Half moon cheese ravioli	combo	320	15	35	2	7	13	6	580
Half moon cheese ravioli	entrée	640	29	73	3	15	25	12	1180
Parmesan cheese topping, incl.	combo	60	4	0	0	0	4	2	180
Parmesan cheese topping, incl.	entrée	90	7	0	0	0	6	3.5	290
Penne w/ marinara	combo	300	12	52	3	6	7	2	350
Penne w/ marinara	entrée	600	23	89	6	15	18	5	900
Pesto cavatappi	combo	600	26	50	3	2	32	14	640
Pesto cavatappi	entrée	1100	49	82	5	5	63	28	1260
SANDWICHES & PANINIS									
California grill panini	combo	350	15	41	4	5	14	6	890
California grill panini	whole	700	30	82	9	11	28	12	1780
Chicken pesto on ciabatta ficelle	combo	380	19	43	2	3	13	2	1220
Chicken pesto on ciabatta ficelle	whole	720	34	89	5	6	23	4	2170
Chicken pomodori panini	combo	380	20	37	2	2	16	7	950
Chicken pomomdori panini	whole	750	41	75	5	3	32	13	1900
Club panini	combo	380	17	35	2	2	18	7	1320
Club panini	whole	760	34	70	4	4	37	15	2640
Corned beef Reuben panini	combo	440	20	40	4	7	21	7	1210
Corned beef Reuben panini	whole	880	40	80	7	15	43	14	2420
D.C. chicken salad on steakhouse rye	combo	275	13	39	2	2	8	1	970
D.C. chicken salad on steakhouse rye	whole	550	25	78	4	13	16	2	1940
Green chili & chicken panini	combo	350	19	37	3	2	14	6	870
Green chili & chicken panini	whole	700	39	73	5	4	28	12	1740

CORNER BAKERY CAFÉ continued

Item	Serving Size	Calories	Protein	Carb	Fiber	Sugar	Total Fat	Sat Fat	Sodium
Grilled ham & Swiss panini	combo	350	21	37	2	3	13	6	1260
Grilled ham & Swiss panini	whole	700	42	73	4	5	26	11	2520
Ham on pretzel bread	combo	340	19	42	2	3	10	4	1780
Ham on pretzel bread	whole	680	39	84	4	7	19	8	3550
Mom's corned beef on caraway rye	combo	240	16	38	3	6	2	0.5	1010
Mom's corned beef on caraway rye	whole	480	32	76	7	12	4	1	2020
Mom's egg salad on white bread	combo	290	10	29	1.5	4	15	4.5	350
Mom's egg salad on white bread	whole	580	21	58	3	8	29	9	1300
Mom's roast beef on sourdough	combo	255	19	36	2	2	3.5	1.5	750
Mom's roast beef on sourdough	whole	510	38	71	4	5	7	2.5	1490
Mom's roasted chicken on harvest bread	combo	200	16	29	3	5	2.5	1	460
Mom's roasted chicken on harvest bread	whole	400	32	57	5	10	5	2	920
Mom's smoked ham on white bread	combo	245	15	28	2	5	7	3	1030
Mom's smoked ham on white bread	whole	490	30	57	3	9	15	6	2050
Mom's turkey on harvest bread	combo	205	18	29	3	6	1	0.5	580
Mom's turkey on harvest bread	whole	410	36	59	5	11	2	1	1160
Poblano fresco chicken on poblano cheese bread	combo	390	20	36	4	3	18	6	930
Poblano fresco chicken on poblano cheese bread	whole	780	40	73	7	5	37	12	1860
Poblano fresco roast beef on poblano cheese bread	combo	415	22	76	4	3	20	4	1050
Poblano fresco roast beef on poblano cheese bread	whole	830	44	71	7	6	40	13	2090
Poblano fresco vegetarian on poblano cheese bread	combo	385	13	36	4	2	21	7	820

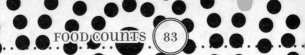

CORNER BAKERY CAFÉ continued

Item	Serving Size	Calories	Protein	Carb	Fiber	Sugar	Total Fat	Sat Fat	Sodium
Poblano fresco vegetarian on poblano cheese bread	whole	770	25	71	8	5	42	15	1640
Tomato mozzarella on ciabatta ficelle	combo	350	14	40	3	5	13	7	850
Tomato mozzarella on ciabatta ficelle	whole	700	29	81	6	10	26	13	1690
Tuna salad on harvest bread	combo	285	16	30	3	5	11	2	510
Tuna salad on harvest bread	whole	570	32	59	6	11	22	4	1010
Turkey Frisco on Asiago cheese bread	combo	365	28	33	3	3	13	5	1040
Turkey Frisco on Asiago cheese bread	whole	730	56	67	6	6	26	9	2080
Turkey on pretzel bread	combo	335	22	43	2	3	8	3	1410
Turkey on pretzel bread	whole	670	43	87	4	6	15	7	2820
Uptown turkey on harvest bread	combo	290	19	31	4	5	9	2	950
Uptown turkey on harvest bread	whole	580	38	63	8	11	19	4	1900

DRESSINGS & SANDWICH SPREADS

Item	Serving Size	Calories	Protein	Carb	Fiber	Sugar	Total Fat	Sat Fat	Sodium
Asian dressing	entrée size	130	2	30	0	16	10	1	1280
Balsamic vinaigrette	entrée size	130	0	10	0	8	8	1	330
Balsamic vinaigrette dressing	whole serving	50	0	2	0	3	3	0.5	120
Caesar dressing	side size	80	0	1	0	0	8	1	130
CBC mayonnaise	whole serving	40	0	<1	0	0	4	0.5	150
Caesar dressing	entrée size	460	2	3	0	2	48	8	790
Country dijon mustard	whole serving	5	1	1	0	0	0	0	120
House dressing	entrée size	280	0	8	0	2	27	4	680
House dressing	side size	70	0	2	0	1	7	1	170
House dressing	whole serving	140	0	4	0	1	14	2	340
Light ranch dressing	entrée size	160	2	2	0	2	16	3	440
Pesto mayo for chicken pesto	whole serving	110	0	2	0	0	11	1.5	380
Pesto mayo for chicken pomodori	whole serving	50	0	1	0	0	4	0.5	140

CORNER BAKERY CAFÉ continued

Item	Serving Size	Calories	Protein	Carb	Fiber	Sugar	Total Fat	Sat Fat	Sodium
Roasted garlic mayo	whole serving	35	0	0	0	0	3.5	0.5	120
Spicy chipotle lime mayo spread	whole serving	80	0	2	0	0	7	1	270
Stone ground mustard mayo spread	whole serving	50	0	2	0	0	4	0.5	160
Sun-dried tomato pesto mayo	whole serving	80	0	2	0	0	7	1	260
Thousand Island	whole serving	160	0	5	0	2	15	2.5	250
White balsamic vinaigrette	entrée size	210	0	15	0	12	15	3	570

KIDS' MENU

Item	Serving Size	Calories	Protein	Carb	Fiber	Sugar	Total Fat	Sat Fat	Sodium
Cheddar broccoli soup	kids'	190	6	10	<1	2	14	8	640
Grilled cheese sandwich	whole serving	660	23	52	2	4	39	18	1040
Half moon cheese ravioli	kids'	320	14	37	2	8	12	6	580
Ham sandwich	whole serving	410	14	52	2	5	13	5	1320
Kids' cheese Scrambler	kids'	490	20	44	3	17	26	10	850
Kids' Scrambler	kids'	430	16	44	3	17	21	8	760
Loaded baked potato soup	kids'	190	5	12	<1	2	12	8	490
Macaroni & cheese	kids'	350	12	48	2	11	11	3	830
Mom's chicken noodle soup	kids'	70	4	9	<1	1	2	1	540
Pasta marinara	kids'	300	10	53	3	8	6	1	310
Peanut butter & jelly sandwich	whole serving	810	20	103	6	45	38	10	860
Roasted poblano corn chowder	kids'	140	2	14	2	3	8	3.5	380
Roasted tomato basil soup	kids'	80	4	13	1	7	2	0	710
Three lentil vegetable soup	kids'	70	4	12	4	2	1.5	0	470
Turkey sandwich	whole serving	410	21	53	1	5	11	5	940
Zesty chicken tortilla soup	kids'	110	4	12	3	3	5	0.5	650

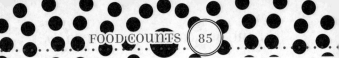

CORNER BAKERY CAFÉ continued

Item	Serving Size	Calories	Protein	Carb	Fiber	Sugar	Total Fat	Sat Fat	Sodium
SIDES									
Baby carrots	as served	30	0	7	2	4	0	0	70
Bakery chips	as served	190	1	22	1	0	12	3	150
Banana	whole	110	1	27	3	14	0	0	0
Focaccia roll	as served	110	3	19	1	0	1.5	0	250
Garlic bread	as served	110	3	17	1	1	3	0.5	240
Grapes	small bunch	40	0	11	<1	9	0	0	0
Harvest crisp	as served	60	2	10	1	1	0.5	0	220
Pickle spear	as served	10	0	1	0	0	0	0	330
Seasonal fruit medley	as served	70	1	19	2	14	0	0	10
DESSERTS									
Apricot-filled shortbread	each	180	1	25	0	12	9	5	120
Apricot walnut rugalach	each	240	2	23	1	12	15	7	120
Banana baby Bundt cake	each	620	6	81	1	50	30	7	540
Chocolate baby Bundt cake	each	580	7	70	2	47	30	7	600
Chocolate chip cookie	each	300	4	46	2	28	13	7	290
Chocolate-truffle-filled shortbread	each	200	2	23	1	12	12	7	120
Cinnamon creme cake	1 slice	770	8	108	2	61	34	12	620
Cinnamon pecan rugalach	each	250	3	24	1	15	16	7	120
Cream cheese brownie	each	590	10	53	2	41	37	21	540
Fudge brownie	each	590	7	86	3	64	28	15	340
Gingerbread pumpkin baby Bundt cake	each	560	6	95	1	72	18	3	440
Lemon bar	each	590	8	90	1	66	24	12	280
Lemon pound cake	1 slice	480	7	64	0	35	22	4.5	500
Maple pecan bar	each	730	7	80	3	51	44	16	490
Monster cookie	each	340	4	51	2	32	14	8	300
Oatmeal raisin cookie	each	290	4	47	2	27	10	5	410
Pumpkin pound cake	1 slice	490	6	73	1	45	19	3.5	560
Raspberry bar	each	530	6	72	2	36	24	13	550
Snickerdoodle cookie	each	290	4	47	1	25	10	5	240
Sugar cookie	each	290	4	47	1	25	10	5	240

CORNER BAKERY CAFÉ continued

Item	Serving Size	Calories	Protein	Carb	Fiber	Sugar	Total Fat	Sat Fat	Sodium
Whoopie Pie, chocolate mocha	each	390	7	45	<1	34	21	9	320
Whoopie Pie, peanut butter	each	440	7	38	2	26	29	11	390
Whoopie Pie, pumpkin	each	400	2	45	1	36	22	11	290
Whoopie Pie, vanilla	each	430	3	43	1	33	26	14	360

HOT BEVERAGES MADE W/ WHOLE MILK

Item	Serving Size	Calories	Protein	Carb	Fiber	Sugar	Total Fat	Sat Fat	Sodium
Cappuccino	12 oz	100	5	8	0	9	5	3	70
Cappuccino	16 oz	140	7	11	0	13	7	4	100
Cappuccino	20 oz	190	10	15	0	17	10	6	130
Caramel latte	12 oz	380	10	61	0	45	11	7	210
Caramel latte	16 oz	490	12	81	0	57	13	8	220
Caramel latte	20 oz	350	16	108	0	76	17	10	280
Latte	12 oz	190	10	15	0	17	10	6	130
Latte	16 oz	250	13	19	0	22	13	8	170
Latte	20 oz	300	16	23	0	27	16	9	210
Truffle hot chocolate w/ whipped cream	12 oz	350	12	50	<1	47	17	10	190
Truffle hot chocolate w/ whipped cream	16 oz	480	16	75	2	72	21	12	250
Truffle hot chocolate w/ whipped cream	20 oz	610	20	100	2	95	24	14	300
Truffle mocha	12 oz	270	10	46	1	45	10	6	150
Truffle mocha	16 oz	380	13	70	2	67	12	7	200
Truffle mocha	20 oz	510	17	95	2	91	16	9	260

COLD BEVERAGES

Item	Serving Size	Calories	Protein	Carb	Fiber	Sugar	Total Fat	Sat Fat	Sodium
Frozen mango lemonade	as served	350	0	91	0	84	0	0	10
Frozen mango pomegranate swirl	as served	320	0	83	0	76	0	0	10
Frozen pomegranate lemonade	as served	290	0	75	0	68	0	0	10
Old-fashioned lemonade	as served	260	0	68	0	63	0	0	15

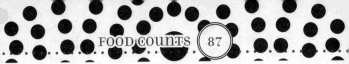

DAIRY QUEEN

Item	Serving Size	Calories	Protein	Carb	Fiber	Sugar	Total Fat	Sat Fat	Sodium
BURGERS & SANDWICHES									
All-beef cheese dog	as served	290	12	19	1	2	19	8	690
All-beef chili cheese dog	as served	430	18	39	2	5	22	10	1010
All-beef chili cheese foot-long hot dog	as served	840	37	52	2	6	54	24	2050
All-beef chili dog	as served	290	11	24	1	5	17	6	930
All-beef foot-long hot dog	as served	560	20	39	2	6	35	14	1600
All-beef hot dog	as served	250	9	21	1	4	14	5	770
Bacon Cheddar GrillBurger™	1/4 lb	650	36	41	2	11	35	15	1410
Barbecue beef sandwich	as served	270	16	43	1	15	4.5	1	830
Barbecue pork sandwich	as served	340	18	41	1	9	12	1.5	840
California GrillBurger™	as served	620	25	39	2	8	39	11	830
Cheeseburger	as served	400	19	34	1	9	18	9	1980
Cheeseburger, double	as served	640	34	34	1	9	34	18	1450
Cheeseburger, double w/ bacon	as served	730	41	35	1	9	41	21	920
Chicken strip basket w/ country gravy	4 pieces	1360	39	103	8	6	63	11	1010
Chicken strip basket w/ country gravy	6 pieces	1640	54	121	10	6	74	12	1600
Classic GrillBurger™	as served	470	24	42	2	11	21	8	680
Classic GrillBurger™ w/ cheese	1/4 lb	560	30	42	2	11	28	12	1090
Classic GrillBurger™ w/ cheese	1/2 lb	910	52	42	2	12	54	25	1540
Corn dog	as served	460	17	56	1	55	19	5	970
Crispy chicken salad	as served	460	29	31	6	8	19	6	3690
Crispy chicken sandwich	as served	560	20	48	3	5	28	3.5	1760
Crispy chicken sandwich w/ cheese	as served	610	22	48	3	6	32	6	1480
Crispy chicken wrap	as served	290	11	17	2	1	16	3	2310
Crispy fish sandwich	as served	430	16	51	2	7	18	2.5	1150
Crispy fish sandwich w/ cheese	as served	480	18	52	2	7	22	5	139

DAIRY QUEEN continued

Item	Serving Size	Calories	Protein	Carb	Fiber	Sugar	Total Fat	Sat Fat	Sodium
Crispy Flame Thrower chicken sandwich	as served	860	30	51	3	6	55	11	690
Crispy Flame Thrower chicken wrap	as served	310	11	17	2	1	19	4	770
Deluxe cheeseburger	as served	400	20	35	1	9	18	9	930
Deluxe double cheeseburger	as served	640	34	35	1	10	34	18	1240
Deluxe double hamburger	as served	540	29	34	1	9	26	13	750
Deluxe hamburger	as served	350	17	34	1	9	14	7	680
DQ Ultimate® burger	as served	780	41	33	1	8	48	22	1390
Flame Thrower GrillBurger™	1/2 lb	1060	54	41	2	9	75	26	1230
Flame Thrower GrillBurger™	1/4 lb	780	34	41	2	9	52	16	740
GrillBurger™	1/2 lb	720	42	42	2	12	40	15	1550
GrillBurger™ w/ cheese	1/4 lb	870	51	42	2	12	51	23	950
Grilled chicken salad	as served	280	31	1	4	8	11	5	3630
Grilled chicken sandwich	as served	370	24	32	1	5	16	2.5	2910
Grilled chicken wrap	as served	200	12	9	1	1	12	3	2470
Grilled Flame Thrower chicken sandwich	as served	590	34	34	1	6	36	9	930
Hamburger	as served	350	17	33	1	8	14	7	1440
Hamburger, double	as served	540	29	33	1	8	26	13	1550
Iron Grilled cheese sandwich	as served	320	13	30	1	2	13	8	1020
Iron Grilled chicken quesadilla basket	as served	1070	34	117	5	8	50	18	2310
Iron Grilled classic club sandwich	as served	580	32	43	2	3	29	9	1750
Iron Grilled supreme BLT sandwich	as served	590	26	42	2	3	33	9	1560
Iron Grilled turkey sandwich	as served	530	29	42	2	2	25	7	980
Iron Grilled veggie quesadilla basket	as served	1020	26	114	9	7	49	19	2470
Mushroom Swiss GrillBurger™	as served	620	29	3	2	8	37	12	910

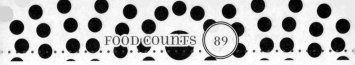

DAIRY QUEEN continued

Item	Serving Size	Calories	Protein	Carb	Fiber	Sugar	Total Fat	Sat Fat	Sodium
Popcorn shrimp basket	as served	990	18	115	8	3	49	26	2050
Pork tenderloin sandwich	as served	610	19	58	3	6	35	6	1330
Shredded chicken sandwich	as served	290	30	30	1	5	7	1.5	560

SALADS, SIDES, & SOUPS

Item	Serving Size	Calories	Protein	Carb	Fiber	Sugar	Total Fat	Sat Fat	Sodium
Breaded mushrooms	as served	250	7	36	2	1	9	1	500
Chili cheese fries	as served	1240	34	119	9	4	71	28	2550
French fries	small	190	2	27	2	0	8	1	400
French fries	regular	310	4	43	3	0	13	2	640
French fries	large	500	6	70	5	0	21	3.5	1040
Onion rings	1 order	360	6	47	2	3	16	2	840
Side salad	as served	45	2	11	3	6	0	0	50
Spicy chili	1 bowl	710	44	81	3	3	24	10	3900
Spicy chili	1 cup	470	29	54	2	2	16	7	2600

KIDS' MEALS

Item	Serving Size	Calories	Protein	Carb	Fiber	Sugar	Total Fat	Sat Fat	Sodium
All-beef hot dog w/ applesauce	as served	380	11	47	2	4	18	7	930
All-beef hot dog w/ fries	as served	470	12	48	3	4	25	8	127
Cheeseburger w/ applesauce	as served	500	20	59	3	9	18	9	930
Cheeseburger w/ fries	as served	590	22	61	3	9	27	10	1290
Chicken strips w/ applesauce	as served	350	15	39	3	0	10	1	780
Chicken strips w/ fries	as served	470	18	44	4	0	18	2.5	1170
Hamburger w/ applesauce	as served	450	17	59	3	8	14	7	690
Hamburger w/ fries	as served	540	19	60	3	6	23	8	1050
Iron Grilled cheese w/ applesauce	as served	420	13	56	3	2	13	8	1050
Iron Grilled cheese w/ fries	as served	510	15	57	3	2	21	9	1410

DAIRY QUEEN continued

Item	Serving Size	Calories	Protein	Carb	Fiber	Sugar	Total Fat	Sat Fat	Sodium
SPECIALTY DRINKS									
Cappuccino MooLatté®	16 oz	500	8	71	0	63	18	15	170
Cappuccino MooLatté®	24 oz	690	12	103	0	91	23	18	230
Caramel MooLatté®	16 oz	630	9	101	0	78	19	15	240
Caramel MooLatté®	24 oz	870	13	143	0	112	24	19	350
French Vanilla MooLatté®	16 oz	560	8	88	0	74	18	14	160
French Vanilla MooLatté®	24 oz	760	12	121	0	103	23	18	230
Mocha MooLatté®	16 oz	590	9	82	0	72	23	15	190
Mocha MooLatté®	24 oz	830	13	118	0	103	31	19	280
DESSERTS									
Arctic Rush®, all flavors	small	240	0	48	0	48	0	0	0
Arctic Rush®, all flavors	medium	310	0	63	0	63	0	0	0
Arctic Rush®, all flavors	large	480	0	96	0	96	0	0	0
Banana Crème Blizzard®	small	580	11	84	0	63	22	13	290
Banana Crème Blizzard®	medium	780	14	115	1	82	30	16	430
Banana Crème Blizzard®	large	1100	20	165	1	116	41	21	630
Banana Split Blizzard®	small	440	11	71	0	58	13	9	190
Banana Split Blizzard®	medium	570	13	93	1	76	16	10	230
Banana Split Blizzard®	large	780	18	129	1	106	22	14	320
Butterfinger Blizzard®	small	470	11	71	0	56	16	10	220
Butterfinger Blizzard®	medium	740	16	114	0	86	26	16	350
Butterfinger Blizzard®	large	990	21	151	0	114	35	21	460
Cappuccino Heath Blizzard®	small	600	11	86	0	75	24	14	310
Cappuccino Heath Blizzard®	medium	870	15	122	1	107	38	22	470
Cappuccino Heath Blizzard®	large	1210	20	171	1	150	52	31	660
Cherry CheeseQuake Blizzard®	small	500	11	68	0	54	20	13	280
Cherry CheeseQuake Blizzard®	medium	690	15	92	0	73	28	17	390
Cherry CheeseQuake Blizzard®	large	960	21	131	0	104	38	24	540
Choco Cherry Love Blizzard®	small	500	11	68	0	57	21	10	190
Choco Cherry Love Blizzard®	medium	730	14	94	1	80	33	15	260

DAIRY QUEEN continued

Item	Serving Size	Calories	Protein	Carb	Fiber	Sugar	Total Fat	Sat Fat	Sodium
Choco Cherry Love Blizzard®	large	1050	19	135	1	114	48	21	360
Chocolate Chip Blizzard®	small	590	11	70	1	59	29	12	190
Chocolate Chip Blizzard®	medium	880	14	96	2	81	50	19	250
Chocolate Chip Blizzard®	large	1220	19	129	2	109	71	26	330
Chocolate Xtreme Blizzard®	small	660	13	88	1	75	29	15	340
Chocolate Xtreme Blizzard®	medium	980	17	130	3	113	44	23	540
Chocolate Xtreme Blizzard®	large	1440	25	189	4	165	67	33	790
Cookie Dough Blizzard®	small	710	13	103	1	76	27	14	350
Cookie Dough Blizzard®	medium	1010	18	148	1	109	40	20	500
Cookie Dough Blizzard®	large	1300	22	189	2	140	51	26	640
French Silk Pie Blizzard®	small	680	12	88	1	68	31	18	260
French Silk Pie Blizzard®	medium	920	16	117	2	87	44	25	350
French Silk Pie Blizzard®	large	1350	22	171	3	126	65	36	520
Georgia Mud Fudge Blizzard®	small	690	13	82	2	69	35	12	400
Georgia Mud Fudge Blizzard®	medium	1010	19	114	4	97	54	16	620
Georgia Mud Fudge Blizzard®	large	1470	27	163	6	139	82	23	900
Hawaiian Blizzard®	small	440	10	67	1	55	15	10	180
Hawaiian Blizzard®	medium	600	13	92	3	75	21	15	240
Hawaiian Blizzard®	large	820	17	125	4	103	29	22	330
Heath Blizzard®	small	600	11	84	1	73	25	16	310
Heath Blizzard®	medium	920	16	126	1	112	41	25	490
Heath Blizzard®	large	1260	2	173	2	154	57	35	670
M&M'S Chocolate Candy Blizzard®	small	660	13	101	1	86	22	14	230
M&M'S Chocolate Candy Blizzard®	medium	840	16	127	1	109	29	19	270
M&M'S Chocolate Candy Blizzard®	large	1140	21	176	2	151	39	25	380
Mint Oreo Blizzard®	small	580	12	89	1	69	20	10	410
Mint Oreo Blizzard®	medium	740	14	116	1	89	25	12	530
Mint Oreo Blizzard®	large	1070	21	168	2	131	36	18	730

DAIRY QUEEN continued

Item	Serving Size	Calories	Protein	Carb	Fiber	Sugar	Total Fat	Sat Fat	Sodium
Mocha Chip Blizzard®	small	570	12	78	1	66	24	18	200
Mocha Chip Blizzard®	medium	810	15	107	3	90	37	29	240
Mocha Chip Blizzard®	large	1110	20	145	5	122	51	40	320
Oreo CheeseQuake® Blizzard®	small	590	12	78	1	58	25	14	410
Oreo CheeseQuake® Blizzard®	medium	820	16	108	1	79	35	19	610
Oreo CheeseQuake® Blizzard®	large	1140	23	151	1	111	49	26	840
Oreo Cookies Blizzard®	small	550	12	81	1	61	20	10	410
Oreo Cookies Blizzard®	medium	680	14	100	1	74	25	12	530
Oreo Cookies Blizzard®	large	980	21	145	2	109	36	18	730
Peanut Butter Butterfinger Blizzard®	small	670	14	83	2	61	32	13	400
Peanut Butter Butterfinger Blizzard®	medium	1050	20	122	5	86	54	20	660
Peanut Butter Butterfinger Blizzard®	large	1510	29	175	8	123	80	28	970
Reese's Peanut Butter Cups Blizzard®	small	530	13	74	1	62	21	11	260
Reese's Peanut Butter Cups Blizzard®	medium	760	18	101	2	85	31	16	380
Reese's Peanut Butter Cups Blizzard®	large	1060	25	140	3	117	45	22	530
Snicker's Blizzard®	small	670	14	99	1	83	25	13	310
Snicker's Blizzard®	medium	850	18	123	2	103	33	17	400
Snicker's Blizzard®	large	1140	24	167	2	140	43	22	530
Strawberry CheeseQuake® Blizzard®	small	510	12	69	0	54	21	13	280
Strawberry CheeseQuake® Blizzard®	medium	690	15	92	0	72	28	18	380
Strawberry CheeseQuake® Blizzard®	large	930	21	124	0	97	37	24	510
Tropical Blizzard®	small	500	11	62	3	48	24	10	220
Tropical Blizzard®	medium	750	15	87	5	67	40	16	340
Tropical Blizzard®	large	1120	22	126	8	96	62	25	510
Turtle Pecan Cluster Blizzard®	small	680	13	86	2	66	32	11	320
Turtle Pecan Cluster Blizzard®	medium	1050	17	127	3	95	54	16	520

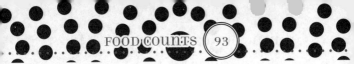

DAIRY QUEEN continued

Item	Serving Size	Calories	Protein	Carb	Fiber	Sugar	Total Fat	Sat Fat	Sodium
Turtle Pecan Cluster Blizzard®	large	1530	24	182	5	136	80	23	750
SHAKES & MALTS									
Banana malt	small	540	16	86	0	68	15	10	260
Banana malt	medium	740	21	120	1	95	20	13	350
Banana malt	large	1090	31	176	2	140	30	19	530
Banana shake	small	450	14	68	1	55	14	9	210
Banana shake	medium	620	19	96	2	76	19	12	280
Banana shake	large	910	28	140	3	111	28	18	410
Caramel malt	small	690	16	116	0	84	18	12	380
Caramel malt	medium	960	22	163	0	117	24	16	530
Caramel malt	large	1380	33	232	0	168	36	23	770
Caramel shake	small	610	15	99	0	70	17	1	320
Caramel shake	medium	850	20	14	0	98	23	15	450
Caramel shake	large	1210	29	196	0	140	34	23	650
Cherry malt	small	590	15	94	3	80	16	10	300
Cherry malt	medium	80	20	130	0	111	22	14	410
Cherry malt	large	1170	30	188	0	160	33	21	610
Cherry shake	small	500	13	76	0	66	15	10	240
Cherry shake	medium	690	18	106	0	92	21	13	330
Cherry shake	large	1000	26	152	0	132	31	20	490
Chocolate malt	small	650	15	110	0	93	16	10	310
Chocolate malt	medium	900	20	154	0	130	22	14	430
Chocolate malt	large	1310	30	220	0	187	33	21	630
Chocolate shake	small	570	13	92	0	79	15	10	250
Chocolate shake	medium	790	18	130	0	112	21	13	350
Chocolate shake	large	1130	26	184	0	158	31	20	510
Hot Fudge malt	small	700	17	105	0	85	23	16	360
Hot Fudge malt	medium	970	22	146	0	118	31	22	490
Hot Fudge malt	large	1390	33	210	0	170	45	32	720
Hot Fudge shake	small	610	15	87	0	71	22	15	300
Hot Fudge shake	medium	850	20	123	0	99	30	22	420
Hot Fudge shake	large	1220	29	174	0	141	43	31	600
Marshmallow malt	small	650	15	112	0	94	16	10	290
Marshmallow malt	medium	900	20	157	0	131	22	14	400
Marshmallow malt	large	1300	30	224	0	188	33	21	580

DAIRY QUEEN continued

Item	Serving Size	Calories	Protein	Carb	Fiber	Sugar	Total Fat	Sat Fat	Sodium
Marshmallow shake	small	560	13	94	0	80	15	10	230
Marshmallow shake	medium	780	18	133	0	113	21	13	320
Marshmallow shake	large	1120	26	188	0	15	31	20	460
Pineapple malt	small	550	15	89	0	76	15	10	280
Pineapple malt	medium	750	20	123	1	105	20	13	380
Pineapple malt	large	1110	30	179	1	153	30	19	560
Pineapple shake	small	480	13	71	0	62	15	10	220
Pineapple shake	medium	650	18	99	1	87	21	13	300
Pineapple shake	large	960	27	143	1	124	31	20	440
Strawberry malt	small	570	15	93	1	80	15	10	290
Strawberry malt	medium	770	21	128	1	111	20	13	390
Strawberry malt	large	1160	31	185	1	161	33	21	58
Strawberry shake	small	470	14	70	0	59	15	10	220
Strawberry shake	medium	650	18	97	1	82	21	13	290
Strawberry shake	large	950	27	140	1	118	31	20	430

SUNDAES

Item	Serving Size	Calories	Protein	Carb	Fiber	Sugar	Total Fat	Sat Fat	Sodium
Banana	small	230	6	37	1	29	7	4.5	90
Banana	medium	330	8	53	1	42	10	6	130
Banana	large	470	12	76	1	59	14	9	190
Caramel	small	300	6	51	0	36	7	5	150
Caramel	medium	430	9	75	0	52	11	7	220
Caramel	large	610	13	104	0	74	15	11	310
Cherry	small	250	5	40	0	34	7	4.5	110
Cherry	medium	350	8	58	0	49	10	6	160
Cherry	large	500	11	82	0	70	14	9	230
Chocolate-covered strawberry waffle bowl sundae	each	790	10	99	2	78	40	27	180
Chocolate	small	280	5	48	0	41	7	4.5	115
Chocolate	medium	400	8	70	0	59	10	6	170
Chocolate	large	570	11	98	0	83	14	9	240
Fab fudge waffle bowl sundae	each	750	10	108	1	79	30	21	230
Fudge brownie temptation waffle bowl sundae	each	970	14	120	3	94	49	21	370
Hot fudge	small	300	6	46	0	37	10	7	140
Hot fudge	medium	440	9	66	0	53	14	11	200

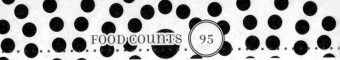

DAIRY QUEEN continued

Item	Serving Size	Calories	Protein	Carb	Fiber	Sugar	Total Fat	Sat Fat	Sodium
Hot fudge	large	610	13	93	0	75	20	15	280
Marshmallow	small	280	5	49	0	42	7	4.5	110
Marshmallow	medium	410	8	72	0	61	10	6	150
Marshmallow	large	570	11	100	0	85	14	9	220
Nut & fudge waffle bowl	each	880	17	99	4	68	47	21	420
Pineapple	small	230	6	38	0	32	7	4.5	100
Pineapple	medium	340	8	54	0	47	10	6	140
Pineapple	large	480	11	77	0	66	14	9	200
Strawberry	small	260	6	44	0	36	7	4.5	105
Strawberry	medium	350	8	56	0	47	10	6	140
Strawberry	large	480	12	76	0	63	14	9	200
Turtle waffle bowl sundae	each	810	12	116	2	76	34	18	320

CONES

Item	Serving Size	Calories	Protein	Carb	Fiber	Sugar	Total Fat	Sat Fat	Sodium
Butterscotch , dipped	kids'	190	4	24	0	18	9	4.5	65
Butterscotch, dipped	small	340	6	35	0	31	16	8	110
Butterscotch, dipped	medium	490	9	59	0	44	23	11	160
Butterscotch, dipped	large	380	12	83	0	62	32	15	220
Cherry, dipped	kids'	190	4	24	0	18	9	6	65
Cherry, dipped	small	330	6	35	0	30	16	11	105
Cherry, dipped	medium	480	9	59	0	43	24	16	150
Cherry, dipped	large	670	12	83	0	60	32	21	220
Chocolate-coated waffle cone w/ soft serve	each	540	10	77	1	57	21	13	170
Chocolate	kids'	150	4	23	0	15	4.5	3	70
Chocolate	small	240	6	32	0	25	7	5	115
Chocolate	medium	340	9	54	0	34	10	7	160
Chocolate	large	490	13	75	0	49	15	10	230
Chocolate, dipped	kids'	190	4	25	0	18	8	3.5	65
Chocolate, dipped	small	330	6	36	0	31	15	6	105
Chocolate, dipped	medium	470	9	60	1	43	22	9	150
Chocolate, dipped	large	660	13	84	1	61	30	13	220
Vanilla	kids'	14	4	22	0	16	4	2.5	60
Vanilla	small	230	6	31	0	26	7	4.5	100
Vanilla	medium	330	9	53	0	36	10	6	140
Vanilla	large	470	12	74	0	52	14	9	200
Waffle cone w/ soft serve	each	420	10	67	0	47	13	7	140

DAIRY QUEEN continued

Item	Serving Size	Calories	Protein	Carb	Fiber	Sugar	Total Fat	Sat Fat	Sodium
OTHER DESSERTS									
Banana split	as served	520	9	94	3	73	13	10	160
Buster Bar Treat	each	480	11	45	2	35	31	15	220
Dilly Bar, butterscotch	each	210	3	24	0	20	11	9	105
Dilly Bar, cherry	each	210	3	24	0	20	12	8	80
Dilly Bar, chocolate	each	240	4	24	1	20	15	9	70
Dilly Bar, chocolate mint	each	240	4	24	1	20	15	9	70
Dilly Bar, Heath	each	220	3	25	0	22	13	10	95
Dilly Bar, no sugar added	each	190	3	24	5	5	13	10	60
DQ fudge bar, no sugar added	each	50	4	13	6	4	0	0	70
DQ sandwich	each	10	4	31	1	18	5	3	135
DQ vanilla orange bar, no sugar added	each	60	2	18	6	4	0	0	40
DQ vanilla Take Home Pack	1/2 cup	140	4	21	0	18	4.5	3	65
Oreo Brownie Earthquake	as served	760	11	117	2	88	27	16	400
Peanut buster parfait	as served	700	16	94	2	72	30	16	360
Starkiss Bar, cherry flavor	each	80	0	21	0	1	0	0	10
Starkiss Bar, Stars & Stripes flavor	each	80	0	21	0	17	0	0	10

DENNY'S

Item	Serving Size	Calories	Protein	Carb	Fiber	Sugar	Total Fat	Sat Fat	Sodium
BREAKFAST ITEMS									
All-American Slam®	as served	820	42	5	1	1	69	26	1520
Bacon avocado burrito	as served	1010	29	91	8	6	59	15	2210
Bacon strips	2 slices	90	7	1	0	1	7	3	350
Bagel & cream cheese	as served	428	11	48	2	8	12	7	560
Belgian waffle Slam®	as served	820	30	32	2	2	64	27	1270
Buttermilk biscuit	1 biscuit	105	2	13	0	0	6	2	285
Buttermilk pancakes	2 pieces	340	2	68	2	12	4	0.5	1180
Buttermilk pancakes	3 pieces	510	12	102	3	18	6	0	1770
Chicken sausage patty	1 1/2 oz	110	7	0	0	1	9	3	460

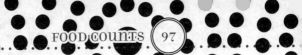

DENNY'S continued

Item	Serving Size	Calories	Protein	Carb	Fiber	Sugar	Total Fat	Sat Fat	Sodium
Chocolate chip pancakes	3 pieces	720	15	129	6	42	18	9	1780
Country fried steak & eggs	as served	660	39	29	3	0	42	15	1620
Egg whites	4 oz	50	11	1	0	0	0	0	180
English muffin	1 piece	180	4	25	1	1	3	1	300
Fabulous French toast platter	as served	1010	43	93	5	16	52	16	2000
French toast Slam®	as served	940	47	68	4	14	53	17	1820
Grand Slamwich® w/o hash browns	as served	1320	52	71	3	9	90	42	3070
Granola w/ 8 oz of milk	as served	690	20	131	9	53	12	3	430
Grits	12 oz	260	5	47	1	0	5	1	840
Ham & Cheddar omelette	as served	590	40	4	0	1	44	17	1330
Hash browns	as served	210	2	26	2	1	12	2.5	650
Hearty wheat pancakes	2 pieces	310	10	64	8	2	1.5	0	950
Hearty wheat pancakes	3 pieces	460	15	96	12	7	2	0	1420
Low fat yogurt	6 oz	160	6	30	0	25	1.5	1	100
Lumberjack Slam®	as served	850	45	60	3	11	46	15	2770
Moons Over My Hammy™	as served	780	46	50	2	3	42	16	2580
Oatmeal w/ 8 oz of milk	16 oz	270	14	37	4	20	7	4	290
Pancake Puppies	6 pieces	390	6	67	2	22	12	2	930
Prime Rib Premium Sizzlin' Breakfast Skillet	as served	850	41	77	6	14	40	15	2110
Sausage links	2 links	182	5	2	1	0	18	6	330
Scrambled eggs	4 oz	250	13	1	0	0	21	5	380
Seasonal fruit	4 oz	70	1	18	3	17	0	0	7
Southwestern Sizzlin' Skillet	as served	990	35	71	6	10	61	21	2140
Southwestern steak burrito	as served	910	33	76	5	4	52	14	1970
T-bone steak & eggs	as served	780	110	4	0	1	36	19	1210
Toast	2 slices	260	6	32	1	4	14	2	110
Turkey bacon	2 slices	76	8	0	0	0	4	0.5	304
Two-egg breakfast	as served	200	13	1	0	0	15	5	330
Ultimate Omelette™	as served	670	36	8	2	3	54	18	740

DENNY'S continued

Item	Serving Size	Calories	Protein	Carb	Fiber	Sugar	Total Fat	Sat Fat	Sodium
Veggie-cheese omelette	as served	500	29	10	2	4	37	12	940
APPETIZERS									
Chicken strips w/ Buffalo sauce	as served	730	57	53	1	1	32	0.5	2940
Chicken wings w/ BBQ sauce	1/2 size	220	12	21	1	19	11	3	700
Chicken wings w/ Buffalo wauce	full size	300	20	5	2	2	21	5	1940
Chicken wings w/ Buffalo wauce	1/2 size	170	11	3	1	1	12	3	1090
Fried shrimp w/ Buffalo sauce	as served	380	17	37	4	10	17	3.5	2690
Mozzarella cheese sticks	as served	750	16	195	1	5	40	17	2270
Sampler	full size	1380	53	139	6	11	71	6	3710
Sampler	1/2 size	870	42	84	3	6	42	5	2420
Smoothered cheese fries	as served	840	24	74	7	3	50	17	1070
Sweet & tangy BBQ chicken strips	as served	820	58	83	2	29	30	0	2160
Sweet & tangy BBQ chicken wings	as served	420	21	41	1	37	19	5	1320
Sweet & tangy BBQ shrimp	as served	460	18	66	4	37	14	3	1850
Tsing Tsing chicken	as served	890	57	92	1	33	31	0	2710
Zesty nachos	full size	1150	46	138	11	11	49	25	2090
Zesty nachos	1/2 size	570	23	67	5	4	24	12	1010
BURGERS & SANDWICHES									
Bacon, lettuce & tomato	as served	520	15	35	2	7	35	8	620
Bacon Cheddar burger	as served	940	64	49	3	11	52	20	1780
Boca burger, w/o fries	as served	420	27	57	8	11	11	3	1300
Cheesy three pack	as served	1930	73	164	8	25	111	21	4120
Chicken ranch melt	as served	800	49	80	4	3	30	9	2540
Chicken sandwich, breaded w/ dressing	as served	1150	41	98	4	22	64	11	2830
Chicken sandwich, grilled w/ dressing	as served	880	36	64	3	23	51	9	1940

DENNY'S continued

Item	Serving Size	Calories	Protein	Carb	Fiber	Sugar	Total Fat	Sat Fat	Sodium
Classic burger w/o cheese	as served	790	55	50	3	11	40	14	1010
Classic cheeseburger	as served	870	59	51	3	12	46	18	1410
Club sandwich	as served	640	27	55	4	9	33	6	1530
Double cheeseburger	as served	1480	110	52	4	12	88	35	2500
Fit-Fare Boca burger w/ fruit	as served	470	26	71	11	22	11	3	1460
Fit-Fare chicken sandwich w/ fruit	as served	450	21	62	4	36	6	1	1380
Grandslamwich w/o side	as served	1320	52	71	3	9	90	42	3070
Mushroom Swiss burger	as served	910	61	55	4	13	49	18	1710
Prime rib Philly melt	as served	730	35	53	4	5	43	12	1820
Slamburger	as served	990	64	59	2	10	54	19	1460
Smoked chicken melt	as served	950	38	72	3	11	55	14	1820
Smokin' Q three pack	as served	2020	79	186	9	35	110	22	3570
Spicy Buffalo Chicken melt	as served	870	45	82	5	3	41	10	3820
The Super Bird®	as served	700	40	53	4	6	37	14	2550
Western burger	as served	1160	63	79	4	19	65	21	1820

SOUPS, SALADS, & SIDES

Item	Serving Size	Calories	Protein	Carb	Fiber	Sugar	Total Fat	Sat Fat	Sodium
Chicken deluxe salad w/ chicken strip (add choicese)	as served	590	42	43	4	7	29	5	1180
Chicken deluxe salad w/ grilled chicken (add choicese)	as served	340	44	13	4	7	13	6	530
Fit-Fare grilled chicken breast salad w/ lemon or lime wedge	as served	340	44	13	4	7	13	6	530
Cranberry apple salad w/ chicken, w/o dressing full size	as served	320	36	22	3	17	10	2	400
Cranberry apple salad w/ chicken, w/o dressing	half size	220	36	5	1	4	6	2	360
Nacho salad	as served	850	48	48	9	19	52	27	2140
Chicken noodle soup	12 oz	140	12	35	2	6	4	2	1150
Broccoli & cheddar soup	12 oz	370	9	48	7	14	16	10	1650

DENNY'S continued

Item	Serving Size	Calories	Protein	Carb	Fiber	Sugar	Total Fat	Sat Fat	Sodium
Vegetable beef soup	12 oz	140	7	17	3	3	5	0	1290
Clam chowder	12 oz	270	5	24	1	12	17	12	1840
Loaded baked potato soup	12 oz	310	5	22	2	5	23	11	1520
Seasoned fries	as served	510	6	48	5	0	33	6	1010
French fries, salted	as served	430	5	50	5	0	23	5	95
Hash browns	1 serving	210	2	26	2	1	12	2.5	650
Onion rings	as served	520	6	48	3	5	36	2	980
Garden salad w/o dressing	as served	120	7	7	2	4	7	5	150
Dippable veggies w/ ranch dressing	as served	210	1	5	1	3	20	4	350
Garlic dinner bread	2 pc	170	4	21	1	0	9	2	350
AMERICAN DINNER CLASSICS™									
Chicken strips	as served	560	45	41	0	2	24	0	1300
Country-fried steak & eggs	as served	660	39	29	3	0	43	15	1620
Country-fried steak w/ gravy	as served	1000	51	54	6	1	65	22	2580
Fit-Fare grilled chicken	as served	380	57	12	2	6	10	2	1280
Grilled chicken	as served	280	55	4	0	2	4	1	1190
Grilled Chicken Sizzlin' Skillet Dinner	as served	770	41	72	5	12	34	12	2020
Homestyle meatloaf w/ gravy	as served	600	33	14	0	4	46	17	1880
Mushroom Swiss chopped steak	as served	940	69	13	1	4	66	24	171
Prime Rib Sizzlin' Skillet Dinner	as served	900	49	77	5	13	42	17	2480
Sweet & Tangy BBQ chicken	as served	650	62	108	3	34	11	3	2290
STEAK & SEAFOOD									
Fit-Fare grilled tilapia	as served	600	59	66	3	7	11	3	1560
Grilled shrimp skewers	as served	370	32	39	2	2	10	2	1140
Lemon pepper tilapia	as served	640	55	41	2	3	27	14	1520
T-Bone steak	12 oz	740	59	0	0	0	56	25	740
T-Bone steak & breaded shrimp	13 oz	920	68	20	2	5	64	27	1490

DENNY'S continued

Item	Serving Size	Calories	Protein	Carb	Fiber	Sugar	Total Fat	Sat Fat	Sodium
T-Bone steak & eggs	16 oz	780	110	4	0	1	36	19	1210
T-Bone steak & shrimp skewer	12 oz	830	72	0	0	0	60	26	900
Tilapia ranchero	as served	470	54	57	4	4	17	5	1090
DINNER SIDES									
Breaded shrimp	6 count	190	9	20	2	4	8	2	750
Coleslaw	as served	260	2	15	3	12	22	3.5	520
Corn	as served	130	4	26	1	3	3	0	250
Cottage cheese	as served	70	9	5	0	3	2	1	300
Country fried potatoes	as served	390	3	30	10	0	28	6	560
Dinner rolls	as served	260	5	38	1	8	9	4	330
Dippable veggies, w/o dressing	as served	30	0	5	1	3	0	0	70
Fiesta corn	as served	135	4	26	1	3	3	0	300
French fries, salted	as served	425	5	50	5	0	23	4	95
Garlic bread	as served	170	4	21	1	0	9	2	350
Green beans, canned	as served	45	2	7	3	1	1	0	480
Green beans, frozen	as served	45	1	4	2	2	2	0	140
Grilled shrimp skewers	as served	90	14	0	0	0	3.5	1	160
Hash browns	as served	210	2	26	2	1	12	2.5	650
Mashed potatoes	as served	17	2	76	1	1	7	1	510
Onion rings	as served	520	6	48	3	5	36	2	980
Ranchero mashed potatoes	as served	140	3	50	1	1	6	2	460
Smoked Cheddar mashed potatoes	as served	120	3	49	1	1	5	2	380
Tomato slices	3 pieces	10	1	2	1	2	0	0	3
Vegetable rice pilaf	as served	200	4	37	1	2	3	0	820
DESSERTS									
Apple crisp à la mode	as served	750	7	134	4	91	21	9	570
Apple pie	as served	510	4	72	3	35	23	9	610
Carrot cake	as served	820	9	100	2	77	45	16	660
Cheesecake	as served	640	9	58	0	44	41	26	350
Cheesecake (no sugar added)	as served	290	6	23	0	2	23	14	340
Cherry topping	as served	57	0	14	0	12	0	0	3

DENNY'S continued

Item	Serving Size	Calories	Protein	Carb	Fiber	Sugar	Total Fat	Sat Fat	Sodium
Chocolate topping	as served	133	2	34	1	32	0.5	0	109
Chocolate vanilla pudding	as served	110	3	32	3	19	1.5	1.5	190
Coconut cream pie	as served	630	6	65	1	43	39	24	370
Double scoop/sundae	as served	280-370	5	38-50	1	32-48	12-18	6-12	80-135
Floats—root beer/cola	as served	430	6	69	0	63	17	9	120
French silk pie	as served	770	6	59	2	38	57	30	400
Fudge topping	as served	201	1	30	1	29	10	7	96
Hershey's chocolate cake	as served	580	6	75	2	55	28	15	400
Hot fudge brownie à la mode	as served	830	9	122	4	95	37	17	520
Milkshake—vanilla/ chocolate/strawberry	as served	560	11	76	<1	65	26	16	272
Oreo Blender Blaster™	as served	890	15	113	3	77	44	20	580
Oreo sundae	as served	760	9	103	3	76	37	21	470
Strawberry topping	as served	77	1	17	1	18	1	0	8

SENIORS

Item	Serving Size	Calories	Protein	Carb	Fiber	Sugar	Total Fat	Sat Fat	Sodium
Senior bacon Cheddar mini burgers	as served	750	49	47	2	7	40	17	1190
Senior Belgian waffle Slam® w/ egg	as served	450	15	29	0	1	31	16	640
Senior club sandwich	as served	570	29	37	4	7	34	7	1340
Senior country-fried steak	as served	530	26	30	3	1	34	12	1460
Senior French toast Slam® w/ egg	as served	300	14	31	1	6	14	4	530
Senior grilled cheese deluxe sandwich	as served	520	16	49	2	5	28	11	1430
Senior grilled chicken	as served	140	28	2	0	1	2	0	590
Senior grilled shrimp skewer	as served	290	18	39	2	2	6	2	980
Senior homestyle meatloaf	as served	280	16	5	0	2	23	17	760
Senior lemon pepper tilapia	as served	450	51	5	1	1	24	14	700
Senior omelette	as served	480	27	6	1	3	37	15	820
Senior scrambled eggs & Cheddar	as served	800	33	58	3	10	47	18	2060

DENNY'S continued

Item	Serving Size	Calories	Protein	Carb	Fiber	Sugar	Total Fat	Sat Fat	Sodium
Senior Starter™	as served	210	9	1	1	0	19	6	290
ROCK STAR MENU									
All Night Sampler	as served	1120	45	131	11	15	47	21	3470
Basket of Puppies	as served	490	11	98	3	18	5	1	1640
Grandslamwich w/o hash browns	as served	1320	52	71	3	9	90	42	3070
Hooburrito	as served	1430	43	164	9	19	67	15	2360
Jewel's smoked chicken quesadilla	as served	720	18	60	5	6	46	16	1350
Los Lonely Boys Texican burger	as served	1020	55	64	3	24	57	19	1430
Nachitos	as served	570	23	67	5	4	24	12	1010
Rascal Flatts Unstoppable Breakfast	as served	1130	54	68	5	5	73	29	3120
Southwestern steak burrito	as served	910	33	76	5	4	52	14	1970
Tsing Tsing chicken	as served	890	57	92	1	33	31	0	2710
KIDS' MEALS									
Apple Dunkers w/ caramel sauce	as served	130	0	30	2	23	0	0	55
Breakaway brownie	as served	310	3	42	1	31	16	6	210
Cheesy @ The Plate	as served	380	15	32	1	3	21	13	670
Chocolate Chip-In pancakes	as served	420	11	61	3	17	18	7	1160
Finish Line fries	as served	450	6	57	6	0	23	4	250
Game on grapes	as served	55	1	29	4	13	0	0	0
Fishing Goldfish® crackers	as served	260	7	38	0	2	9	2	490
High Diving veggies w/ dip	as served	280	2	11	1	3	25	5	540
Home Plate mashed potatoes w/ gravy	as served	140	2	52	1	2	6	1	650
Jr. Glam Slam®	as served	38	15	39	2	7	19	6	1000
Jump-Shot Jell-O	as served	70	1	22	0	17	0	0	40
Kid's Oreo Blender Blaster	as served	680	12	88	3	65	33	17	450
Pit Stop pizza	as served	320	11	38	2	3	14	4	470

DENNY'S continued

Item	Serving Size	Calories	Protein	Carb	Fiber	Sugar	Total Fat	Sat Fat	Sodium
Power Play pudding	as served	110	3	32	3	19	1.5	1.5	190
Slam® dribblers	as served	410	9	74	2	41	11	3	750
Slap Shot slider	2 each	310	20	22	1	3	15	6	470
Slap Shot slider	as served	620	41	43	1	5	30	12	930
Soccer Shake—all flavors	as served	400–580	10	54–63	1	40–69	17–31	17–13	120–170
Softball pancake w/ meat	as served	250	7	30	1	5	11	4	730
Spaghetti, Set, Go!	as served	260	7	40	3	4	7	2	470
Sundae Sundae Sundae!	as served	300	4	36	1	16	16	11	90
Track & Cheese	as served	340	12	48	2	11	11	3	830
Triple Play Nuggets w/ BBQ sauce	as served	340	16	43	1	29	13	3	1020
Tumbling vanilla yogurt	as served	160	6	30	0	25	1.5	1	100

CONDIMENTS

Item	Serving Size	Calories	Protein	Carb	Fiber	Sugar	Total Fat	Sat Fat	Sodium
BBQ sweet & spicy	1.5 oz	110	0	30	1	28	0	0	470
Balsamic vinaigrette	1 oz	120	0	5	0	0	12	2	190
Bleu cheese dressing	1 oz	130	1	1	0	0	13	3	230
Butter roll	2 pieces	260	5	38	1	8	9	4	330
Caesar dressing	1 oz	100	1	0	0	0	10	0	300
Cherry topping	3 oz	86	0	21	0	12	0	0	7
Croutons	0.25 oz	90	3	15	0	0	3	0	240
Fat-free Italian dressing	1 oz	9	0	3	0	2	0	0	367
Fat-free ranch dressing	1 oz	25	0	5	1	1	0	0	230
French dressing	1 oz	74	0	8	0	4	5	0	248
Garlic dinner bread	2 pieces	170	4	21	1	0	9	2	350
Honey mustard dressing	1 oz	160	0	5	0	4	15	0	140
Maple-flavored syrup	3 tbsp	143	0	36	0	28	0	0	26
Maple-flavored syrup, sugar-free	3 tbsp	23	0	9	0	1	0	0	71
Pico de gallo	3 oz	21	1	5	1	3	0	0	125
Ranch dressing	1 oz	129	0	1	0	4	14	0	189
Sour cream	1.5 oz	91	1	2	0	0	9	0	23
Thousand Island dressing	1 oz	107	0	5	0	4	10	0	275
Whipped margarine	1 tbsp	50	0	0	0	0	6	2	40

DOMINO'S PIZZA

Item	Serving Size	Calories	Protein	Carb	Fiber	Sugar	Total Fat	Sat Fat	Sodium
PIZZAS, 12"									
America's Favorite Feast®	1/4 pizza	508	22	57	4	5	22	9.2	1340
Bacon Cheeseburger Feast®	1/4 pizza	549	25	55	3	5	25.9	11.6	1274
Barbecue Bacon Feast®	1/4 pizza	506	22	62	3	9	19.7	9.1	1206
Cheese	1/4 pizza	375	15	55	3	5	11.1	4.8	776
Deluxe Feast®	1/4 pizza	465	20	57	4	5	18	8	1063
ExtravaganZZa Feast®	1/4 pizza	576	27	59	4	5	26.9	11.6	1511
Hawaiian Feast®	1/4 pizza	450	21	58	3	7	15.6	7.2	1102
Pepperoni Feast®	1/4 pizza	534	24	56	3	5	24.7	10.9	1349
Ultimate Deep Dish®, cheese	1/4 pizza	450	16	54	6	5	24	7	1050
Ultimate Deep Dish®, pepperoni	1/4 pizza	530	20	54	6	5	31	9	1330
Veggie Feast®	1/4 pizza	439	19	57	4	5	15.8	7.1	987
SIDES									
Breadsticks, cheesy	1 stick	142	4	18	1	1	6.2	2	183
Chocolate Lava Crunch Cakes	2 cakes	690	8	93	3	62	34	20	340
Cinna Stix®	1 stick	122	2	15	1	3	6.1	1.2	110
Dipping sauce, garlic	1 pack	440	0	5	1	0	50	10	390
Dipping sauce, sweet icing	1 pack	250	0	57	0	55	3	2.5	0
Fried chicken Buffalo wings	1 wing	50	6	2	0	1	2.4	0.7	175
Garden fresh salad	1 salad	140	7	9	4	4	7	4.5	160
Grilled chicken Caesar salad	1 salad	170	19	9	4	3	7	3.5	590

DON PABLO'S

Item	Serving Size	Calories	Protein	Carb	Fiber	Sugar	Total Fat	Sat Fat	Sodium
APPETIZERS									
Don's boneless wings	3 strips	623	21	28	3	n/a	48	8	n/a
Don's wings	4 wings	874	45	17	1	n/a	67	16	n/a
Flautas	2 pieces	188	9	13	2	n/a	12	2	n/a
Taquitos	2 pieces	209	8	9	1	n/a	15	7	n/a
The Don's sampler	1/4 of plate	497	25	35	3	n/a	29	14	n/a
QUESADILLAS									
Cheese, large	2 wedges	358	15	24	1	n/a	23	13	n/a
Cheese, small	2 wedges	497	19	27	2	n/a	35	18	n/a
Mesquite grilled chicken, large	2 wedges	389	15	30	1	n/a	23	11	n/a
Mesquite grilled chicken, Small	2 wedges	413	16	31	1	n/a	25	12	n/a
Mesquite grilled steak, large	2 wedges	407	20	26	1	n/a	25	12	n/a
Mesquite grilled steak, small	2 wedges	431	21	27	1	n/a	27	13	n/a
NACHOS									
Acapulco, beef	3 chips	462	27	23	4	n/a	29	15	n/a
Acapulco, chicken	3 chips	430	25	23	3	n/a	27	14	n/a
Bean & cheese	3 chips	364	18	20	3	n/a	23	13	n/a
Cheese	3 chips	381	20	13	1	n/a	28	17	n/a
Fajita, chicken	3 chips	451	31	25	3	n/a	25	14	n/a
Fajita, steak	3 chips	473	31	25	3	n/a	28	15	n/a
DIPS									
Border dip	2 oz	170	10	6	2	n/a	12	6	n/a
Chips & salsa	1 order	125	3	21	2	n/a	4	1	n/a
Dip sampler	1/4 plate	151	7	7	2	n/a	11	5	n/a
Guacamole, appetizer	1/4 plate	115	2	11	3	n/a	8	1	n/a
Guacamole	1 side	153	2	8	4	n/a	13	2	n/a
Pico de gallo	as served	7	0	2	0	n/a	0	0	n/a
Prairie Fire bean dip	Bowl (1/6th)	120	5	9	2	n/a	7	3	n/a
Prairie Fire bean dip	Cup (1/3rd)	119	5	9	2	n/a	7	3	n/a
Prairie Fire bean dip	1 side	138	6	9	2	n/a	9	4	n/a

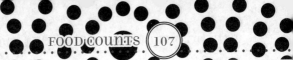

DON PABLO'S continued

Item	Serving Size	Calories	Protein	Carb	Fiber	Sugar	Total Fat	Sat Fat	Sodium
Queso blanco	Bowl (1/6th)	180	10	2	0	n/a	15	9	n/a
Queso blanco	Cup (1/3rd)	180	10	2	0	n/a	15	9	n/a
Queso blanco	1 side	180	10	2	0	n/a	15	9	n/a
Queso	Bowl (1/6th)	124	7	5	0	n/a	8	5	n/a
Queso	Cup (1/3rd)	124	7	5	0	n/a	8	5	n/a
Queso	1 side	124	7	5	0	n/a	8	5	n/a
Salsa, chili, macho	2 oz	18	1	3	1	n/a	0	0	n/a
Salsa, table, regular	2 oz	15	0	3	1	n/a	0	0	n/a
Shrimp queso blanco	2 oz	198	10	3	0	n/a	17	10	n/a

TORTILLAS & CHIPS

Item	Serving Size	Calories	Protein	Carb	Fiber	Sugar	Total Fat	Sat Fat	Sodium
7" flour tortillas	3 tortillas	374	8	60	2	n/a	11	5	n/a
Corn tortillas	4 tortillas	59	1	12	1	n/a	1	0	n/a
Tortilla chips	13 chips	135	2	20	2	n/a	5	1	n/a

FRESH SALADS

Item	Serving Size	Calories	Protein	Carb	Fiber	Sugar	Total Fat	Sat Fat	Sodium
Caesar salad	as served	1047	20	89	11	n/a	68	12	1264
Caesar salad, w/ chicken	as served	1285	37	114	11	n/a	76	13	2107
Caesar salad, w/ steak	as served	1358	57	99	11	n/a	82	18	2081
Fajita taco salad, w/ chicken	as served	1169	77	104	15	n/a	49	23	2497
Fajita taco salad, w/ steak	as served	1236	76	104	15	n/a	57	28	2457
Margarita shaker salad	as served	900	16	52	14	n/a	71	15	310
Red River salad	as served	758	53	47	8	n/a	41	7	1263
Side salad	as served	120	6	14	3	n/a	5	3	104
Sizzling fajita salad, w/ chicken	as served	841	36	81	14	n/a	45	15	1268
Sizzling fajita salad, w/ steak	as served	831	52	69	14	n/a	41	18	1150
Taco salad, w/ beef	as served	1380	79	102	18	n/a	73	32	2593
Taco salad, w/ chicken	as served	1235	68	103	16	n/a	63	27	3126
Tortilla salad shell	as served	351	10	52	2	n/a	11	4	412
Tortilla salad w/ fried shell	as served	482	16	69	6	n/a	16	6	470

DON PABLO'S continued

Item	Serving Size	Calories	Protein	Carb	Fiber	Sugar	Total Fat	Sat Fat	Sodium
SALAD DRESSINGS									
Bleu cheese	2 oz	359	2	2	0	n/a	38	7	6
Caesar dressing	2 oz	274	2	0	0	n/a	29	5	548
Cilantro lemon vinaigrette	2 oz	142	0	2	0	n/a	15	2	248
Cilantro ranch	2 oz	149	1	2	0	n/a	16	2	121
Honey lime	2 oz	272	0	16	0	n/a	24	3	152
Honey mustard	2 oz	302	2	16	0	n/a	28	5	418
Low-fat French	2 oz	143	0	14	0	n/a	9	1	718
Ranch	2 oz	145	1	1	0	n/a	16	2	119
Red wine vinegar & oil	2 oz	241	0	0	0	n/a	28	4	2
Strawberry margarita	2 oz	128	0	5	0	n/a	11	2	8
SOUPS									
Tortilla soup	1 bowl	330	20	40	5	n/a	12	4	3691
Tortilla soup	1 cup	165	10	20	3	n/a	6	2	1844
White chicken chili	1 bowl	487	30	64	9	n/a	11	3	1347
White chicken chili	1 cup	252	15	32	4	n/a	6	2	674
CLASSIC FAJITAS									
Chipotle portabella mushroom	as served	562	10	39	9	n/a	46	8	545
Classic combo— steak & chicken	as served	627	44	47	3	n/a	31	8	1263
Fajita trio—shrimp & chicken	as served	732	44	48	4	n/a	43	10	1858
Grilled shrimp	as served	423	4	22	4	n/a	38	6	1209
Mesquite-grilled chicken	as served	572	29	58	3	n/a	27	4	1283
Mesquite-grilled steak	as served	681	59	36	3	n/a	36	11	1244
Mexican rice	as served	119	1	4	1	n/a	2	0	431
Pecos Valley veggie	as served	334	7	39	8	n/a	20	3	315
Refritos	as served	214	13	50	7	n/a	7	2	614
Shrimp & chicken	as served	498	16	40	4	n/a	32	5	1246
Shrimp & steak	as served	552	32	29	4	n/a	37	9	1226

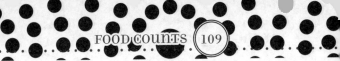

DON PABLO'S continued

Item	Serving Size	Calories	Protein	Carb	Fiber	Sugar	Total Fat	Sat Fat	Sodium
FAJITA COMBOS									
Chicken fajitas & enchilada	as served	604	30	60	4	n/a	28	8	1619
Shrimp fajitas & enchilada	as served	585	11	23	4	n/a	52	16	2629
Steak fajitas & enchilada	as served	650	55	33	3	n/a	34	14	1573
Ultimate Tex-Mex chicken	as served	892	45	55	4	n/a	63	16	1590
Ultimate Tex-Mex steak	as served	947	60	44	4	n/a	68	19	2570
TASTES OF TEXAS									
Big Tex ribeye	as served	1045	60	2	0	n/a	87	33	1958
Rio Grande ribs	as served	1568	73	116	13	n/a	105	29	6001
Shrimp skewer	as served	102	0	0	0	n/a	11	2	96
Side ribs	as served	500	29	16	1	n/a	42	12	1939
Texas Two Step	as served	1808	125	130	12	n/a	100	29	6232
SANDWICH & BURGERS									
Don's burger	as served	1456	53	113	8	n/a	87	30	1657
Don's chicken sandwich	as served	1515	41	128	16	n/a	95	26	1627
Pulled pork sandwich	as served	988	39	121	7	n/a	41	11	3337
MESQUITE GRILLED FAVORITES									
Grilled chicken	as served	877	49	113	3	n/a	25	5	3292
Grilled chicken & shrimp	as served	943	33	128	8	n/a	33	6	3973
Grilled shrimp	as served	735	12	93	7	n/a	36	6	3621
BURRITOS & CHIMICHANGAS									
Burrito, beef, & bean	as served	1285	69	97	12	n/a	68	30	2000
Burrito, chicken	as served	1181	60	105	11	n/a	58	26	2411
Burrito, fajita chicken	as served	1077	70	102	8	n/a	43	19	2939
Burrito, steak	as served	1144	68	102	8	n/a	52	24	2899
Chimichanga, beef	as served	1477	74	112	16	n/a	80	28	2530
Chimichanga, chicken	as served	1110	49	91	8	n/a	61	21	2209

DON PABLO'S continued

Item	Serving Size	Calories	Protein	Carb	Fiber	Sugar	Total Fat	Sat Fat	Sodium
CARNITAS									
Pork	as served	987	53	120	13	n/a	34	12	3048
TACOS									
AYCE taco, 3 beef, soft	as served	1113	62	98	8	n/a	98	22	2302
AYCE taco, 3 beef, crispy	as served	871	57	65	9	n/a	65	18	1639
Buffalo chicken taco trio	as served	1156	43	117	7	n/a	59	21	3586
Chipotle pork taco trio	as served	927	48	92	6	n/a	41	18	2392
Fish tacos, fried	as served	1137	55	100	5	n/a	58	16	2756
Fish tacos, grilled	as served	989	49	71	3	n/a	57	16	1683
Fried chicken taco trio	as served	1052	42	116	7	n/a	48	18	2630
Grilled chicken taco trio	as served	1113	48	129	5	n/a	45	17	2865
Shrimp, fried	as served	859	23	98	5	n/a	42	13	2445
Shrimp, grilled	as served	742	17	69	4	n/a	45	13	1871
Taco, 3 chicken, crispy	as served	724	46	66	6	n/a	31	13	2172
Taco, 3 chicken, soft	as served	968	51	99	6	n/a	40	18	2835
ENCHILADAS									
3 Amigos	as served	812	47	50	4	n/a	47	22	2521
3 beef	as served	900	66	46	5	n/a	49	19	2131
3 cheese	as served	722	34	50	4	n/a	43	25	1800
3 chicken	as served	814	42	55	3	n/a	48	23	1700
3 Mama's Skinny	as served	470	29	48	4	n/a	17	7	1271
Cadillac Enchiladas, chicken	as served	1088	73	87	4	n/a	48	26	1712
Cadillac Enchiladas, steak	as served	1155	72	88	4	n/a	57	31	1672
DESSERTS									
Chocolate Volcano	as served	1139	10	126	4	n/a	70	21	1143
Fried ice cream	as served	686	7	96	3	n/a	29	9	627
Iron Skillet apple pie	as served	1303	6	147	4	n/a	80	29	1027
Sopapillas	as served	1252	12	154	3	n/a	65	20	1324

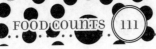

DON PABLO'S continued

Item	Serving Size	Calories	Protein	Carb	Fiber	Sugar	Total Fat	Sat Fat	Sodium
LITTLE AMIGOS									
Beef taco	as served	493	28	51	8	n/a	20	8	808
Cheese enchilada	as served	530	27	41	5	n/a	29	16	1335
Chicken stix	as served	978	26	80	4	n/a	66	11	2622
Corn dog	as served	832	18	107	9	n/a	39	9	3114
Dogs in a blanket	as served	613	12	83	6	n/a	27	6	2323
Grilled cheese crisp	as served	873	23	80	4	n/a	52	19	1591
COOL AMIGOS									
Cheeseburger	as served	1080	36	96	6	n/a	62	20	1496
Chicken fajitas	as served	1201	45	145	12	n/a	49	20	2594
Chicken nachos	as served	754	49	43	6	n/a	43	23	1306
Chicken quesadilla	as served	1095	33	112	7	n/a	58	26	1838
Chicken sandwich	as served	1028	21	102	11	n/a	61	16	1296
Chicken tenders	as served	1007	33	109	8	n/a	51	10	3144
Fried ice cream	as served	300	4	53	1	n/a	7	3	324
Kids' ice cream	as served	120	1	18	0	n/a	5	3	35
Kids' queso dip	as served	124	7	5	0	n/a	8	5	690
Steak fajitas	as served	1260	60	135	12	n/a	54	24	2575

DUNKIN' DONUTS

Item	Serving Size	Calories	Protein	Carb	Fiber	Sugar	Total Fat	Sat Fat	Sodium
BAGELS & BAGEL TWISTS									
Blueberry bagel	each	330	11	65	5	10	3	1	620
Cheddar cheese bagel twist	each	400	17	63	5	5	9	4.5	800
Chocolate chip bagel twist	each	340	10	66	4	19	4	1.5	530
Cinnamon raisin bagel	each	330	11	65	5	13	3.5	0.5	450
Cinnamon raisin bagel twist	each	350	11	72	5	19	3.5	0.5	460
Everything bagel	each	350	13	66	5	5	4.5	0.5	660
French Toast bagel twist	each	330	10	66	4	16	2.5	0	540
Garlic bagel	each	340	12	68	6	5	2.5	0.5	330
Multigrain bagel	each	390	14	65	9	7	8	0.5	560
Onion bagel	each	310	11	63	3	3	2	0	380
Plain bagel	each	320	11	63	5	5	2.5	0.5	660

DUNKIN' DONUTS continued

Item	Serving Size	Calories	Protein	Carb	Fiber	Sugar	Total Fat	Sat Fat	Sodium
Poppy seed bagel	each	350	13	64	5	5	6	0.5	660
Salt bagel	each	320	11	63	5	5	2.5	0.5	3420
Sesame seed bagel	each	360	13	63	5	5	6	0.5	660
Tomato basil bagel twist	each	360	15	55	4	6	9	4.5	760
Wheat bagel	each	320	12	61	5	4	3.5	0	550

CREAM CHEESE

Item	Serving Size	Calories	Protein	Carb	Fiber	Sugar	Total Fat	Sat Fat	Sodium
Blueberry, reduced fat	1 unit (50g)	150	2	15	0	11	9	6	210
Onion & chive, reduced fat	1 unit (50g)	130	3	6	0	3	11	7	250
Plain	1 unit (50g)	150	3	3	0	3	15	9	250
Plain, reduced fat	1 unit (50g)	100	4	5	0	2	8	5	250
Smoked salmon, reduced fat	1 unit (50g)	140	4	6	0	3	11	7	260
Strawberry, reduced fat	1 unit (50g)	150	2	15	0	11	10	6	200
Veggie, reduced fat	1 unit (50g)	120	2	6	0	2	10	6	240

COOKIES, DANISH, MUFFINS, & OTHER

Item	Serving Size	Calories	Protein	Carb	Fiber	Sugar	Total Fat	Sat Fat	Sodium
Apple cheese danish	1 Danish	330	4	41	1	18	16	7	270
Apple pie		230	3	34	1	14	10	4.5	150
Biscuit		280	5	32	1	2	14	8	620
Blueberry muffin	1 muffin	480	6	81	2	46	25	1.5	470
Blueberry muffin, reduced fat	1 muffin	430	6	80	2	41	9	1	650
Brownie	each	440	3	58	1	49	23	5	250
Cheese danish	1 Danish	330	5	39	1	17	17	8	270
Chocolate chip muffin	1 muffin	590	7	92	3	54	22	6	490
Coffee Cake Muffin	1 muffin	630	7	95	1	55	25	7	510
Corn Muffin	1 muffin	490	6	80	1	34	16	1.5	820
English Muffin	each	160	5	31	1	1	2	0	350
Honey Bran Raisin Muffin	1 muffin	480	6	82	5	46	13	1.5	430
Oatmeal Raisin Cookie	1 cookie	350	5	54	3	33	9	4.5	210
Plain Croissant	each	310	7	35	1	4	16	7	350
Pumpkin Muffin	1 muffin	600	7	83	3	44	26	6	520
Reverse Chocolate Chunk Cookie	1 cookie	380	5	50	2	34	18	10	320

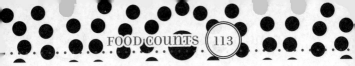

DUNKIN' DONUTS continued

Item	Serving Size	Calories	Protein	Carb	Fiber	Sugar	Total Fat	Sat Fat	Sodium
Strawberry Cheese Danish	1 danish	320	4	40	1	18	16	7	260
Triple Chocolate Chunk Cookie	1 cookie	360	5	53	2	31	15	8	380
COOLATTA DRINKS									
Coffee Coolatta® w/ cream	small	400	3	49	0	43	23	14	75
Coffee Coolatta® w/ cream	medium	600	5	73	0	65	35	22	110
Coffee Coolatta® w/ cream	large	80	7	98	0	87	46	29	150
Coffee Coolatta® w/ milk	small	240	4	50	0	49	4	2.5	90
Coffee Coolatta® w/ milk	medium	360	6	75	0	73	6	3.5	130
Coffee Coolatta® w/ milk	large	480	8	100	0	98	8	5	180
Coffee Coolatta® w/ skim milk	small	210	4	51	0	49	0	0	90
Coffee Coolatta® w/ skim milk	medium	310	7	76	0	73	0	0	135
Coffee Coolatta® w/ skim milk	large	420	9	102	0	98	0	0	180
Strawberry Fruit Coolatta®	small	310	0	75	0	68	0	0	45
Strawberry Fruit Coolatta®	medium	460	1	112	0	102	0	0	65
Strawberry Fruit Coolatta®	large	610	1	150	0	135	0	0	85
Tropicana Orange Coolatta®	small	230	1	57	0	54	0	0	40
Tropicana Orange Coolatta®	medium	350	2	85	0	82	0	0	0
Tropicana Orange Coolatta®	large	470	2	113	0	109	0	0	80
Vanilla Bean Coolatta®	small	430	3	91	0	86	6	3.5	170
Vanilla Bean Coolatta®	medium	650	4	136	0	129	9	5	260
Vanilla Bean Coolatta®	large	860	6	181	0	172	12	7	350
FLAVORED COFFEES									
Blueberry Coffee	small	15	0	2	0	0	0	0	5
Caramel Coffee	small	10	0	2	0	0	0	0	5
Cinnamon Coffee	small	15	0	2	0	0	0	0	5
Coconut Coffee	small	10	0	1	0	0	0	0	5

DUNKIN' DONUTS continued

Item	Serving Size	Calories	Protein	Carb	Fiber	Sugar	Total Fat	Sat Fat	Sodium
French Vanilla Coffee	small	10	0	1	0	0	0	0	5
Hazelnut Coffee	small	10	0	1	0	0	0	0	5
Mocha Coffee	small	110	1	23	1	23	0	0	
Mocha Coffee	medium	170	2	39	2	34	0.5	0	30
Mocha Coffee	large	230	3	52	2	46	1	0	40
Mocha Coffee	extra large	280	3	65	3	57	1	0.5	50
Mocha Coffee w/ cream	small	170	2	27	1	23	6	4	30
Mocha Coffee w/ cream	medium	260	3	41	2	34	9	6	45
Mocha Coffee w/ cream	large	34	4	54	2	46	12	8	60
Mocha Coffee w/ cream	extra large	430	5	68	3	57	16	10	75
Raspberry Coffee	small	15	0	2	0	0	0	0	5
Toasted Almond Coffee	small	10	0	1	0	0	0	0	5

ESPRESSO DRINKS—HOT OR ICED

Item	Serving Size	Calories	Protein	Carb	Fiber	Sugar	Total Fat	Sat Fat	Sodium
Cappuccino	small	80	4	7	0	7	4	2.5	70
Cappuccino w/ sugar	small	140	4	24	0	24	4	2.5	70
Caramel Apple Latte	small	230	8	35	0	33	6	3.5	180
Caramel Apple Latte	medium	340	11	52	0	49	9	6	270
Caramel Apple Latte	large	450	15	70	0	66	12	7	360
Caramel Swirl Latte	small	220	8	35	0	34	6	3.5	150
Espresso	1.75 oz	5	0	1	0	1	0	0	5
Espresso w/ sugar	1.75 oz	30	0	7	0	7	0	0	5
Latte	small	120	6	10	0	10	6	3.5	105
Latte Lite	small	80	7	13	0	10	0	0	110
Latte Lite	medium	120	10	19	0	15	0	0	170
Latte Lite	large	160	14	25	0	20	0	0	220
Latte w/ sugar	small	170	6	27	0	27	6	3.5	100
Mocha Raspberry Latte	small	230	7	36	1	32	6	4	110
Mocha Raspberry Latte	medium	340	10	54	2	48	9	6	160
Mocha Raspberry Latte	large	450	13	73	2	64	12	8	220
Mocha Spice Latte	medium	330	10	53	2	48	9	6	140
Mocha Spice Latte	large	450	13	70	2	64	12	8	190
Mocha Spice Latte	small	220	7	35	1	32	6	4	95
Mocha Swirl Latte	small	220	7	35	1	32	6	4	115
Pumpkin Latte	small	210	8	32	0	32	6	4	140
Pumpkin Latte	medium	320	11	49	0	48	9	6	210

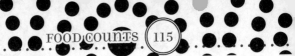

DUNKIN' DONUTS continued

Item	Serving Size	Calories	Protein	Carb	Fiber	Sugar	Total Fat	Sat Fat	Sodium
Pumpkin Latte	large	430	15	65	0	64	12	8	280
Vanilla Latte Lite	small	90	7	14	0	10	0	0	110
Vanilla Latte Lite	medium	130	10	20	0	15	0	0	170
Vanilla Latte Lite	large	170	14	28	0	20	0	0	220
ICED COFFEE									
Iced Coffee	small	10	1	2	0	0	0	0	5
Iced Coffee	medium	15	1	2	0	0	0	0	10
Iced Coffee	large	20	1	3	0	0	0	0	15
Iced Coffee w/ milk	small	30	2	3	0	1	1	1	20
Iced Coffee w/ milk & sugar	small	90	2	21	0	19	1	1	20
Iced Coffee w/ skim milk	small	20	2	3	0	2	0	0	25
Iced Coffee w/ skim milk & sugar	small	80	2	21	0	19	0	0	25
Iced Coffee w/ sugar	small	70	1	19	0	17	0	0	5
Iced Dunkin' Dark® Roast Coffee w/ cream & sugar	small	130	1	20	0	17	6	3.5	20
Iced Dunkin' Dark® Roast Coffee w/ cream & sugar	medium	190	2	30	0	26	9	5	30
Iced Dunkin' Dark® Roast Coffee w/ cream & sugar	large	250	3	40	0	35	12	7	40
Iced Dunkin' Dark® Roast Coffee w/ skim milk & Splenda	small	30	2	5	0	1	0	0	25
Iced Dunkin' Dark® Roast Coffee w/ skim milk & Splenda	medium	40	3	8	0	2	0	0	35
Iced Dunkin' Dark® Roast Coffee w/ skim milk & Splenda	large	60	3	10	0	3	0	0	50
Iced Pumpkin Coffee w/ cream	small	170	3	25	0	23	6	3.5	60
Iced Pumpkin Coffee w/ cream	medium	250	5	38	0	34	9	6	90
Iced Pumpkin Coffee w/ cream	large	330	6	51	0	45	12	7	125
Mocha Iced Coffee w/ cream	small	180	2	28	1	23	6	4	35

DUNKIN' DONUTS continued

Item	Serving Size	Calories	Protein	Carb	Fiber	Sugar	Total Fat	Sat Fat	Sodium
Mocha Iced Coffee w/ cream	medium	260	3	42	2	34	9	6	50
Mocha Iced Coffee w/ cream	large	350	5	56	2	46	12	8	70
OTHER DRINKS									
Apple Cider, hot or iced	small	120	0	31	0	31	0	0	40
Apple Cider, hot or iced	medium	180	0	45	0	45	0	0	55
Apple Cider, hot or iced	large	260	0	66	0	66	0	0	85
Apple Cider, hot or iced	extra large	320	0	80	0	80	0	0	100
Dunkaccino	small	240	2	35	1	26	11	9	220
Hot Chocolate	small	220	2	39	2	30	7	7	270
Hot Tea, unsweetened	medium	5	0	2	0	0	0	0	0
Hot Tea, unsweetened	large	10	0	2	0	0	0	0	5
Sweet Tea	16 oz	120	0	29	0	28	0	0	5
Turbo Shot™	small	5	0	1	0	1	0	0	5
Turbo Shot™	medium	5	0	1	0	1	0	0	10
Turbo Shot™	large	10	0	2	0	2	0	0	15
Turbo Shot™	extra large	10	0	2	0	2	0	0	15
Vanilla Chai	14 oz	330	11	53	1	45	8	8	180
White Hot Chocolate	small	230	2	38	1	32	8	8	310
White Hot Chocolate	medium	340	3	56	1	47	12	11	460
White Hot Chocolate	large	470	4	79	1	65	17	16	650
DONUTS & SWEETS									
Apple Crumb Donut	1 donut	490	4	80	2	49	18	9	35
Apple Fritter	1 fritter	410	6	60	2	27	17	7	380
Apple n' Spice Donut	1 donut	27	3	32	1	8	14	5	350
Bavarian Kreme Donut	1 donut	270	4	31	1	9	15	7	350
Blueberry Cake Donut	1 donut	340	4	44	1	21	17	8	579
Blueberry Crumb Donut	1 donut	500	4	84	2	52	18	9	350
Boston Kreme Donut	1 donut	310	3	39	1	16	16	7	370
Bow Tie Donut	1 donut	310	4	39	1	15	15	7	400
Chocolate Coconut Donut	1 donut	550	5	47	2	22	39	25	39
Chocolate Frosted Cake Donut	1 donut	370	4	45	1	20	23	10	320

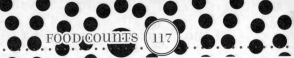

DUNKIN' DONUTS continued

Item	Serving Size	Calories	Protein	Carb	Fiber	Sugar	Total Fat	Sat Fat	Sodium
Chocolate Frosted Coffee Roll	1 coffee roll	410	7	53	3	19	19	8	420
Chocolate Frosted Donut	1 donut	270	3	31	1	13	15	7	340
Chocolate Glazed Cake Donut	1 donut	370	3	35	1	17	24	11	390
Chocolate Iced Bismark	1 Bismark	390	5	52	2	21	19	8	360
Chocolate Kreme Filled Donut	1 donut	370	4	42	1	21	21	10	370
Cinnamon Cake Donut	1 donut	340	3	38	1	13	22	10	300
Coffee Roll	1 coffee roll	400	7	53	3	19	18	7	400
Double Chocolate Cake Donut	1 donut	380	4	36	2	17	25	11	410
Dulce de Chocolate Donut	1 donut	350	4	45	1	21	17	7	360
Dulce de Leche Donut	1 donut	290	4	31	1	10	16	7	340
Éclair	1 Éclair	390	5	52	2	21	19	8	360
Fall Harvest Donut	1 donut	290	3	35	1	15	15	7	340
French Crulller	1 donut	250	2	18	0	10	20	9	105
Glazed Cake Donut	1 donut	360	3	44	1	19	22	10	300
Glazed Donut	1 donut	260	3	31	1	12	14	6	330
Glazed Fritter	1 Fritter	410	6	60	2	27	17	7	380
Guayaba Burst Donut	1 donut	300	4	38	1	15	15	7	330
Jelly Filled Donut	1 donut	290	3	36	1	6	14	7	340
Maple Frosted Coffee Roll	1 coffee roll	410	7	54	3	20	19	8	410
Maple Frosted Donut	1 donut	270	3	32	1	14	15	7	340
Marble Frosted Donut	1 donut	270	3	32	1	13	15	7	340
Monkey See Monkey Donut	1 donut	340	5	43	2	22	17	8	360
Old Fashioned Cake Donut	1 donut	320	3	33	1	9	22	10	300
Piña Boom Donut	1 donut	270	4	32	1	12	15	7	350
Piña Colada Donut	1 donut	330	4	42	1	20	17	9	380
Powdered Cake Donut	1 donut	340	4	38	1	13	22	10	300
Pumpkin Donut	1 donut	340	3	38	1	19	19	9	260
Strawberry Frosted Donut	1 donut	280	3	32	1	14	15	7	340

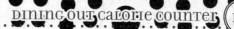

DUNKIN' DONUTS continued

Item	Serving Size	Calories	Protein	Carb	Fiber	Sugar	Total Fat	Sat Fat	Sodium
Sugar Raised Donut	1 donut	230	3	22	1	4	14	6	330
Vanilla Frosted Coffee Roll	1 coffee roll	410	7	54	3	20	19	8	410
Vanilla Kreme Filled Donut	1 donut	390	4	42	1	22	23	10	370

MUNCHKINS

Item	Serving Size	Calories	Protein	Carb	Fiber	Sugar	Total Fat	Sat Fat	Sodium
Cinnamon Cake Munchkin	1 Munchkin	60	1	6	0	3	3.5	1.5	65
Fall Munchkin	1 Munchkin	90	1	12	0	9	3.5	1.5	65
Glazed Cake Munchkin	1 Munchkin	70	1	8	0	4	3.5	1.5	65
Glazed Chocolate Cake Munchkin	1 Munchkin	70	1	8	0	4	3.5	1.5	85
Glazed Munchkin	1 Munchkin	70	1	7	0	3	4	2	80
Jelly Filled Munchkin	1 Munchkin	80	1	9	0	2	4	2	85
Plain Cake Munchkin	1 Munchkin	60	1	6	0	2	3.5	1.5	65
Powdered Cake Munchkin	1 Munchkin	60	1	7	0	3	3.5	1.5	65
Sugared Munchkin	1 Munchkin	60	1	6	0	2	3.5	1.5	65

DONUT STICKS

Item	Serving Size	Calories	Protein	Carb	Fiber	Sugar	Total Fat	Sat Fat	Sodium
Cinnamon Cake Stick	1 stick	350	4	44	2	19	18	8	420
Glazed Cake Stick	1 stick	370	4	48	1	23	18	8	420
Glazed Chocolate Cake Stick	1 stick	390	3	40	2	17	25	11	540
Jelly Stick	1 stick	450	4	60	1	20	18	8	440
Plain Cake Stick	1 stick	330	4	36	1	12	18	8	420
Powdered Cake Stick	1 stick	360	5	43	2	18	18	8	420

SANDWICHES & FLATBREADS

Item	Serving Size	Calories	Protein	Carb	Fiber	Sugar	Total Fat	Sat Fat	Sodium
Chicken Bruschetta Sandwich	1 sandwich	580	37	49	2	4	26	7	1200
Chipotle Chicken Sandwich	1 sandwich	600	43	50	3	5	25	8	1380
Grilled Cheese Flatbread	1 sandwich	380	16	35	1	2	18	9	850
Ham & Cheese Flatbread	1 sandwich	320	20	34	1	2	11	5	960

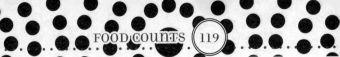

DUNKIN' DONUTS continued

Item	Serving Size	Calories	Protein	Carb	Fiber	Sugar	Total Fat	Sat Fat	Sodium
Pastrami Supreme Sandwich	1 sandwich	750	48	51	3	4	39	16	2060
Pressed Cuban Sandwich	1 sandwich	680	46	50	2	6	33	13	2000
Steak and Cheese Sandwich	1 sandwich	470	3	50	2	3	16	6	2040
Toasted Italian Sandwich	1 sandwich	560	33	52	3	5	25	9	2630
Tuna (albacore) Sandwich	1 sandwich	660	31	56	3	9	1	2.5	1280
Tuna Melt Sandwich	1 sandwich	770	36	57	3	8	30	7	1560
Tuna Salad Sandwich on Plain Bagel	1 sandwich	540	18	69	5	6	20	3	1070
Turkey, Cheddar & Bacon Flatbread	1 sandwich	410	21	36	1	2	20	7	1110
Turkey & Bacon Club Sandwich	1 sandwich	440	35	51	3	5	13	3	1800
Turkey & Cheese Sandwich	1 sandwich	450	35	52	3	4	13	4.5	1500
SOUPS & SALADS									
Broccoli Cheddar Soup	8 oz	190	10	14	2	5	11	6	90
Caesar Salad	as served	320	6	11	3	2	29	6	790
Chicken Caesar Salad	as served	440	25	11	3	2	33	7	1020
Chicken Noodle Soup	8 oz	130	7	1	1	1	3	1	970
Garden Salad	as served	180	8	21	4	6	6	3	500
BREAKFAST ITEMS (BREAKFAST SANDWICHES & SIDES)									
Bacon, Egg & Cheese on Bagel	1 sandwich	560	24	66	5	7	19	7	1340
Bacon, Egg & Cheese on Biscuit	1 sandwich	490	18	35	1	4	30	14	1300
Bacon, Egg & Cheese on Croissant	1 sandwich	560	20	38	2	6	33	13	1030
Bacon, Egg & Cheese on English Muffin	1 sandwich	370	18	34	1	3	18	6	1030
Bacon, Egg & Cheese Wake-Up Wrap	1 wrap	210	10	14	1	1	12	5	580
Bacon, Egg White & Cheese on English Muffin	1 sandwich	300	19	33	1	3	10	4.5	1040

DUNKIN' DONUTS continued

Item	Serving Size	Calories	Protein	Carb	Fiber	Sugar	Total Fat	Sat Fat	Sodium
Bacon, Egg White & Cheese on Wheat English Muffin	1 sandwich	290	20	32	2	3	10	4.5	1050
Bacon, Egg White & Cheese Wake-Up Wrap	1 wrap	170	10	13	1	1	8	3.5	580
Chicken Biscuit	1 sandwich	500	20	48	2	5	25	10	1260
Egg & Cheese on Bagel	1 sandwich	480	20	66	5	6	15	5	1130
Egg & Cheese on Biscuit	1 sandwich	440	14	35	1	3	27	13	1090
Egg & Cheese on Croissant	1 sandwich	480	16	38	2	6	29	12	820
Egg & Cheese on English Muffin	1 sandwich	320	14	34	1	3	15	5	820
Egg & Cheese Wake-Up Wrap	1 wrap	180	8	14	1	1	11	4	470
Egg White & Cheese on English Muffin	1 sandwich	250	15	33	1	2	7	3	830
Egg White & Cheese on Wheat English Muffin	1 sandwich	250	15	32	2	3	7	3	840
Egg White & Cheese Wake-Up Wrap	1 wrap	150	8	13	1	1	7	3	480
Egg White Turkey Sausage Flatbread	1 sandwich	290	21	34	3	6	8	3	600
Egg White Veggie Flatbread	1 sandwich	330	20	35	4	5	12	5	820
Ham, Egg & Cheese on Bagel	1 sandwich	510	26	66	5	7	16	6	1390
Ham, Egg & Cheese on Biscuit	1 sandwich	480	19	35	1	4	28	14	1350
Ham, Egg & Cheese on Croissant	1 sandwich	510	21	38	2	6	31	12	1080
Ham, Egg & Cheese on English Muffin	1 sandwich	360	20	34	1	3	16	6	1080
Ham, Egg & Cheese Wake-Up Wrap	1 wrap	200	11	14	1	1	11	4.5	600

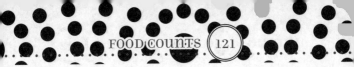

DUNKIN' DONUTS continued

Item	Serving Size	Calories	Protein	Carb	Fiber	Sugar	Total Fat	Sat Fat	Sodium
Ham, Egg White & Cheese on English Muffin	1 sandwich	280	21	33	1	3	8	3.5	1090
Ham, Egg White & Cheese on Wheat English Muffin	1 sandwich	280	21	32	2	3	8	3.5	1110
Ham, Egg White & Cheese Wake-Up Wrap	1 wrap	160	11	13	1	1	7	3.5	610
Hash Browns	9 pieces	200	2	22	3	0	11	1.5	730
Maple Cheddar Breakfast Sandwich	1 sandwich	720	26	42	2	9	49	20	1140
Sausage Biscuit	1 sandwich	450	12	33	1	2	28	14	1020
Sausage, Egg & Cheese on Bagel	1 sandwich	680	29	67	5	7	32	12	1590
Sausage, Egg & Cheese on Biscuit	1 sandwich	640	22	36	1	4	44	19	1550
Sausage, Egg & Cheese on Croissant	1 sandwich	680	24	39	2	6	4	18	1280
Sausage, Egg & Cheese on English Muffin	1 sandwich	520	23	34	1	3	31	12	1280
Sausage, Egg & Cheese Wake-Up Wrap	1 wrap	280	12	14	1	1	19	7	700
Sausage, Egg White & Cheese on English Muffin	1 sandwich	450	24	34	1	3	23	9	1290
Sausage, Egg White & Cheese on Wheat English Muffin	1 sandwich	450	24	33	2	3	23	9	1310
Sausage, Egg White & Cheese Wake-Up Wrap	1 wrap	250	13	14	1	1	15	6	710

EINSTEIN BROS.

Item	Serving Size	Calories	Protein	Carb	Fiber	Sugar	Total Fat	Sat Fat	Sodium
BAGELS, BAGEL PRETZELS, & BREADS									
Asiago cheese bagel	each	310	14	56	2	5	5	3	630
Asiago cheese bagel pretzel	each	300	11	52	2	5	7	2.5	710
Blueberry bagel	each	300	10	65	3	11	1	0	480
Braided challah roll	each	220	8	41	1	5	3.5	0.5	200
Chocolate chip bagel	each	280	9	56	3	10	2.5	1	430
Ciabatta roll	each	290	10	60	2	1	2.5	0	640
Cinnamon raisin swirl bagel	each	290	10	63	3	13	1	0	450
Cinnamon sugar bagel, Chicago style	each	310	10	66	3	12	2.5	0.5	510
Cinnamon sugar bagel pretzel	each	320	8	66	3	18	5	1	630
Cranberry bagel	each	270	9	60	2	12	1	0	420
Dutch apple bagel	each	350	8	66	3	15	7	2	530
Egg bagel	each	300	12	54	2	6	5	1.5	490
Everything bagel	each	270	9	56	2	5	2	0	620
Garlic dip'd bagel	each	270	9	56	2	5	2.5	0	460
Good grains bagel	each	280	10	58	3	8	2.5	0	440
Green chili bagel	each	350	15	58	2	6	8	4.5	680
Honey whole wheat bagel	each	260	9	57	3	8	1	0	440
Multi grain bread	each	130	5	23	2	3	2.5	0	220
Onion bagel	each	270	9	59	2	5	1	0	460
Onion dip'd bagel	each	270	9	56	2	5	2.5	0	460
Plain bagel	each	260	9	56	2	5	1	0	460
Plain bagel pretzel	each	270	8	52	2	5	5	1	630
Poppy dip'd bagel	each	280	10	56	2	5	3	0	460
Potato bagel	each	270	8	52	2	5	4	0.5	500
Power bagel, fruit & nut	each	310	11	61	4	1	5	0.5	280
Pumpernickel bagel	each	240	9	53	3	4	1.5	0	490
Salt bagel pretzel	each	270	8	52	2	5	5	1	1740
Sesame dip'd bagel	each	280	10	56	2	5	3	0	460
Six-cheese bagel	each	330	15	56	2	5	6	3.5	650
Spinach florentine bagel	each	340	15	57	2	5	8	4	590
Sun-dried tomato bagel	each	260	9	54	3	3	1.5	0	530

EINSTEIN BROS. continued

Item	Serving Size	Calories	Protein	Carb	Fiber	Sugar	Total Fat	Sat Fat	Sodium
CREAM CHEESE									
Whipped blueberry reduced fat	2 tbsp	70	1	6	0	5	5	3.5	50
Whipped garden vegetable reduced fat	2 tbsp	60	1	3	0	1	5	3.5	100
Whipped garlic herb reduced fat	2 tbsp	60	1	3	0	1	5	3.5	100
Whipped honey almond reduced fat	2 tbsp	70	1	6	0	4	5	3	45
Whipped jalapeño salsa reduced fat	2 tbsp	60	1	3	0	1	5	3.5	105
Whipped onion & chive	2 tbsp	70	1	3	0	1	6	4	60
Whipped plain	2 tbsp	70	1	1	0	1	7	4.5	65
Whipped plain reduced fat	2 tbsp	60	1	2	0	1	5	3.5	100
Whipped smoked salmon	2 tbsp	60	1	2	0	1	6	3.5	120
Whipped strawberry reduced fat	2 tbsp	70	1	5	0	4	5	3.5	50
Whipped sun-dried tomato basil reduced fat	2 tbsp	60	1	2	0	1	5	3.5	100
SPECIALTY COFFEES									
Americano	large	1	0	0	0	0	0	0	0
Americano	small	1	0	0	0	0	0	0	0
Café latte	medium	140	4	13	0	13	5	3.5	20
Café latte	large	200	6	20	0	19	8	5	30
Café latte	regular	250	8	24	0	23	9	6	35
Café latte, nonfat	medium	100	4	14	0	14	1	0	5
Café latte, nonfat	large	140	6	20	0	19	1	0.5	5
Café latte, nonfat	regular	180	8	25	0	23	1	0.5	10
Café latte, whole milk	medium	200	0	16	0	16	10	6	30
Café latte, whole milk	large	250	0	21	0	21	12	7	35
Café latte, whole milk	regular	320	0	26	0	26	16	9	50
Cappuccino	medium	90	2	9	0	8	3.5	2	15
Cappuccino	large	190	4	19	0	18	7	4.5	30
Cappuccino	regular	230	6	23	0	22	9	5	35
Cappuccino, nonfat	medium	130	6	19	0	18	1	0	5
Cappuccino, nonfat	regular	90	4	13	0	13	0	0	5
Cappuccino, nonfat	large	170	8	23	0	22	1	0.5	10

EINSTEIN BROS. continued

Item	Serving Size	Calories	Protein	Carb	Fiber	Sugar	Total Fat	Sat Fat	Sodium
Cappuccino, whole milk	medium	150	0	13	0	13	8	4.5	25
Cappuccino, whole milk	large	190	0	17	0	17	9	5	25
Cappuccino, whole milk	regular	250	0	21	0	21	12	7	35
Chai tea w/ 2% milk	small	220	3	47	0	45	2	1	65
Chai tea w/ 2% milk	regular	290	4	63	0	60	2.5	1.5	85
Chai tea w/ 2% milk	large	360	5	78	0	75	3	2	105
Chai tea w/ skim milk	small	210	3	47	0	45	0	0	65
Chai tea w/ skim milk	regular	270	4	63	0	60	0	0	85
Chai tea w/ skim milk	large	340	6	79	0	75	0	0	105
Chai tea w/ whole milk	regular	230	3	47	0	45	3	1.5	55
Chai tea w/ whole milk	large	310	4	63	0	60	4	2.5	75
Chai tea w/ whole milk	regular	380	5	78	0	74	4.5	2.5	85
Espresso	regular	1	0	0	0	0	0	0	0
Hot chocolate	8 oz	290	9	39	0	33	11	8	160
Hot chocolate w/ whole milk	regular	320	9	39	0	33	14	10	160
Iced Americano	12 oz	1	0	0	0	0	0	0	0
Iced coffee	16 oz	0	0	0	0	0	0	0	0
Iced latte	16 oz	120	8	12	0	11	4.5	3	125
Iced mocha	16 oz	210	7	33	0	31	6	4	120
Iced nonfat latte	16 oz	90	8	12	0	11	0	0	130
Low fat iced mocha	16 oz	180	7	32	0	30	2.5	2	115
Low fat mocha	12 oz	190	8	34	0	31	2.5	2	130
Low fat mocha	medium	240	7	29	0	27	10	6	135
Low fat mocha	large	350	10	42	1	38	15	9	180
Low fat mocha	regular	420	13	56	1	50	16	9	240
Mocha	medium	230	2	34	0	32	6	4.5	15
Mocha	large	390	4	42	1	39	20	12	75
Mocha	regular	470	13	56	1	50	22	13	230
Mocha, whole milk	medium	270	8	38	0	33	9	5	150
Mocha, whole milk	large	400	10	67	0	57	10	6	210
Mocha, whole milk	regular	480	14	72	0	63	14	8	260
Whole milk iced latte	12 oz	190	9	17	0	17	9	5	150
Whole milk iced latte	16 oz	390	9	66	0	56	9	5	200

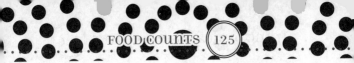

EINSTEIN BROS. continued

Item	Serving Size	Calories	Protein	Carb	Fiber	Sugar	Total Fat	Sat Fat	Sodium
FROZEN BLENDED DRINKS									
Café caramel	18 oz	620	8	100	0	66	9	2.5	140
Café caramel	24 oz	660	10	128	0	86	11	2.5	180
Café latte	18 oz	400	9	65	0	29	10	2.5	140
Café latte	24 oz	440	10	73	0	33	11	2.5	160
Café mocha	18 oz	510	7	102	0	64	8	2.5	160
Café mocha	24 oz	740	10	149	0	94	11	2.5	230
Cookies & cream	18 oz	680	11	101	1	89	36	25	200
Cookies & cream	24 oz	870	15	129	1	114	46	32	260
Strawberry	18 oz	450	6	75	3	64	19	14	95
Strawberry	24 oz	620	7	109	5	92	23	17	125
Vanilla	18 oz	600	10	92	0	89	31	23	150
Vanilla	24 oz	860	15	133	0	129	44	32	210
Wild berry	18 oz	290	6	66	5	50	0	0	105
Wild berry	24 oz	410	8	91	7	70	0.5	0	140
POURED DRINKS									
Fresh squeezed orange juice	10 oz	143	1	34	2	31	0	0	71
Harney & Sons tropical berry green tea	8 oz	0	0	0	0	0	0	0	0
Harney & Sons tropical green tea	8 oz	0	0	0	0	0	0	0	0
Lemonade	16 oz	200	2	48	1	48	0	0	0
Lemonade blackberry	16 oz	310	2	74	0	74	0	0	5
Spontaneitea	24 oz	100	0	25	0	25	0	0	0
SIDES									
Bagel croutons	1.2 oz	150	1	9	0	1	12	12	160
Bagel croutons	1 oz	100	2	15	1	1	4	4	220
Candied walnuts	1.5 oz	260	4	9	3	7	22	22	20
Cole slaw	5 oz	230	2	12	3	8	21	21	135
Fruit & yogurt parfait	as served	230	12	42	4	25	1.5	1.5	200
Fruit salad	5 oz	60	1	16	1	14	0	0	15
Fruit salad	large	140	2	36	3	30	0	0	35
Kettle Classic natural potato chips	1 oz	150	2	15	1	0	9	9	120
Potato salad	as served	160	1	13	1	1	12	12	360

EINSTEIN BROS. continued

Item	Serving Size	Calories	Protein	Carb	Fiber	Sugar	Total Fat	Sat Fat	Sodium
SOUPS									
Chicken noodle soup	cup	120	5	14	1	1	3.5	1	770
Corn crab chowder	cup	280	8	18	1	7	18	15	940
Italian wedding soup	cup	160	11	15	2	2	6	1.5	1060
Seafood minestrone	cup	130	8	16	2	4	4.5	1	1010
Turkey chili	cup	220	20	24	5	5	7	1.5	930
Vegetarian broccoli cheese	cup	290	14	16	2	6	20	10	990
SALADS									
Bros bistro salad	full	820	14	38	7	29	68	68	320
Bros bistro salad	half	410	7	19	3	15	34	34	160
Bros bistro salad w/ chicken	full	940	36	39	7	30	71	71	810
Bros bistro salad w/ chicken	half	480	19	19	3	15	36	36	440
Caesar salad	full	690	18	18	4	4	63	63	1730
Caesar salad	half	280	6	7	2	2	27	27	680
Caesar salad w/ chicken	full	820	42	20	4	4	66	66	2290
Caesar salad w/ chicken	half	350	18	8	2	2	28	28	960
Chicken chipotle salad	full	710	34	54	10	15	41	41	1960
Chicken chipotle salad	half	360	18	27	5	7	21	21	970
Chipotle salad	full	590	13	53	10	14	38	38	1470
Chipotle salad	half	290	6	26	5	7	18	18	730
SALAD DRESSINGS									
Caesar dressing	2 tbsp	150	1	1	0	1	16	16	350
Chile lime dressing	2 tbsp	60	1	5	0	3	3.5	3.5	650
Raspberry vinaigrette dressing	2 tbsp	160	0	8	0	8	14	14	0
BREAKFAST SANDWICHES & WRAPS									
Bacon & spinach panini	each	860	27	66	6	5	51	51	1610
Egg Way w/ bacon	each	580	33	59	2	8	24	24	1030
Egg Way w/ black forest ham	each	570	37	62	2	7	21	21	1270
Egg Way w/ sausage	each	600	38	63	2	8	24	24	1020
Egg Way, original	each	530	30	62	2	7	20	20	840
Egg Way, spinach mushroom & swiss omelette	each	540	29	65	3	8	20	20	860

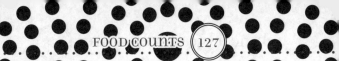

EINSTEIN BROS. continued

Item	Serving Size	Calories	Protein	Carb	Fiber	Sugar	Total Fat	Sat Fat	Sodium
Santa Fe wrap	each	720	37	60	7	8	37	37	1290
Sausage ranchero panini	each	680	32	64	4	5	29	29	1360
Spicy Elmo wrap	each	720	34	56	6	6	41	41	1050
Vegetable breakfast panini	each	730	26	68	4	6	36	36	1300
SANDWICHES									
California chicken wrap	each	630	33	63	8	6	28	8	1170
Chipotle turkey wrap	each	730	34	70	9	11	37	12	1990
Club Mex on challah	each	750	36	46	2	8	49	49	1530
Deli bacon	each	830	39	52	4	10	52	52	1930
Deli chicken salad	each	460	28	47	4	7	18	18	890
Deli ham	each	520	26	48	4	7	26	26	1550
Deli pastrami	each	630	34	53	5	8	33	33	1860
Deli tuna salad	each	440	29	50	4	7	15	15	920
Deli turkey & swiss	each	690	36	59	4	7	41	41	1510
Grilled chicken, bacon & swiss	each	750	40	45	2	7	46	46	1220
Ham deli melt	each	510	36	62	3	7	16	16	1700
Italian chicken panini	each	800	35	66	5	3	40	12	2450
Lox & bagels	each	500	24	62	3	11	21	11	950
Pastrami deli melt	each	540	38	64	3	7	17	17	1690
Rachel	regular	910	36	51	2	15	64	64	2210
Rachel	overstuffed	1030	54	53	2	15	68	68	3320
Reuben	regular	650	34	47	3	9	38	38	2360
Reuben	overstuffed	760	51	49	3	10	42	42	3380
Roasted turkey & swiss	each	690	35	49	4	7	41	41	1460
Tasty Turkey on Asiago bagel	each	580	37	69	3	9	20	20	1500
Tuna salad deli melt	each	590	38	64	3	7	23	23	1140
Turkey club panini	each	790	34	66	6	5	41	11	2200
Turkey deli melt	each	510	38	62	3	7	15	15	1430
Turkey rachel	regular	870	38	49	1	14	62	62	1860
Turkey rachel	each	1100	59	54	2	15	74	74	3400
Turkey reuben	regular	610	36	45	3	8	36	36	2040
Turkey reuben	overstuffed	680	54	45	3	8	37	37	2740
Veg Out on sesame seed bagel	each	440	17	66	4	9	14	7	760

EINSTEIN BROS. continued

Item	Serving Size	Calories	Protein	Carb	Fiber	Sugar	Total Fat	Sat Fat	Sodium
Veggie deli melt	each	640	24	76	5	12	29	29	1350

CONDIMENTS & SPREADS

Item	Serving Size	Calories	Protein	Carb	Fiber	Sugar	Total Fat	Sat Fat	Sodium
Ancho lime salsa	1 oz	15	0	2	0	1	0.5	0	270
Ancho mayo	1.5 oz	310	0	1	0	1	34	5	240
Butter blend	1 oz	170	0	0	0	0	18	5	220
Creamy mustard spread	1.5 oz	270	0	1	0	1	29	4.5	220
Deli mustard	1 tsp	5	0	0	0	0	0	0	65
Feta pinenut spread	1 oz	70	4	2	0	0	5	3.5	190
Honey butter	1 tbsp	170	0	0	0	0	18	5	220
Hummus	1 oz	70	4	6	4	0	3	0	150
Peanut butter, creamy	2 oz	330	14	12	4	5	28	6	260
Roasted garlic horseradish spread	2 tbsp	15	0	4	1	1	0	0	340
Spicy roasted tomato spread	2 tbsp	140	0	3	1	1	14	2	240
Whole kosher pickle	1	5	0	1	1	0	0	0	650
Yellow mustard	1 tbsp	0	0	0	0	0	0	0	80

BAGEL DOGS

Item	Serving Size	Calories	Protein	Carb	Fiber	Sugar	Total Fat	Sat Fat	Sodium
Original Asiago bagel dog	each	490	22	56	2	7	21	8	1230
Original Asiago bagel dog w/ cheese	each	560	26	56	2	7	27	12	1350
Original bagel dog	each	470	20	56	2	7	20	7	1190
Original bagel dog w/ cheese	each	550	25	56	2	7	26	11	1310

PIZZA BAGELS

Item	Serving Size	Calories	Protein	Carb	Fiber	Sugar	Total Fat	Sat Fat	Sodium
Cheese pizza bagel	each	420	23	63	3	7	12	7	980
Cheesy garlic and herb pizza bagel	each	500	24	65	2	7	19	12	1010
Pepperonio pizza bagel	each	470	24	63	3	7	16	8	1120
Spinach and mushroom pizza bagel	each	580	26	70	4	8	25	13	1250

DESSERTS

Item	Serving Size	Calories	Protein	Carb	Fiber	Sugar	Total Fat	Sat Fat	Sodium
Blueberry muffin	each	480	6	65	2	36	22	4.5	480
Chocolate chip coffee cake	each	760	6	110	2	58	34	13	270
Chocolate mudslide cookie	each	320	4	46	1	38	17	9	75

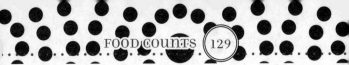

EINSTEIN BROS. continued

Item	Serving Size	Calories	Protein	Carb	Fiber	Sugar	Total Fat	Sat Fat	Sodium
Cinnamon stix	each	370	5	41	2	18	21	10	120
Cinnamon walnut strudel	each	630	9	56	4	20	42	17	360
Fudge brownie	each	510	6	74	2	62	25	13	115
Heavenly chocolate chunk cookie	each	360	4	48	2	29	18	9	290
Iced sugar cookie	each	480	4	76	1	46	15	6	26
Lemon pound cake	each	440	7	69	1	47	16	8	390
Marshmallow crispy treat	each	220	3	48	0	20	3.5	1	60
Mini Chocolate Mudslide cookie	each	160	2	23	1	19	8	4.5	40
Mini Heavenly chocolate chunk cookie	each	180	2	24	1	14	9	4.5	150
Mini iced sugar cookie	each	230	2	39	1	24	7	3	130
Mini oatmeal raisin cookie	each	160	2	27	1	16	5	2.5	160
Mixed berry coffee cake	each	710	5	110	2	59	29	10	270
Oatmeal raisin cookie	each	320	5	54	2	31	11	5	310
Strawberry white chocolate muffin	each	550	7	78	1	49	25	7	510

FAZOLI'S

Item	Serving Size	Calories	Protein	Carb	Fiber	Sugar	Total Fat	Sat Fat	Sodium
ENTRÉES									
Baked spaghetti	as served	640	29	80	7	13	22	12	1340
Baked spaghetti w/ meatballs	as served	890	41	86	7	13	39	20	204
Cheesy baked ziti	as served	670	34	71	7	12	27	15	1630
Chicken broccoli penne	as served	900	52	76	6	11	40	23	2360
Chicken carbonara	as served	790	43	87	4	9	26	13	1840
Chicken Parmigano	as served	920	51	106	8	15	32	14	2420
Classic Sampler Platter	as served	890	39	122	9	16	25	11	2270
Fettuccine w/ Alfredo	as served	800	26	108	5	11	26	15	1480
Fettuccine w/ meat sauce	as served	680	28	113	10	17	12	3.5	1640
Fettuccine w/ marinara	as served	560	19	111	9	17	2.5	0	970

FAZOLI'S continued

Item	Serving Size	Calories	Protein	Carb	Fiber	Sugar	Total Fat	Sat Fat	Sodium
Penne w/ Alfredo	as served	800	26	108	5	11	26	15	1480
Penne w/ creamy basil chicken	as served	970	52	73	4	9	51	24	2430
Penne w/ marinara	as served	560	19	111	9	17	2.5	0	970
Penne w/ meat sauce	as served	680	28	113	10	17	12	3.5	1640
Ravioli w/ marinara	as served	490	21	69	7	13	15	8	1080
Ravioli w/ meat sauce	as served	570	27	70	8	12	21	10	1530
Rigatoni Romano	as served	880	44	76	7	12	44	20	2460
Spaghetti w/ Alfredo	as served	800	26	108	5	11	26	15	1480
Spaghetti w/ marinara	as served	560	19	111	9	17	2.5	0	970
Spaghetti w/ meat sauce	as served	680	28	113	10	17	12	3.5	1640
Tortellini & sun-dried tomato rustico	as served	850	30	81	6	9	46	15	1380
Tortellini robusto	as served	1000	59	79	5	9	49	27	2560
Twice baked lasagne	as served	700	41	47	6	11	39	20	2420
Ultimate Sampler Platter	as served	1150	50	166	12	21	29	13	2810
PASTA TOPPINGS									
Broccoli	1 serving	25	3	5	3	1	0	0	10
Broccoli & fire-roasted tomatoes	1 serving	35	1	5	2	3	0	0	85
Grilled chicken	1 serving	100	18	1	0	1	2.5	0	570
Italian sausage	1 serving	200	10	3	0	1	16	5	680
Meatballs	1 serving	250	13	6	1	1	18	8	700
PIZZA									
Cheese	1 slice	290	14	32	2	2	12	6	730
Four Meatza	1 slice	330	16	33	2	2	14	6	880
Margherita	1 slice	330	14	33	2	3	15	6	710
Pepperoni	1 slice	300	14	32	2	2	13	6	810
Supremo	1 slice	320	15	33	2	3	14	6	870
OVEN-BAKED SUBMARINOS®									
Club Italiano	each	780	39	68	3	8	36	10	2800
Fazoli's Original	each	880	34	68	3	7	50	14	2890
Ham & swiss Supremo	each	690	33	68	3	9	31	8	2390

FAZOLI'S continued

Item	Serving Size	Calories	Protein	Carb	Fiber	Sugar	Total Fat	Sat Fat	Sodium
Smoked turkey basil	each	750	36	68	3	5	37	10	2550
Ultimate Meatball Smasher	each	1070	40	76	4	7	65	22	2970
SIDES & SALADS									
Breadstick, garlic	each	150	3	20	1	1	7	1.5	290
Breadstick, plain	each	100	3	2	0	1	2	0	160
Chicken & pasta Caesar	as served	440	35	37	3	8	13	5	1680
Cranberry & walnut chicken	as served	340	31	25	4	18	12	2	910
Crispy chicken BLT	as served	410	31	29	4	4	19	6	1390
Grilled chicken artichoke	as served	210	30	10	3	4	3.5	2	960
Side Caesar salad	as served	40	4	4	2	1	2	1	7
Side garden salad	as served	30	2	6	2	4	0	0	20
Side pasta salad	as served	300	8	38	1	7	12	3.5	970
DRESSINGS									
Caesar	1.5 oz	230	1	1	0	0	25	4	350
Creamy Parmesan peppercorn ranch	1.5 oz	230	1	2	0	2	24	4	380
Croutons	1 pack	70	2	8	0	0	3	0	100
Fat free Italian	1.5 oz	25	0	6	0	3	0	0	390
Honey French	1.5 oz	220	0	14	0	13	18	3	310
House Italian	1.5 oz	160	0	7	0	7	14	2	760
Lemon basil	1.5 oz	110	0	5	0	3	11	1.5	380
Lite ranch	1.5 oz	120	1	2	0	1	12	2	350
Ranch	1.5 oz	220	1	2	0	2	24	4	420
Red wine vinaigrette	1.5 oz	110	0		0	2	10	1.5	410
KIDS' MEALS									
Cheese pizza	as served	290	14	32	2	2	12	6	730
Fettuccine Alfredo	as served	290	8	42	2	4	8	4.5	470
Meat lasagne	as served	260	14	21	3	4	13	6	910
Pepperoni pizza	as served	300	14	32	2	2	13	6	810
Ravioli w/ marinara sauce	as served	250	10	35	3	6	7	4	540
Ravioli w/ meat sauce	as served	290	14	35	4	6	10	5	770

FAZOLI'S continued

Item	Serving Size	Calories	Protein	Carb	Fiber	Sugar	Total Fat	Sat Fat	Sodium
Spaghetti w/ marinara sauce	as served	220	7	43	3	6	1	0	330
Spaghetti w/ meat sauce	as served	260	10	44	4	6	4	1	560
Spaghetti w/ meatballs	as served	300	12	45	3	6	7	2.5	570

DRINKS & DESSERTS

Item	Serving Size	Calories	Protein	Carb	Fiber	Sugar	Total Fat	Sat Fat	Sodium
Chocolate chunk cookie	1 serving	510	5	68	3	39	26	15	350
Chocolate layer cake	1 serving	700	7	87	4	63	38	17	550
Italian lemon ice	regular	170	0	46	0	46	0	0	15
Italian lemon ice	large	250	0	65	0	65	0	0	20
Italian lemon ice w/ strawberry	large	270	0	70	0	70	0	0	55
NY style cheesecake w/ strawberry topping	1 serving	630	8	49	1	32	45	26	630
Turtle cheesecake	1 serving	590	7	56	2	34	37	17	330

FIVE GUYS

Item	Serving Size	Calories	Protein	Carb	Fiber	Sugar	Total Fat	Sat Fat	Sodium

BURGERS, SANDWICHES, & DOGS

Item	Serving Size	Calories	Protein	Carb	Fiber	Sugar	Total Fat	Sat Fat	Sodium
Bacon burger	each	279	43	39	2	8	50	22.5	690
Bacon cheese dog	each	200	26	40.5	2	8.5	48	22	1700
Bacon cheeseburger	each	317	51	40	2	9	62	29.5	1310
Bacon dog	each	181	22	40	2	8	42	18.5	1390
Cheese dog	each	186	22	40.5	2	8.5	41	19	1440
Cheeseburger	each	303	47	40	2	9	55	26.5	1050
Grilled cheese	each	110	11	41	2.5	10	26	9	715
Hamburger	each	265	39	39	2	8	43	19.5	430
Hot dog	each	167	18	40	2	8	35	15.5	1130
Little bacon burger	each	185	27	39	2	8	3	14.5	640
Little bacon cheeseburger	each	204	31	39.5	2	8.5	39	18	950
Little cheeseburger	each	190	27	39.5	2	8.5	2	15	690
Little hamburger	each	171	23	39	2	8	26	11.5	380
Veggie sandwich	each	209	16	60	2	14	15	6	1040

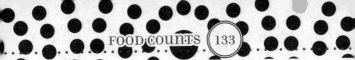

FIVE GUYS continued

Item	Serving Size	Calories	Protein	Carb	Fiber	Sugar	Total Fat	Sat Fat	Sodium
SIDES AND TOPPINGS									
Bacon	topping	79	4	0	0	0	7	3	260
Cheese	topping	74	4	1	0	1	6	3.5	310
Fries	regular	244	10	78	6	2	30	6	90
Fries	large	454	24	184	14	5	71	14	213

FRIENDLY'S

Item	Serving Size	Calories	Protein	Carb	Fiber	Sugar	Total Fat	Sat Fat	Sodium
MUNCHIES & STARTERS									
Chicken quesadilla	as served	570	35	29	3	29	35	18	1340
Jumbo Fronions	as served	1430	14	140	7	31	90	13	2970
Kickin™ Buffalo chicken strips	as served	1090	35	39	4	5	88	21	2740
Loaded waffle fries	as served	1650	31	123	9	123	112	28	4720
Mini mozzarella cheesesticks	as served	680	23	55	3	55	40	14	1870
CREATE YOUR OWN MUNCHIE MANIA™									
Cheese quesadilla	as served	530	20	31	3	5	36	16	940
Cheeseburger sliders	as served	500	20	57	6	18	21	7	1440
Chicken quesadilla	as served	640	35	32	3	5	40	17	1410
Chicken sliders	as served	740	23	69	7	15	42	9	1210
Jumbo Fronions	as served	700	6	63	3	12	47	7	1300
Loaded waffle fries	as served	920	17	67	4	4	64	15	2510
Mini mozzarella cheesesticks	as served	350	13	30	2	3	20	7	1010
Waffle fries	as served	570	6	71	4	13	29	4	1840
SUPERMELTS™ SANDWICHES									
Bruschetta mozzarella	each	1140	57	105	7	6	54	17	1870
Cheddar Jack chicken	each	1070	56	98	6	5	49	18	2270
Grilled chicken pesto	each	1360	59	98	6	7	82	26	2060
Honey BBQ chicken	each	1400	49	134	8	23	75	22	2160
Kickin™ Buffalo chicken	each	1430	45	118	7	7	86	25	2520
Reuben	each	1130	54	105	6	10	56	18	2910
Steak 'n' mushroom	each	1150	44	108	7	9	61	19	2120

FRIENDLY'S continued

Item	Serving Size	Calories	Protein	Carb	Fiber	Sugar	Total Fat	Sat Fat	Sodium
Tuna	each	1140	39	98	7	6	66	15	1700
Turkey club	each	990	44	102	7	9	46	13	2220
QUESADILLAS									
Chicken	each	1330	29	97	4	10	82	41	3350
Chicken Fajita	each	1540	74	106	7	13	91	42	3870
ENTRÉE SALADS W/O DRESSING									
Apple walnut chicken	each	390	38	22	5	9	18	7	1140
Asian chicken	each	490	36	41	6	21	20	3	1200
Chipotle chicken	each	550	37	8	8	7	22	3	1440
Crispy chicken	each	630	35	38	6	5	38	10	820
Kickin™ Buffalo chicken	each	710	29	42	7	5	47	9	1370
Steak & bleu cheese	each	640	44	41	8	9	34	11	1240
SIDE SALADS									
Side Caesar	each	410	9	15	1	5	36	7	640
Side garden salad w/o dressing	each	60	2	10	2	2	1	0	110
SALAD DRESSINGS									
Balsamic viniagrette	1 serving	180	0	5	0	9	15	2	1230
Bleu cheese	1 serving	470	6	2	0	3	48	11	720
Honey mustard	1 serving	360	0	12	0	18	30	5	420
Italian	1 serving	410	0	3	0	6	42	0	690
LF Dijon vinaigrette	1 serving	110	0	11	0	21	3	0	1560
Lite peppercorn parmesan	1 serving	230	3	2	0	3	21	5	630
Ranch	1 serving	330	3	8	0	3	33	6	750
Salsa ranch	1 serving	170	2	2	1	3	17	3	620
Sesame oriental	1 serving	270	0	18	0	30	14	2	960
Thousand Island	1 serving	390	0	2	0	12	36	6	840
SOUPS									
Broccoli cheddar	1 cup	200	7	14	1	3	13	7	780
Broccoli cheddar	1 bowl	390	13	28	2	6	25	14	1560
Chili	1 cup	270	14	18	3	3	16	6	910
Chili	1 bowl	540	27	36	7	5	33	12	1820
Chuncky chicken noodle	1 cup	280	20	31	2	4	10	3	1970

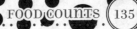

FRIENDLY'S continued

Item	Serving Size	Calories	Protein	Carb	Fiber	Sugar	Total Fat	Sat Fat	Sodium
Chunky chicken noodle	1 bowl	560	40	62	4	8	18	6	3940
Homestyle clam chowder	1 cup	270	11	17	1	3	18	10	890
Homestyle clam chowder	1 bowl	540	21	34	2	6	36	20	1790
Minestrone	1 cup	90	4	15	2	2	1	0	620
Minestrone	1 bowl	170	7	31	5	5	3	0	1230
WRAPS & SANDWICHES									
Buffalo chicken	each	1510	42	123	9	6	94	19	2640
Crispy chicken	each	1140	31	132	10	14	54	8	1610
Crispy chicken Caesar	each	1500	43	123	9	7	94	18	2300
Grilled chicken deluxe	each	1000	43	108	8	15	45	9	1810
BIG BEEF® BURGERS									
All American w/o cheese	each	1190	43	103	8	12	68	19	1170
BBQ Fronion	each	1560	55	134	8	21	91	30	2020
Mushroom Swiss bacon	each	1570	61	109	7	15	100	33	2040
Soft pretzel bacon	each	1420	58	119	7	11	79	29	1360
The Vermonter	each	1420	89	102	7	4	87	32	1530
Ultimate bacon cheese	each	1400	55	103	7	11	86	29	2040
BIG BEEF® BURGERMELTS									
Big beef burger	each	390	29	0	0	0	30	12	110
Boca burger patty	each	180	20	8	5	0	7	2	410
Deluxe cheese	each	1180	44	83	7	5	75	25	1310
Grilled chicken breast	each	170	29	2	0	0	5	1	720
Swiss patty	each	1360	56	110	8	12	78	27	1220
Ultimate grilled cheese	each	1500	54	101	9	4	97	38	2090
Zesty questo	each	1380	53	117	7	8	79	26	2410
STEAK & SEAFOOD									
Clamboat basket	as served	1710	28	170	11	19	102	15	3340
Grilled flounder	as served	980	38	100	7	10	48	10	3070
New England fish 'n chips	as served	1150	25	106	9	15	70	10	2120
Shrimp basket	as served	1090	27	110	9	17	60	7	3290
Sirloin steak tips	as served	1140	77	92	13	28	51	19	3350
SIGNATURE CHICKEN ENTRÉES									
Chicken strips basket	5 strips	1030	37	93	8	9	58	8	1330

FRIENDLY'S continued

Item	Serving Size	Calories	Protein	Carb	Fiber	Sugar	Total Fat	Sat Fat	Sodium
Honey BBQ chicken strips	5 strips	1560	38	188	8	88	74	11	2240
Kickin' Buffalo chicken strips	5 strips	1530	40	97	8	10	109	13	2860
FRIENDLY'S SIDES									
Apple slices	as served	100	1	26	1	20	0	0	26
Applesauce	as served	110	0	27	0	25	0	0	27
Broccoli	as served	80	3	5	2	2	6	5	80
Cole slaw	as served	160	1	13	1	8	12	2	260
Corn	as served	160	4	20	9	9	7	3	70
Fries	as served	330	4	48	4	0	14	1	160
Mashed potatoes	as served	240	4	29	4	4	12	7	160
Mixed vegetables	as served	110	3	13	6	6	6	3	110
Rice	as served	210	3	41	2	2	3	0	900
Spanish rice	as served	330	7	41	7	2	15	6	1200
Waffle fries	as served	590	7	67	1	1	33	5	1430
FRIENDLY'S ORIGINALS									
Fishamajig	as served	970	30	99	7	5	51	14	1520
Frendly Frank	as served	750	15	73	5	5	44	13	1070
Friendly's BLT	as served	990	21	99	7	7	57	13	1110
Grilled cheese	as served	790	20	96	6	4	37	12	1280
Tuna roll	as served	920	28	73	6	5	57	10	1080
FOR GUESTS OVER 60									
Clamboat platter	as served	1380	21	136	10	17	84	12	2460
Fishamajig	as served	970	30	99	7	5	51	14	1520
Friendly's big beef burger	as served	1190	39	55	4	12	54	18	1210
Grilled chicken deluxe	as served	1000	43	108	8	15	45	9	1810
Happy Ending sundae	as served	330	5	40	1	30	17	11	110
Tuna roll	as served	920	28	73	6	5	57	10	1080
Turkey club Supermelt™	as served	990	45	53	3	10	35	14	2290
SUNDAE CREATIONS									
Butterfinger sundae	as served	830	9	117	2	81	36	23	370
Caramel cone crunch	as served	690	10	91	3	54	27	13	280

FRIENDLY'S continued

Item	Serving Size	Calories	Protein	Carb	Fiber	Sugar	Total Fat	Sat Fat	Sodium
Caramel fudge brownie	as served	1410	19	186	2	124	118	64	620
Chocolate Lava cake	as served	820	10	137	3	86	52	32	580
Forbidden Fudge brownie	as served	940	13	131	4	85	41	51	340
Giant crowd pleaser	as served	2480	41	317	4	233	121	65	930
Hunka Chunka PB fudge	as served	1700	36	157	14	103	56	24	1060
Jim Dandy w/ pineapple	as served	1100	14	158	1	124	47	27	270
Jim Dandy w/ strawberry	as served	1090	14	156	2	121	47	27	270
Kit Kat sundae	as served	740	10	91	1	65	37	25	210
Mint chocolate chip Lava	as served	1240	16	175	7	118	66	40	670
Mint cookie crunch	as served	660	11	81	1	56	33	19	270
Mocha Java Lava	as served	1230	19	171	3	109	104	33	710
Nuts over caramel	as served	1370	21	197	5	114	53	34	970
Reese's peanut butter cup	5-scoop	1190	21	123	7	86	70	62	460
Reese's peanut butter cup	3-scoop	890	17	90	7	59	52	50	380
Reese's pieces sundae	5-scoop	1330	23	152	4	112	71	38	460
Reese's pieces sundae	3-scoop	930	18	95	4	67	53	26	360
Royal banana Split	as served	880	10	132	2	102	35	20	200
Strawberry shortcake	as served	580	8	79	2	63	27	16	190
Sweet cinnamon roll	as served	910	11	141	1	82	32	20	540
Ultimate cookies & cream	as served	690	11	86	1	59	33	20	330
FRIBBLES									
Chocolate	as served	590	19	94	1	78	17	11	420
Coffee	as served	630	16	102	0	85	19	12	360
Strawberry	as served	630	16	103	0	86	19	12	460
Vanilla	as served	620	16	100	0	88	19	12	360
DOUBLE THICK MILKSHAKE									
Chocolate	each	700	21	85	1	73	32	21	300
Coffee	each	770	15	107	0	89	32	18	270

FRIENDLY'S continued

Item	Serving Size	Calories	Protein	Carb	Fiber	Sugar	Total Fat	Sat Fat	Sodium
Cookie Jar	each	1050	21	141	2	100	26	150	430
Make Your Own Malt	each	90	2	15	0	10	2	1	100
Mint chocolate chip	each	860	18	114	2	99	37	24	270
Oreo mocha crunch	each	1090	19	146	3	117	49	32	450
Strawberry	each	740	16	110	0	93	27	16	390
Vanilla	each	770	15	106	0	92	32	21	270

SMOOTHIES

Item	Serving Size	Calories	Protein	Carb	Fiber	Sugar	Total Fat	Sat Fat	Sodium
Banana	each	520	17	104	1	71	4	2	280
Pineapple	each	590	16	122	1	91	4	2	290
Strawberry	each	520	17	105	2	76	4	2	290
Strawberry banana	each	520	17	105	2	73	4	2	290

FOUNTAIN BEVERAGES

Item	Serving Size	Calories	Protein	Carb	Fiber	Sugar	Total Fat	Sat Fat	Sodium
Barq's float	each	590	6	98	0	89	21	14	150
Orange slammer	each	600	3	138	0	115	4	3	80
Watermelon slammer	each	450	3	100	0	76	4	3	80

FRIEND-Z

Item	Serving Size	Calories	Protein	Carb	Fiber	Sugar	Total Fat	Sat Fat	Sodium
Heath	each	680	9	88	0	78	34	19	410
M&M'S	each	560	10	80	2	70	23	52	260
Oreo	each	580	9	84	2	62	23	12	470
Reese's peanut butter cup	each	860	20	96	4	71	45	18	520

GODFATHER'S PIZZA

Item	Serving Size	Calories	Protein	Carb	Fiber	Sugar	Total Fat	Sat Fat	Sodium
ORIGINAL CRUST PIZZAS									
All meat combo	1/4 mini	220	12	21	1	2	9	3.5	470
All meat combo	1/6 small	240	18	32	2	2	14	6	760
All meat combo	1/8 medium	370	20	35	2	3	15	6	840
All meat combo	1/10 large	410	22	37	2	3	17	7	920
All meat combo	1/12 jumbo	500	27	46	3	3	21	9	1140
Bacon cheeseburger	1/4 mini	210	11	21	1	2	9	4.5	540
Bacon cheeseburger	1/6 small	320	17	32	2	2	14	7	700
Bacon cheeseburger	1/8 medium	330	16	35	2	3	13	6	810
Bacon cheeseburger	1/10 large	390	21	37	2	3	17	8	890

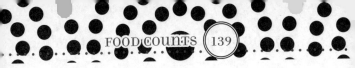

GODFATHER'S PIZZA continued

Item	Serving Size	Calories	Protein	Carb	Fiber	Sugar	Total Fat	Sat Fat	Sodium
Bacon cheeseburger	1/12 jumbo	480	25	45	3	4	21	10	1140
Cheese	1/4 mini	150	7	20	1	1	4	2	250
Cheese	1/6 small	240	11	31	1	2	7	3	420
Cheese	1/8 medium	260	12	34	2	2	7	3	470
Cheese	1/10 large	290	14	36	2	2	9	4	530
Cheese	1/12 jumbo	350	17	44	2	3	10	5	640
Combo	1/4 mini	200	10	21	2	2	8	3	500
Combo	1/6 small	320	15	33	2	3	13	5	780
Combo	1/8 medium	350	17	36	2	3	14	6	890
Combo	1/10 large	390	19	38	3	3	16	7	970
Combo	1/12 jumbo	480	24	47	3	4	20	8	1200
Hawaiian	1/4 mini	160	7	22	1	4	4	2	270
Hawaiian	1/6 small	240	11	32	2	3	7	3	430
Hawaiian	1/8 medium	270	13	36	2	4	7	3	530
Hawaiian	1/10 large	300	15	37	2	4	9	4	600
Hawaiian	1/12 jumbo	370	18	46	2	5	11	5	740
Hot Stuff	1/4 mini	210	10	21	1	2	9	3.5	490
Hot Stuff	1/6 small	330	15	32	2	3	14	6	810
Hot Stuff	1/8 medium	360	17	35	2	3	15	6	870
Hot Stuff	1/10 large	400	19	37	2	3	18	7	960
Hot Stuff	1/12 jumbo	490	23	46	3	4	22	9	1190
Humble	1/4 mini	220	10	21	1	2	11	4	430
Humble	1/6 small	340	15	32	2	3	16	6	680
Humble	1/8 medium	360	16	35	2	3	16	6	780
Humble	1/10 large	410	19	37	2	3	19	8	900
Humble	1/12 jumbo	510	23	46	3	4	24	9	1110
Pepperoni	1/4 mini	160	7	20	1	1	5	2	310
Pepperoni	1/6 small	270	12	31	2	2	9	4	530
Pepperoni	1/8 medium	290	13	34	2	2	10	5	580
Pepperoni	1/10 large	330	15	36	2	2	12	5	650
Pepperoni	1/12 jumbo	400	19	44	2	3	15	6	800
Super combo	1/4 mini	220	11	22	2	2	9	4	520
Super combo	1/6 small	330	17	33	2	3	14	6	850
Super combo	1/8 medium	350	18	36	2	3	14	8	820
Super combo	1/10 large	430	22	39	3	4	19	9	1060
Super combo	1/12 jumbo	520	27	48	4	4	23	10	1310

GODFATHER'S PIZZA continued

Item	Serving Size	Calories	Protein	Carb	Fiber	Sugar	Total Fat	Sat Fat	Sodium
Super Hawaiian	1/4 of mini	170	9	21	1	3	5	2	270
Super Hawaiian	1/6 small	60	13	32	2	3	8	3.5	430
Super Hawaiian	1/8 medium	290	15	36	2	4	9	4	530
Super Hawaiian	1/10 large	330	17	38	2	4	11	4.5	600
Super Hawaiian	1/12 jumbo	410	21	47	2	6	13	6	740
Super taco	1/4 mini	230	11	22	2	2	10	5	520
Super taco	1/6 small	340	17	33	2	3	15	8	720
Super taco	1/8 medium	390	19	36	3	4	18	9	880
Super taco	1/10 large	450	22	39	3	4	22	12	980
Super taco	1/12 jumbo	530	26	48	3	5	26	13	1190
Taco	1/4 mini	210	11	22	2	2	9	4	490
Taco	1/6 small	320	16	32	2	3	14	7	680
Taco	1/8 medium	350	18	36	2	4	16	8	830
Taco	1/10 large	420	22	38	3	4	19	10	930
Taco	1/12 jumbo	500	25	47	3	5	22	11	1120
Veggie	1/4 mini	160	7	21	1	2	4.5	2	300
Veggie	1/6 small	250	11	32	2	3	7	3	490
Veggie	1/8 medium	270	12	36	2	3	8	3.5	550
Veggie	1/10 large	300	14	38	2	3	9	4	610
Veggie	1/12 jumbo	370	17	46	3	4	11	5	750

GOLDEN CRUST PIZZAS

Item	Serving Size	Calories	Protein	Carb	Fiber	Sugar	Total Fat	Sat Fat	Sodium
All meat combo	1/6 small	310	16	26	2	2	14	6	710
All meat combo	1/8 medium	300	15	26	2	2	14	5	670
All meat combo	1/10 large	340	17	29	2	2	16	6	760
Bacon cheeseburger	1/6 small	290	15	26	2	2	14	6	650
Bacon cheeseburger	1/8 medium	270	13	26	2	2	12	5	640
Bacon cheeseburger	1/10 large	330	15	29	2	3	17	7	750
Cheese	1/6 small	200	9	25	1	2	6	2.5	360
Cheese	1/8 medium	220	10	25	1	2	8	3	380
Cheese	1/10 large	250	11	28	1	2	9	3.5	440
Combo	1/6 small	300	14	27	2	2	14	5	750
Combo	1/8 medium	290	13	27	2	2	13	5	680
Combo	1/10 large	330	15	30	2	2	15	6	740
Hawaiian	1/6 small	220	10	26	1	3	7	3	380
Hawaiian	1/8 medium	230	11	27	1	3	8	3.5	450
Hawaiian	1/10 large	260	12	30	1	4	9	3.5	510

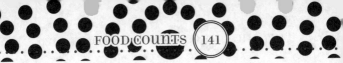
GODFATHER'S PIZZA continued

Item	Serving Size	Calories	Protein	Carb	Fiber	Sugar	Total Fat	Sat Fat	Sodium
Hot stuff	1/6 small	300	14	26	2	2	14	6	760
Hot stuff	1/8 medium	290	13	2	2	2	14	6	670
Hot stuff	1/10 large	330	15	29	2	2	16	6	780
Humble	1/6 small	320	13	26	2	2	16	6	630
Humble	1/8 medium	300	13	26	2	2	15	6	630
Humble	1/10 large	340	15	29	2	2	17	7	730
Pepperoni	1/6 small	240	11	25	1	2	10	4	480
Pepperoni	1/8 medium	250	11	26	2	2	11	4.5	500
Pepperoni	1/10 large	290	12	28	1	2	12	4.5	560
Super combo	1/6 small	300	15	27	2	3	14	8	780
Super combo	1/8 medium	320	16	28	1	2	15	8	760
Super combo	1/10 large	370	18	31	2	3	18	8	880
Super Hawaiian	1/6 small	240	11	27	1	3	9	3.5	380
Super Hawaiian	1/8 medium	250	12	27	2	3	9	3.5	450
Super Hawaiian	1/10 large	280	14	30	2	4	11	4	510
Super taco	1/6 small	290	14	27	2	3	14	7	650
Super taco	1/8 medium	330	15	28	1	3	17	10	670
Super taco	1/10 large	370	17	30	2	3	20	10	780
Taco	1/6 small	280	14	26	2	3	12	6	600
Taco	1/8 medium	300	15	27	2	3	14	8	630
Taco	1/10 large	350	17	30	2	3	17	8	740
Veggie	1/6 small	210	10	27	2	3	6	3	430
Veggie	1/8 medium	230	10	27	2	2	8	3	430
Veggie	1/10 large	260	11	30	2	3	10	3.5	500

MOZZA LOADED PIZZAS

Item	Serving Size	Calories	Protein	Carb	Fiber	Sugar	Total Fat	Sat Fat	Sodium
All meat combo	1/8 medium	350	17	27	2	2	18	7	800
All meat combo	1/10 large	390	20	30	2	2	21	8	890
Bacon cheeseburger	1/8 medium	320	15	27	2	2	17	7	770
Bacon cheeseburger	1/10 large	380	17	29	2	3	21	9	880
Cheese	1/8 medium	270	12	26	1	2	12	5	510
Cheese	1/10 large	300	13	29	1	2	14	6	560
Combo	1/8 medium	340	15	28	2	2	17	7	810
Combo	1/10 large	380	17	30	2	2	20	8	570
Hawaiian	1/8 medium	230	11	27	1	3	8	3	450
Hawaiian	1/10 large	320	14	31	1	4	14	6	640
Hot stuff	1/8 medium	340	15	27	2	2	18	7	800

GODFATHER'S PIZZA continued

Item	Serving Size	Calories	Protein	Carb	Fiber	Sugar	Total Fat	Sat Fat	Sodium
Hot stuff	1/10 large	360	16	28	2	3	21	8	940
Humble	1/8 medium	350	15	27	2	2	19	8	760
Humble	1/10 large	400	17	30	2	2	22	9	860
Pepperoni	1/8 medium	300	13	26	1	2	15	6	620
Pepperoni	1/10 large	340	14	29	1	2	17	7	690
Super combo	1/8 medium	370	18	28	2	2	20	9	880
Super combo	1/10 large	420	2	31	2	3	23	10	1010
Super Hawaiian	1/8 medium	300	14	28	1	3	13	6	580
Super Hawaiian	1/10 large	330	16	30	2	4	15	6	640
Super taco	1/8 medium	380	17	28	2	2	21	10	800
Super taco	1/10 large	430	20	31	2	3	25	12	910
Taco	1/8 medium	350	17	28	2	2	19	9	760
Taco	1/10 large	400	19	30	2	3	22	10	870
Veggie	1/8 medium	280	12	27	2	2	12	5	560
Veggie	1/10 large	310	13	30	2	3	14	6	630

THIN CRUST PIZZAS

Item	Serving Size	Calories	Protein	Carb	Fiber	Sugar	Total Fat	Sat Fat	Sodium
All meat combo	1/8 medium	270	14	18	1	1	15	5	520
All meat combo	1/10 large	300	16	19	1	1	17	6	610
Bacon cheeseburger	1/8 medium	260	12	18	1	1	14	6	500
Bacon cheeseburger	1/10 large	280	14	18	1	2	16	7	570
Cheese	1/8 medium	170	8	15	1	1	8	3	230
Cheese	1/10 large	210	9	17	1	1	10	3.5	270
Combo	1/8 medium	240	11	17	1	1	13	3	530
Combo	1/10 large	280	13	20	2	1	16	6	630
Hawaiian	1/8 medium	190	9	16	1	1	8	3	330
Hawaiian	1/10 large	230	11	21	1	4	10	3	380
Hot Stuff	1/8 medium	260	11	18	1	1	15	5	530
Hot Stuff	1/10 large	290	13	19	1	1	17	5	620
Humble	1/8 medium	260	11	16	1	1	15	5	480
Humble	1/10 large	300	13	19	1	1	18	6	570
Pepperoni	1/8 medium	210	9	15	1	1	11	4	350
Pepperoni	1/10 large	240	10	18	1	1	13	5	400
Super combo	1/8 medium	290	14	19	2	1	16	6	620
Super combo	1/10 large	330	17	20	2	2	19	6	730
Super Hawaiian	1/8 medium	220	11	19	1	2	10	3.5	330
Super Hawaiian	1/10 large	240	13	19	1	3	11	4	380

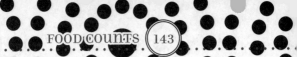

GODFATHER'S PIZZA continued

Item	Serving Size	Calories	Protein	Carb	Fiber	Sugar	Total Fat	Sat Fat	Sodium
Super taco	1/8 medium	300	13	19	1	2	18	8	530
Super taco	1/10 large	330	15	20	2	2	21	8	620
Taco	1/8 medium	260	13	16	1	2	15	7	480
Taco	1/10 large	300	15	19	2	2	18	7	580
Veggie	1/8 medium	180	8	16	1	1	8	3	280
Veggie	1/10 large	220	9	19	1	2	10	3.5	340

DESSERTS & SIDES

Item	Serving Size	Calories	Protein	Carb	Fiber	Sugar	Total Fat	Sat Fat	Sodium
Apple dessert, golden crust	1/6 alum pan	150	3	28	1	4	2.5	0.5	160
Apple dessert, golden crust	1/8 medium	200	4	38	1	6	4	1	220
Apple dessert, golden crust	1/10 large	230	5	42	1	6	4.5	1	240
Breadsticks	1 each	110	3	20	1	1	2	0	160
Breadsticks w/ cheese	1 each	140	5	20	1	1	4	1.5	220
Calzone, cheese	1 each	1660	81	200	9	11	51	24	2920
Calzone, combo	1 each	1450	63	199	10	12	40	16	2900
Calzone, pepperoni	1 each	1410	60	195	9	11	39	16	2540
Cheesesticks	1/6 alum pan	130	7	18	1	1	3.5	1.5	210
Cheesesticks	1/8 medium	200	8	24	1	1	7	2.5	300
Cheesesticks	1/10 large	220	9	26	1	1	8	3	340
Cherry dessert, golden crust	1/6 alum pan	150	3	28	1	1	2.5	0.5	160
Cherry dessert, golden crust	1/8 medium	210	4	39	1	2	4	1	210
Cherry dessert, golden crust	1/10 large	230	5	43	1	2	4.5	1	230
Cinnamon streusel, golden crust	1/6 alum pan	160	3	29	1	4	3	0.5	160
Cinnamon streusel, golden crust	1/8 medium	230	5	40	1	5	5	1	220
Cinnamon streusel, golden crust	1/10 large	260	5	45	1	6	6	1.5	250
Garlic toast	1 each	150	3	15	1	1	9	2	260
Garlic toast w/ cheese	1 each	210	7	16	1	1	12	3.5	360
Hot wings, breaded	1 each	45	3	1	0	0	3	1	90
Monkey bread, cinnamon	1 each	830	18	190	4	37	24	4.5	970
Monkey bread, Italian	1 each	690	19	105	4	5	23	4.5	970

GODFATHER'S PIZZA continued

Item	Serving Size	Calories	Protein	Carb	Fiber	Sugar	Total Fat	Sat Fat	Sodium
Potato wedges	16 oz	690	11	96	11	3	32	8	1440

GLUTEN-FREE MENU

Item	Serving Size	Calories	Protein	Carb	Fiber	Sugar	Total Fat	Sat Fat	Sodium
Gluten-free beef	1/6	170	7	18	1	2	7	3	500
Gluten-free cheese	1/6	140	5	18	1	2	4.5	2	380
Gluten-free classic combo	1/6	180	7	19	1	2	8	3	570
Gluten-free meat combo	1/6	190	9	18	1	2	8	3.5	570
Gluten-free pepperoni	1/6	170	6	18	1	2	7	3	480
Gluten-free sausage	1/6	170	7	18	1	2	6	2.5	510

HARDEE'S

Item	Serving Size	Calories	Protein	Carb	Fiber	Sugar	Total Fat	Sat Fat	Sodium
BREAKFAST									
Bacon, egg, & cheese biscuit	each	530	15	36	0	4	36	11	1390
Big Country breakfast platter, bacon	each	910	27	91	4	12	48	12	2210
Biscuit 'N' Gravy™	each	530	9	48	1	3	33	8	1510
Breaded pork chop biscuit	each	640	25	46	1	4	39	7	1270
Chicken fillet biscuit	each	620	24	47	1	3	37	8	1560
Cinnamon 'N' Raisin biscuit™	each	300	3	40	1	17	15	3	680
Country ham biscuit	each	440	14	36	0	3	26	6	1710
Country steak biscuit	each	590	13	43	1	4	40	10	1290
Frisco Breakfast Sandwich®	each	420	25	39	2	4	18	7	1250
Ham, egg, & cheese biscuit	each	540	23	36	0	4	33	10	1830
Jelly biscuit	each	520	5	44	0	10	34	7	1020
Loaded breakfast burrito	each	780	39	39	1	2	49	21	1700
Loaded omelet biscuit	each	610	20	36	0	4	42	14	1540
Low carb Breakfast Bowl®	each	620	36	6	2	2	50	21	1380
Made from Scratch biscuit™	each	370	5	35	0	3	23	5	890
Monster Biscuit™	each	770	29	37	0	4	55	18	2310
Pancakes (3)	one order	300	8	55	2	12	5	1	830

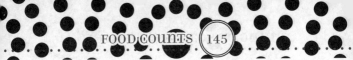

HARDEE'S continued

Item	Serving Size	Calories	Protein	Carb	Fiber	Sugar	Total Fat	Sat Fat	Sodium
Pork Chop 'N' Gravy biscuit	each	680	26	48	1	4	42	8	1400
Sausage and egg biscuit	each	590	16	36	0	4	42	11	1300
Sausage biscuit	each	530	11	36	0	4	38	10	1240
Smoked sausage biscuit	each	620	14	37	0	5	46	15	1680
Sunrise Croissant® w/ ham	each	400	21	27	1	4	23	10	1070
Texas toast breakfast sandwich, sausage	each	480	20	32	2	3	30	10	960
BREAKFAST SIDES									
Grits	as served	110	2	16	1	0	5	1	490
Hash Rounds	small	250	3	25	2	1	16	3.5	360
Hash Rounds	medium	390	3	36	4	0	26	4.5	490
Hash Rounds	large	530	5	49	5	0	35	6	670
THICKBURGERS® & SANDWICHES									
1/3 Lb bacon cheese burger	each	850	38	49	3	7	57	19	1650
1/3 Lb Cheeseburger Thickburger®	each	620	5	51	3	10	33	13	1580
1/3 Lb Frisco Thickburger®	each	930	44	42	2	6	64	2	1840
1/3 Lb Low carb Thickburger®	each	420	30	5	2	3	32	12	1010
1/3 Lb Mushroom & Swiss Thickburger®	each	650	39	47	3	5	36	14	1620
1/3 Lb Original Thickburger®	each	860	35	52	4	10	58	17	1630
2/3 Lb Double bacon cheese Thickburger®	each	1200	65	50	3	7	84	30	2450
2/3 Lb Double Thickburger®	each	1150	62	53	4	10	78	28	2410
2/3 Lb Monster Thickburger®	each	1320	70	46	2	6	95	36	3020
Big chicken fillet sandwich	each	710	33	62	5	6	38	7	1610
Big hot ham 'N' cheese	each	160	36	40	2	4	20	8	2040
Big roast beef	each	400	25	28	1	3	21	7	1180

HARDEE'S continued

Item	Serving Size	Calories	Protein	Carb	Fiber	Sugar	Total Fat	Sat Fat	Sodium
Charbroiled BBQ chicken sandwich	each	400	27	62	5	21	6	1	1370
Charbroiled chicken club sandwich	each	630	32	54	4	16	32	8	173
Double cheeseburger	each	530	27	34	1	8	32	6	1070
Fish Supreme sandwich	each	360	22	51	3	14	38	7	1310
Hand-breaded chicken tenders™	3 pieces	260	25	13	2	0	13	2.5	770
Hand-breaded chicken tenders™	5 pieces	440	41	21	3	0	21	4.5	1290
Hot Ham 'N' Cheese™	each	280	18	29	1	4	12	4	1090
Jumbo chili dog	each	400	16	25	1	6	26	9	1170
Kids Meal, cheeseburger	each	560	19	59	3	6	29	6	1260
Kids Meal, Chicken tenders	each	380	19	36	3	0	18	4	1050
Kids Meal, hamburger	each	520	16	59	3	6	25	6	1040
Little Thick cheeseburger	each	450	24	38	3	10	23	9	1180
Little Thickburger®	each	570	24	35	3	7	39	12	1140
Low carb charbroiled chicken club sandwich	each	360	24	14	1	8	23	7	1290
Regular roast beef sandwich	each	310	17	28	1	3	15	5	840
Small cheeseburger	each	350	16	32	1	6	19	4	730
Small hamburger	each	310	14	32	1	6	15	4	500
Spicy chicken sandwich	each	440	11	41	3	3	21	5	1140
The Six Dollar Thickburger®	each	930	46	57	4	15	59	21	1960

SIDES

Item	Serving Size	Calories	Protein	Carb	Fiber	Sugar	Total Fat	Sat Fat	Sodium
Beer battered onion rings	one side	410	3	45	3	5	24	4.5	470
Crispy curls	small	340	4	43	4	0	17	4	840
Crispy curls	medium	410	5	52	4	0	20	5	1020
Crispy curls	large	480	6	60	5	0	23	6	1190
Natural-cut French fries	kids'	200	2	28	2	0	9	2	450
Natural-cut French fries	small	320	4	45	3	0	14	3	710
Natural-cut French fries	medium	430	5	60	4	0	19	4	960
Natural-cut French fries	large	470	5	65	5	0	21	4	1640
Side salad, w/o dressing	each	120	7	7	2	4	7	5	160

HARDEE'S continued

Item	Serving Size	Calories	Protein	Carb	Fiber	Sugar	Total Fat	Sat Fat	Sodium
FRIED CHICKEN & SIDES									
Cole slaw	small	170	1	2	2	16	10	2	140
Fried chicken breast	each	370	29	29	0	0	15	4	1190
Fried chicken leg	each	170	13	15	0	0	7	2	570
Fried chicken thigh	each	330	19	3	0	0	15	4	1000
Fried chicken wing	each	200	10	23	0	0	8	2	740
Mashed potatoes	small	90	1	17	0	1	2	0	410
DESSERTS									
Apple turnover w/o topping	as served	270	3	35	1	11	13	3.5	260
Chocolate cake	as served	300	4	56	2	43	12	3	420
Chocolate chip cookie	each	290	4	44	0	26	11	5	280
Chocolate chip cookie, fresh baked	each	250	2	30	1	17	14	5	180
Hand-Scooped Ice Cream Malt™	as served	780	17	98	0	76	35	24	330
Hand-Scooped Ice Cream Shake™	as served	705	14	86	0	68	33	23	260
Peach cobbler	1 small	285	1	56	1	45	7	1	230
Single scoop ice cream	1 cone	285	6	37	0	26	13	8	140
Single scoop ice cream	1 bowl	235	5	27	0	22	13	8	85

IHOP

Item	Serving Size	Calories	Protein	Carb	Fiber	Sugar	Total Fat	Sat Fat	Sodium
HEARTY OMELETTES									
Avocado, bacon & cheese omelette	as served	840	49	17	5	3	65	26	1080
Bacon Temptation omelette	as served	980	62	17	2	5	75	30	1900
Big steak omelette	as served	120	69	54	8	9	82	29	2270
Chicken fajita omelette	as served	960	74	22	4	8	65	26	1850
Colorado omelette	as served	1120	71	24	3	10	82	33	2240
Corned beef hash & cheese omelette	as served	990	57	30	4	4	72	31	1860
Country omelette	as served	1140	58	50	6	8	80	31	2060
Create Your Own Omelette, plain	as served	440	28	10	2	3	32	9	500
Create Your Own Omelette, plain w/ egg substitute	as served	140	23	2	0	0	4	0.5	320
w/ 2 bacon strips	2 strips	80	6	<1	0	0	6	2	300
w/ 2 pork sausage links	2 links	180	6	1	0	0	16	6	290
w/ American cheese	1 slice	160	8	2	0	1	13	8	690
w/ Cheddar cheese	1 slice	240	14	2	0	0	20	14	270
w/ diced ham	as served	30	5	1	0	1	1	0	320
w/ fresh spinach	as served	15	2	2	1	0	0	0	45
w/ green peppers & onions	as served	10	0	2	0	<1	0	0	0
w/ Jack & Cheddar cheese blend	1 slice	230	14	2	0	0	19	12	290
w/ mushrooms	as served	10	2	2	<1	<1	0	0	0
w/ oven-roasted tomatoes	as served	90	0	12	4	0	4	0	170
w/ Provolone cheese	1 slice	160	10	0	0	0	12	8	380
w/ Swiss cheese	1 slice	160	11	<1	0	0	13	8	100
w/ tomatoes	as served	10	<1	2	<1	1	0	0	0
Garden omelette	as served	840	45	18	4	6	66	26	890
Hearty ham & cheese omelette	as served	870	65	18	2	8	60	25	2270
International omelette	as served	740	48	19	3	7	53	23	1410
Spinach & mushroom omelette	as served	910	45	23	5	7	71	26	1580

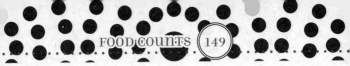

IHOP continued

Item	Serving Size	Calories	Protein	Carb	Fiber	Sugar	Total Fat	Sat Fat	Sodium
HEARTY OMELETTES SIDES									
Chocolate chip pancakes	3 each	550	15	85	6	25	19	8	1550
Cinnamon apple pancakes	3 each	510	14	86	5	28	13	4.5	1620
CINN-A-STACK™ pancakes	3 each	690	14	106	4	46	23	8	1700
Double Blueberry pancakes	3 each	640	14	117	9	50	13	4.5	1630
Harvest Grain 'N Nut® pancakes	3 each	700	18	71	8	17	39	10	1380
New York cheesecake pancakes	3 each	850	19	118	6	42	34	16	1830
Original buttermilk pancakes	3 each	490	13	69	4	13	18	8	1610
Seasonal fresh Fruit	as served	80	<1	21	2	16	0	0	0
Seasoned hash browns	as served	320	3	31	3	<1	20	3.5	590
Strawberry banana pancakes	3 each	600	15	109	8	34	13	4.5	1560
Strawberry pancakes	3 each	520	14	87	5	22	13	4.5	1560
SIMPLE & FIT OMELETTES									
SIMPLE & FIT spinach, mushroom & tomato omelette w/ fresh fruit	as served	330	28	30	5	19	12	5	690
SIMPLE & FIT Turkey Bacon omelette w/ fresh fruit	as served	420	36	24	2	17	21	10	730
SIMPLE & FIT Veggie omelette w/ fresh fruit	as served	320	21	40	8	19	10	1	420
BREAKFAST COMBINATIONS									
Big country breakfast	as served	1790	48	156	10	18	110	2	3910
Big two-egg breakfast	as served	880	28	80	6	9	50	1	1870
Biscuits & gravy combo w/ country gravy	as served	1420	39	99	5	7	95	0.5	3080
Biscuits & gravy combo w/ sausage gravy	as served	1530	41	105	5	8	103	0.5	3410
Breakfast Sampler	as served	1180	49	82	6	11	74	1	3160
Chicken fried chicken & eggs w/ country gravy	as served	1240	51	105	9	10	69	1.5	2950

IHOP continued

Item	Serving Size	Calories	Protein	Carb	Fiber	Sugar	Total Fat	Sat Fat	Sodium
Chicken fried chicken & eggs w/ sausage gravy	as served	1300	53	107	9	11	73	1.5	3120
Chorizo & eggs	as served	1400	55	111	8	17	82	1.5	3160
Classic Skillet	as served	1460	48	102	8	12	97	1.5	2740
Corned beef hash & eggs	as served	1110	51	91	6	15	61	2.5	2970
Country/chicken fried steak & eggs w/ country gravy	as served	1570	57	139	11	13	87	2	3710
Country/chicken fried steak & eggs w/ sausage gravy	as served	1680	60	145	11	14	95	2	4050
Eggs Benedict	as served	1020	43	80	6	8	57	0	3140
Huevos rancheros	as served	1110	50	83	11	3	65	0.5	1810
Loco Moco	as served	1190	61	108	1	2	56	1.5	1050
Machaca	as served	1270	54	60	6	7	90	1	2110
Migas	as served	1140	43	57	6	5	83	1	1870
Migas w/ chorizo	as served	1400	58	59	6	6	103	1	2240
Pigs in blankets	as served	980	30	95	6	18	54	1	2710
Pork chops & eggs	as served	1090	67	81	6	10	56	1	2370
Quick two-egg breakfast	as served	1080	30	105	7	20	61	1.5	1580
SIMPLE & FIT oatmeal	as served	290	7	58	4	30	4.5	0	25
SIMPLE & FIT two-egg breakfast	as served	350	25	48	7	19	8	0	710
Sirloin tips & eggs	as served	1350	69	99	8	25	76	1.5	3050
Smokehouse combo	as served	1340	47	84	6	11	91	1.5	3180
South-of-the-Border burrito	as served	1380	50	130	10	11	74	1	3330
Split Decision breakfast	as served	1170	46	80	6	16	75	1.5	2280
T-bone steak & eggs	as served	1250	86	74	4	13	6	2	2840
Thick-cut bone-in ham & eggs	as served	1170	70	88	6	15	61	1	4310
Top sirloin steak & eggs	as served	1090	82	73	4	13	53	1.5	2350
Weekday Breakfast Specials: French toast	as served	640	20	59	5	12	36	0.5	750

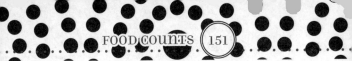

IHOP continued

Item	Serving Size	Calories	Protein	Carb	Fiber	Sugar	Total Fat	Sat Fat	Sodium
Weekday Breakfast Specials: Two eggs, hash browns & toast	as served	1080	30	105	7	20	61	1.5	1580
Weekday Breakfast Specials: Two eggs & two buttermilk pancakes	as served	560	25	49	3	9	31	0.5	1280
Weekday Breakfast Specials: Two-egg cheese omelette w/ two buttermilk pancakes	as served	780	36	52	4	10	49	1	1610

FRENCH TOAST, WAFFLES, & SWEET CREPES

Item	Serving Size	Calories	Protein	Carb	Fiber	Sugar	Total Fat	Sat Fat	Sodium
Belgian waffle combo	as served	640	23	50	2	11	39	18	770
W/ apple cinnamon compote w/ whipped topping	topping	140	0	32	1	28	2.5	2	135
W/ blueberry compote w/ whipped topping	topping	170	<1	37	2	29	2.5	2	80
W/ strawberry topping w/ whipped topping	topping	160	<1	36	2	17	2.5	2	20
Belgian waffle w/ butter	as served	420	8	47	2	11	23	14	580
Belgian waffle, plain	as served	360	8	47	2	11	15	8	520
Cheese blintzes	as served	1000	27	66	4	27	69	30	1260
W/ blueberry compote	topping	150	0	36	2	28	0	0	80
W/ cinnamon apple compote	topping	120	0	31	1	27	0	0	130
W/ strawberry preserves	topping	210	0	55	<1	51	0	0	10
W/ strawberry topping	topping	130	0	35	2	16	0	0	15
CINN-A-STACK™ French Toast	as served	1120	32	126	8	51	54	16	1190
Cinnamon swirl French toast combo	as served	1210	33	102	8	16	75	25	1370
Create Your Own Viva La French Toast Combo, blueberry	as served	1200	40	112	10	28	66	17	1510
Create Your Own Viva La French Toast Combo, cinnamon apple	as served	1180	40	109	10	28	66	17	1540

IHOP continued

Item	Serving Size	Calories	Protein	Carb	Fiber	Sugar	Total Fat	Sat Fat	Sodium
Create Your Own Viva La French Toast Combo, CINN-A-STACK™	as served	1300	40	121	9	39	73	19	1580
Create Your Own Viva La French Toast Combo, original	as served	1170	40	93	9	13	71	20	1530
Create Your Own Viva La French Toast Combo, strawberry	as served	1190	40	111	10	22	66	17	1480
Create Your Own Viva La French Toast Combo, strawberry banana	as served	1210	40	116	10	25	6	17	1480
Create Your Own Viva La French Toast Combo, whole wheat	as served	900	36	88	8	23	45	11	1290
German crepes	as served	830	15	71	5	23	54	15	790
International Crepe Passport, fresh fruit	as served	870	36	71	5	38	50	15	1010
International Crepe Passport, German	as served	930	35	40	3	12	69	23	1170
International Crepe Passport, Nutella	as served	1100	38	83	5	42	71	22	1200
International Crepe Passport, strawberry banana danish	as served	1000	35	68	4	30	67	26	1150
International Crepe Passport, Swedish	as served	1030	35	48	2	20	77	28	1180
Nutella crepes	as served	910	16	109	7	57	48	13	620
Original French toast	as served	920	31	88	8	18	50	15	1100
SIMPLE & FIT seasonal fresh fruit crepes	as served	590	12	84	7	43	24	4.5	430
SIMPLE & FIT whole wheat French toast combo	as served	490	33	56	5	23	15	4	930
Strawberry Banana Danish fruit crepes	as served	970	16	106	7	49	57	26	730
Strawberry Banana French toast	as served	1060	32	135	11	41	45	12	1050
Stuffed French toast	full order	900	18	120	4	45	39	17	740
Stuffed French toast	side order	450	9	60	2	23	19	9	370

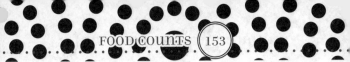

IHOP continued

Item	Serving Size	Calories	Protein	Carb	Fiber	Sugar	Total Fat	Sat Fat	Sodium
Stuffed French toast combo	as served	950	28	92	5	22	52	14	1150
Swedish Crepes	as served	930	15	78	5	31	61	20	790
PANCAKES									
Chocolate chip pancakes	4	720	20	112	8	32	24	10	2070
CINN-A-STACK™ pancakes	4	890	19	138	6	58	29	10	2260
Double blueberry pancakes	4	800	19	144	11	57	17	5	2150
Harvest Grain 'N Nut® pancakes	4	920	25	95	10	22	49	11	1810
w/ apple cinnamon compote w/ whipped topping	topping	140	0	32	1	28	2.5	2	135
w/ blueberry compote w/ whipped topping	topping	100	0	19	1	15	2.5	2	45
New York cheesecake pancakes	4	1100	26	152	8	53	44	21	2430
Original buttermilk pancakes	5	770	22	115	7	22	25	9	2640
Original buttermilk pancakes, short stack	3	490	13	69	4	13	18	8	1610
Pancake Platter	as served	490	13	69	4	13	18	8	1610
Pick-A-Pancake Combo, chocolate chip	as served	910	29	92	8	19	49	15	1810
Pick-A-Pancake Combo, cinnamon apple	as served	890	28	94	7	24	45	12	1850
Pick-A-Pancake Combo, CINN-A-STACK™	as served	1010	29	109	6	35	51	14	1920
Pick-A-Pancake Combo, double blueberry	as served	1020	29	124	10	44	45	12	1890
Pick-A-Pancake Combo, Harvest Grain 'N Nut®	as served	1020	31	81	9	12	64	16	120
Pick-A-Pancake Combo, New York cheesecake	as served	1130	32	119	8	32	59	20	2000
Pick-A-Pancake Combo, original	as served	880	28	80	6	9	50	15	1870
Pick-A-Pancake Combo, strawberry	as served	900	29	98	7	18	45	12	1820
Pick-A-Pancake Combo, strawberry banana	as served	970	29	114	9	27	45	12	1820

IHOP continued

Item	Serving Size	Calories	Protein	Carb	Fiber	Sugar	Total Fat	Sat Fat	Sodium
Rooty Tooty Fresh 'N Fruity®	as served	750	36	51	3	9	45	14	1810
w/ apple cinnamon compote w/ whipped topping	topping	90	0	17	<1	15	2.5	2	70
w/ blueberry compote w/ whipped topping	topping	170	<1	37	2	29	2.5	2	80
w/ strawberry topping w/ whipped topping	topping	90	0	19	<1	15	2.5	2	10
SIMPLE & FIT blueberry Harvest Grain 'N Nut® Combo	as served	560	25	64	8	21	23	3.5	1040
SIMPLE FIT Two x Two x Two	as served	400	25	48	3	10	12	2.5	1450
Strawberry banana pancakes	4	760	20	137	10	41	17	5	2070
Three eggs & pancakes	as served	810	37	73	4	13	42	15	1880
Three eggs & pancakes w/ hashbrowns	as served	1130	40	104	8	14	62	18	2480
Two x Two x Two	as served	560	25	49	3	9	31	11	1280
SAVORY CREPES									
Bacon & Cheddar stuffed crepes	as served	1130	54	43	2	13	82	37	1500
Chicken Florentine crepes	as served	880	53	47	5	16	54	21	1810
Garden stuffed crepes	as served	1040	39	50	5	16	76	27	142
TAKE TWO COMBOS									
1/2 double BLT sandwich	as served	390	12	21	2	3	28	6	1180
1/2 pot roast melt sandwich	as served	530	28	43	3	5	28	15	1580
1/2 Turkey sandwich	as served	290	18	15	4	2	18	4.5	117
Broccoli cheese soup	as served	340	12	19	2	6	23	14	1440
Chicken noodle soup	as served	170	12	18	1	3	5	1.5	1110
Chicken tortilla soup	as served	190	9	23	3	3	7	2	1450
Dressing, balsamic vinaigrette	as served	260	0	5	0	5	26	3.5	240

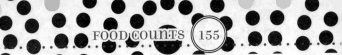

IHOP continued

Item	Serving Size	Calories	Protein	Carb	Fiber	Sugar	Total Fat	Sat Fat	Sodium
Dressing, blue cheese	as served	350	2	2	0	2	37	7	400
Dressing, buttermilk ranch	as served	290	0	3	0	2	30	4.5	540
Dressing, creamy Caesar	as served	310	2	1	0	0	33	6	550
Dressing, honey mustard	as served	270	1	16	<1	15	23	3.5	200
Dressing, reduced-fat Italian	as served	15	0	1	0	<1	1	0	105
House salad	as served	90	3	15	3	6	3	0	170
Loaded potato & bacon soup	as served	430	13	30	1	5	29	17	1310
Minestrone soup	as served	170	7	28	2	3	2	0	1290
New England clam chowder	as served	460	13	25	1	4	34	19	1060
Seasonal fresh fruit	as served	80	<1	21	2	1	0	0	0
Side Caesar salad	as served	440	11	13	3	3	40	8	870

SIGNATURE SOUPS

Item	Serving Size	Calories	Protein	Carb	Fiber	Sugar	Total Fat	Sat Fat	Sodium
Broccoli cheese soup	as served	340	12	19	2	6	23	14	1440
Chicken noodle soup	as served	170	12	18	1	3	5	1.5	1110
Chicken tortilla soup	as served	190	9	23	3	3	7	2	1450
Loaded potato & bacon soup	as served	430	13	30	1	5	29	17	1310
Minestrone soup	as served	170	7	28	2	3	2	0	1290
New England clam chowder	as served	460	13	25	1	4	34	19	1060

SANDWICHES & BURGERS

Item	Serving Size	Calories	Protein	Carb	Fiber	Sugar	Total Fat	Sat Fat	Sodium
Bacon cheddar chicken sandwich	as served	680	38	40	3	5	42	18	1580
Bacon 'N Beef™ bacon & egg cheeseburger w/ bacon patty	as served	970	52	43	3	6	65	30	1380
Bacon 'N Beef™ bacon & egg cheeseburger w/ beef patty	as served	930	55	42	3	5	62	29	1290
Bacon 'N Beef™ Bacon cheeseburger w/ bacon patty	as served	820	48	40	3	5	54	27	1200

IHOP continued

Item	Serving Size	Calories	Protein	Carb	Fiber	Sugar	Total Fat	Sat Fat	Sodium
Bacon 'N Beef™ Bacon cheeseburger w/ beef patty	as served	860	45	42	3	6	57	28	1290
Bacon 'N Beef™ cheeseburger w/ bacon patty	as served	790	39	41	3	6	51	26	990
Bacon 'N Beef™ cheeseburger w/ beef patty	as served	740	42	40	3	5	48	25	890
Bacon 'N Beef™ Mega mushroom burger w/ bacon patty	as served	930	41	45	3	8	64	28	960
Bacon 'N Beef™ Mega mushroom burger w/ beef patty	as served	880	44	43	3	7	61	27	870
Chicken Clubhouse Super Stacker	as served	1180	53	55	4	9	81	33	2690
Double BLT	as served	660	23	39	2	5	45	10	1460
Ham & egg melt	as served	1090	64	78	3	5	58	30	2930
Monster Bacon 'N Beef™ cheeseburger w/ bacon patty	as served	1250	68	44	3	8	85	42	1590
Monster Bacon 'N Beef™ cheeseburger w/ beef patty	as served	1160	74	41	3	5	79	40	1410
Patty Melt	as served	940	43	44	5	7	67	31	1500
Philly Cheese Steak Stacker	as served	820	47	56	3	9	43	18	2300
Pot roast melt	as served	1050	57	83	3	10	55	30	2350
SIMPLE & FIT Simply Chicken sandwich w/ fresh fruit	as served	470	42	59	5	20	9	3	980
Turkey & Bacon club sandwich	as served	720	40	49	2	6	39	10	2030
Tuscan Chicken Griller	as served	900	47	54	7	5	56	19	2270
ADD SOUPS & SIDES									
Broccoli cheese soup	as served	340	12	19	2	6	23	14	1440
Chicken noodle soup	as served	170	12	18	1	3	5	1.5	1110
Chicken tortilla soup	as served	190	9	23	3	3	7	2	1450
Dill pickle spear	as served	5	0	1	1	0	0	0	410

IHOP continued

Item	Serving Size	Calories	Protein	Carb	Fiber	Sugar	Total Fat	Sat Fat	Sodium
House salad	as served	90	3	15	3	6	3	0	170
Loaded potato & bacon soup	as served	430	13	30	1	5	29	17	1310
Minestrone soup	as served	170	7	28	2	3	2	0	1290
New England clam chowder	as served	460	13	25	1	4	34	19	1060
Onion rings	as served	620	8	70	3	9	34	6	550
Seasonal fresh fruit	as served	80	<1	21	2	16	0	0	0
Seasoned fries	as served	300	3	44	4	0	12	2.5	490
Side Caesar salad	as served	440	11	13	3	3	40	8	870

APPETIZERS

Item	Serving Size	Calories	Protein	Carb	Fiber	Sugar	Total Fat	Sat Fat	Sodium
Appetizer Sampler	as served	1780	60	163	12	28	99	23	3120
Chicken fajita quesadilla	as served	1060	69	70	5	8	57	29	2410
Crispy chicken strips & fries	as served	1230	41	117	9	15	67	12	1330
Monster Mozza sticks	as served	770	39	68	7	6	36	16	2680
Onion rings	as served	1250	17	140	7	18	69	12	1110
Seasoned fries	as served	590	6	87	9	0	24	4.5	980
Steak fajita quesadilla	as served	1040	60	71	5	8	59	30	2540
Wings	as served	680	57	15	<1	7	44	11	1960
w/ blue cheese	side	350	2	2	0	2	37	7	400
w/ buttermilk ranch	side	290	0	3	0	2	30	4.5	540

FRESH SALADS

Item	Serving Size	Calories	Protein	Carb	Fiber	Sugar	Total Fat	Sat Fat	Sodium
Chicken & spinach salad	as served	1600	63	72	7	15	118	32	2340
Chicken fajita salad	as served	790	51	49	9	14	44	21	1600
Chicken fajita salad w/ avocado	as served	870	52	54	12	15	52	22	1600
Crispy chicken salad w/ fried chicken	as served	1450	63	93	10	32	94	26	2110
Crispy chicken salad w/ grilled chicken	as served	1260	56	59	8	32	90	25	2430
Grilled chicken Caesar salad	as served	960	42	39	6	7	72	15	2140
Grilled chicken Caesar salad, no chicken	as served	870	23	39	6	7	71	15	1720

IHOP continued

Item	Serving Size	Calories	Protein	Carb	Fiber	Sugar	Total Fat	Sat Fat	Sodium
House salad	as served	90	3	15	3	6	3	0	17
Side Caesar salad	as served	440	11	13	3	3	40	8	870
SIMPLE & FIT fresh fruit & yogurt bowl	as served	330	7	75	7	46	3	0	40
SIMPLE & FIT fruit bowl	as served	130	1	33	4	25	0	0	0
SIMPLE & FIT house salad	as served	50	2	9	3	5	1.5	0	140

SALAD DRESSINGS

Item	Serving Size	Calories	Protein	Carb	Fiber	Sugar	Total Fat	Sat Fat	Sodium
Balsamic vinaigrette	side	260	0	5	0	5	26	3.5	240
Blue cheese	side	350	2	2	0	2	37	7	400
Buttermilk ranch	side	290	0	3	0	2	30	4.5	540
Creamy Caesar	side	310	2	1	0	0	33	6	550
Honey mustard	side	270	1	16	<1	15	23	3.5	200
Reduced-fat Italian	side	15	0	1	0	<1	1	0	105

HEARTY DINNER FAVORITES

Item	Serving Size	Calories	Protein	Carb	Fiber	Sugar	Total Fat	Sat Fat	Sodium
Country/chicken fried steak dinner w/ country gravy	as served	830	39	82	7	5	38	14	2300
Country/chicken fried steak dinner w/ sausage gravy	as served	940	41	88	7	6	46	17	2630
Crispy chicken strips	as served	1010	40	89	9	18	56	14	1680
French onion pot roast	as served	790	42	73	3	23	39	15	2770
Fried chicken w/ country gravy	as served	690	29	74	5	11	33	11	2160
Fried chicken w/ sausage gravy	as served	750	30	77	5	12	37	12	2330
Grilled liver	as served	810	59	63	4	13	39	13	1370
Grilled tilapia Hollandaise	as served	810	51	46	8	4	46	13	1890
Maui-style crunchy shrimp	as served	720	26	95	9	33	27	6	1570
Mediterranean lemon chicken	as served	780	57	44	7	4	41	13	1350
Savory pork chops	as served	620	61	41	7	3	23	6	890
SIMPLE & FIT grilled balsamic-glazed chicken	as served	440	39	25	8	13	22	3.5	940

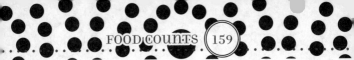

IHOP continued

Item	Serving Size	Calories	Protein	Carb	Fiber	Sugar	Total Fat	Sat Fat	Sodium
SIMPLE & FIT grilled tilapia	as served	490	49	27	8	14	23	4	1270
Sirloin steak tips dinner	as served	800	46	69	4	26	40	13	2250
Smoked sausage	as served	830	25	40	6	7	64	22	2650
T-bone steak	as served	760	57	40	7	2	41	14	1160
Thick-cut bone-in ham dinner	as served	680	48	73	4	30	25	10	3580
Top sirloin steak	as served	810	66	48	9	6	38	15	2100
ADD HEARTY DINNER SIDES									
Baked potato	as served	340	7	63	7	4	7	1	30
Broccoli cheese soup	as served	340	12	19	2	6	23	14	1440
Chicken noodle soup	as served	170	12	18	1	3	5	1.5	1110
Chicken tortilla soup	as served	190	9	23	3	3	7	2	1450
Garlic bread	as served	150	3	15	<1	0	8	2	250
House salad	as served	90	3	15	3	6	3	0	170
Loaded potato & bacon soup	as served	430	13	30	1	5	29	17	1310
Minestrone soup	as served	170	7	28	2	3	2	0	1290
New England clam chowder	as served	460	13	25	1	4	34	19	1060
Side Caesar salad	as served	440	11	13	3	3	40	8	870
DELICIOUS DESSERTS									
Crispy strawberry banana cheesecake	as served	580	8	77	3	30	27	14	660
w/ ice cream, chocolate	1 scoop	90	2	11	0	9	4	2.5	45
w/ ice cream, strawberry	1 scoop	80	1	11	0	9	3.5	2.5	30
w/ ice cream, vanilla	1 scoop	90	1	10	0	8	5	3.5	30
Fruit crepe w/ blueberry compote	as served	480	6	66	3	44	21	10	310
Fruit crepe w/ cinnamon apple compote	as served	390	6	45	2	29	21	10	300
Fruit crepe w/ strawberry topping	as served	460	6	65	3	31	21	10	250
Ice cream sundae (ice cream, whipped topping & cherry)	as served	300	4	26	0	22	20	15	80

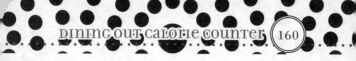

IHOP continued

Item	Serving Size	Calories	Protein	Carb	Fiber	Sugar	Total Fat	Sat Fat	Sodium
w/ hot fudge	topping	190	2	26	1	22	9	9	75
w/ strawberry topping	topping	70	0	17	<1	8	0	0	5
Ice cream, chocolate	1 scoop	90	2	11	0	9	4	2.5	45
Ice cream, strawberry	1 scoop	80	1	11	0	9	3.5	2.5	30
Ice cream, vanilla	1 scoop	90	1	10	0	8	5	3.5	30
Old fashioned chocolate cake	as served	460	4	72	3	25	18	10	320

55+ SPECIALTY ENTRÉES

Item	Serving Size	Calories	Protein	Carb	Fiber	Sugar	Total Fat	Sat Fat	Sodium
Rise 'N Shine	as served	1080	30	105	7	20	61	25	1580
Senior crispy chicken Strips	as served	900	28	87	8	17	49	13	1560
Senior French toast	as served	640	20	59	5	12	36	12	750
Senior grilled chicken breast	as served	640	42	54	7	2	28	6	870
w/ Hollandaise sauce	side	60	0	2	0	<1	6	3	120
w/ barbecue sauce	side	50	0	12	<1	7	0	0	300
Senior grilled liver	as served	790	35	74	5	13	42	13	1530
Senior grilled tilapia Hollandaise	as served	780	32	58	8	4	46	11	1530
Senior Mediterranean lemon chicken	as served	760	35	59	8	4	42	13	1140
Senior omelette, plain	as served	550	22	51	4	10	30	11	1320
Senior omelette, plain w/ egg substitute	as served	420	20	47	3	9	17	7	1250
w/ 2 bacon strips	2 strips	80	6	<1	0	0	6	2	300
w/ 2 pork sausage links	2 links	180	6	1	0	0	16	6	290
w/ American cheese	1 slice	160	8	2	0	1	13	8	690
w/ Cheddar cheese	1 slice	240	14	2	0	0	20	14	270
w/ diced ham	as served	30	5	1	0	1	1	0	320
w/ fresh spinach	as served	15	2	2	1	0	0	0	45
w/ green peppers & onions	as served	10	0	2	0	<1	0	0	0
w/ Jack & Cheddar cheese blend	1 slice	230	14	2	0	0	19	12	290
w/ mushrooms	as served	10	2	2	<1	<1	0	0	0
w/ oven-roasted tomatoes	as served	90	0	12	4	0	4	0	170
w/ Provolone cheese	1 slice	160	10	0	0	0	12	8	380

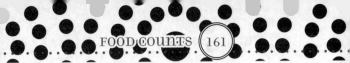

IHOP continued

Item	Serving Size	Calories	Protein	Carb	Fiber	Sugar	Total Fat	Sat Fat	Sodium
w/ Swiss cheese	1 slice	160	11	<1	0	0	13	8	100
w/ tomatoes	as served	10	<1	2	<1	1	0	0	0
Senior pork chop	as served	610	37	55	7	3	27	6	790
Senior pot roast	as served	630	20	72	4	15	31	12	1880
Senior Rooty Tooty Fresh 'N Fruity®	as served	370	18	25	1	5	22	7	910
w/ apple cinnamon compote w/ whipped topping	as served	90	0	17	<1	15	2.5	2	70
w/ blueberry compote w/ whipped topping	as served	100	0	19	1	15	2.5	2	45
w/ strawberry topping w/ whipped topping	as served	90	0	19	<1	9	2.5	2	10
Senior Sampler	as served	780	26	57	5	6	51	16	1910
Senior smoked sausage dinner	as served	750	18	53	7	7	52	17	2240
Senior Steakhouse Combo	as served	860	25	58	5	6	59	19	1920
Senior Two x Two x Two	as served	560	25	49	3	9	31	11	1280
SIMPLE & FIT senior buttermilk pancakes 3 pancakes		490	13	69	4	13	18	8	1610

IN-N-OUT BURGER

Item	Serving Size	Calories	Protein	Carb	Fiber	Sugar	Total Fat	Sat Fat	Sodium
BURGERS & FRIES									
Cheeseburger w/ onion	each	480	22	39	3	10	27	10	1000
Cheeseburger w/ onion, protein style	each	330	18	11	3	7	25	9	720
Cheeseburger w/ onion w/ mustard & ketchup instead of spread	each	400	22	41	3	10	18	9	1080
Double-Double w/ onion	each	670	37	39	3	10	41	18	1440
Double-Double w/ onion, protein style	each	520	33	11	3	7	39	17	1160
Double-Double w/ onion w/ mustard & ketchup instead of spread	each	590	37	41	3	10	32	17	1520

IN-N-OUT BURGER continued

Item	Serving Size	Calories	Protein	Carb	Fiber	Sugar	Total Fat	Sat Fat	Sodium
French fries	each	400	7	54	2	0	18	5	245
Hamburger w/ onion	each	390	16	39	3	10	19	5	650
Hamburger w/ onion, protein style	each	240	13	11	3	7	17	4	370
Hamburger w/ onion w/ mustard & ketchup instead of spread	each	310	16	41	3	10	10	4	730

BEVERAGES

Item	Serving Size	Calories	Protein	Carb	Fiber	Sugar	Total Fat	Sat Fat	Sodium
Chocolate shake	15 oz	690	9	83	0	62	36	24	350
Coffee	10 oz	5	0	1	0	0	0	0	3
Iced Tea	16 oz	0	0	0	0	0	0	0	0
Lemonade	16 oz	180	0	40	0	3	0	0	20
Minute Maid Light Lemonade	16 oz	8	0	1	0	0	0	0	7
Root Beer	16 oz	222	0	60	0	60	0	0	48
Strawberry shake	15 oz	690	9	91	0	75	33	22	280
Vanilla shake	15 oz	680	9	78	0	57	37	25	390

JACK IN THE BOX

Item	Serving Size	Calories	Protein	Carb	Fiber	Sugar	Total Fat	Sat Fat	Sodium
BURGERS									
Cheeseburger	each	350	18	31	1	7	17	8	790
Cheeseburger deluxe	each	460	21	33	2	7	28	11	930
Double bacon cheeseburger	each	840	34	51	2	9	56	19	1610
Hamburger	each	310	16	30	1	6	14	6	600
Hamburger w/ ciabatta	each	720	25	67	3	5	42	13	1280
Jumbo Jack® cheeseburger	each	690	25	54	3	12	42	16	1310
Junior bacon cheeseburger	each	430	20	30	1	6	25	9	820
Ultimate bacon cheeseburger	each	1090	46	53	2	12	77	30	2040
Ultimate cheeseburger	each	1010	40	53	2	12	71	28	1580

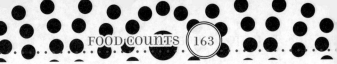

JACK IN THE BOX continued

Item	Serving Size	Calories	Protein	Carb	Fiber	Sugar	Total Fat	Sat Fat	Sodium
SNACKS & SIDES									
Bacon cheddar potato wedges	2 pieces	710	20	58	5	2	45	12	810
Beef taco	small	180	6	17	2	3	10	2.5	270
Egg roll	1 piece	150	5	15	2	2	7	1.5	320
Egg roll	3 pieces	440	16	46	7	6	22	5	950
French fries	small	290	3	39	3	0	13	1	580
French fries	medium	410	5	56	4	0	19	1.5	750
French fries	large	560	6	76	6	1	20	2.5	1020
Fruit cup	1 order	50	1	14	1	11	0	0	10
Mozzarella cheese sticks	3 pieces	260	12	22	2	1	16	6	690
Mozzarella cheese sticks	6 pieces	500	24	43	3	1	33	11	1190
Onion rings	each	450	6	45	3	5	28	2	620
Pita snack, crispy chicken	each	410	16	43	3	2	18	4	850
Pita snack, fish	each	390	13	40	3	2	20	4	760
Pita snack, grilled chicken	each	330	19	31	3	2	14	3.5	730
Pita snack, steak	each	350	19	31	3	2	16	4.5	640
Sampler Trio	1 order	790	28	75	7	6	43	13	1950
Seasoned curly fries	small	280	3	30	3	0	16	1.5	610
Seasoned curly fries	medium	43	5	48	4	0	25	2	940
Seasoned curly fries	large	580	7	63	5	0	34	3	1260
Stuffed jalapeños	3 pieces	220	6	21	1	2	12	4.5	730
Stuffed jalapeños	7 pieces	310	14	49	3	5	29	10	1690

JAMBA JUICE

Item	Serving Size	Calories	Protein	Carb	Fiber	Sugar	Total Fat	Sat Fat	Sodium
3G Charger™ Boost	1 serving	5	n/a	2	2	n/a	0	n/a	n/a
Acai Super-Antioxidant™	sixteen	260	4	53	3	45	4	1	45
Acai Super-Antioxidant™	original	380	5	77	5	65	6	2	55
Acai Super-Antioxidant™	power	520	8	107	6	92	7	2	105
Acai Topper™	twelve	440	9	84	9	48	10	1.5	40
Acai Topper™	sixteen	490	9	96	11	57	10	1.5	40
Aloha Pineapple®	sixteen	290	5	67	3	63	1	0	50
Aloha Pineapple®	original	410	6	97	4	91	1.5	0.5	55

JAMBA JUICE continued

Item	Serving Size	Calories	Protein	Carb	Fiber	Sugar	Total Fat	Sat Fat	Sodium
Aloha Pineapple®	power	550	7	130	5	123	2	1	70
Antioxidant Power™ Boost	per serving	n/a	n/a	n/a	n/a	n/a	n/a	n/a	n/a
Apple cinnamon oatmeal	as served	290	8	60	5	25	4	1	25
w/ brown sugar crumble	serving	40	0	8	0	7	1	0	0
w/ fruit	serving	70	0	16	1	13	0	0	0
Apple cinnamon pretzel	per serving	380	11	76	4	14	4	0	250
Banana Berry™	sixteen	270	3	64	3	57	1	0	60
Banana Berry™	power	560	6	131	5	115	2	0.5	160
Banana Berry™	original	400	4	94	4	82	1.5	0.5	90
Berry Cherry Pecan	as served	340	9	62	7	27	9	1.5	55
w/ brown sugar crumble	serving	40	0	8	0	7	1	0	0
w/ dried fruit medley	serving	60	0	14	1	13	0	0	0
w/ glazed pecan	serving	60	1	3	1	2	5	0	30
Berry Fulfilling®	sixteen	150	6	32	4	24	0.5	0	200
Berry Fulfilling®	power	320	9	71	8	53	1	0	290
Berry Fulfilling®	original	230	7	51	6	38	1	0	240
Berry Topper™	twelve	300	9	59	7	37	4.5	0.5	85
Berry Topper™	sixteen	460	13	85	10	50	9	1	115
Blackberry Bliss™	sixteen	230	1	55	5	49	1	0	25
Blackberry Bliss™	original	340	2	82	6	72	1.5	0	35
Blackberry Bliss™	power	480	3	113	9	100	2	1	50
Blueberry & Blackberry Oatmeal	as served	290	8	58	6	24	3.5	1	30
w/ brown sugar crumble	serving	40	0	8	0	7	1	0	0
w/ fruit	serving	60	0	15	1	13	0	0	5
Caribbean Passion®	sixteen	250	2	57	2	51	1	0	35
Caribbean Passion®	power	490	4	112	5	101	2	1	70
Caribbean Passion®	original	360	3	82	3	73	1.5	0.5	50
Carrot juice	twelve	100	3	22	0	20	0.5	0	170
Carrot juice	sixteen	130	4	30	0	26	0.5	0	230
Cheddar Tomato Twist	per serving	240	8	41	2	3	4.5	1.5	430

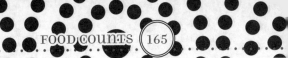

JAMBA JUICE continued

Item	Serving Size	Calories	Protein	Carb	Fiber	Sugar	Total Fat	Sat Fat	Sodium
Chill-icious Chai™	sixteen	310	10	65	0	58	0	0	240
Chill-icious Chai™	original	440	13	92	0	82	0	0	340
Chocolate Moo'd®	original	570	15	116	3	103	5	2.5	380
Chocolate Moo'd®	sixteen	430	11	86	2	77	4	2	270
Chunky Strawberry Topper™	twelve	520	14	82	9	46	17	2.5	160
Chunky Strawberry Topper™	sixteen	570	16	92	10	54	17	2.5	180
Classic hot chocolate	twelve w/ 2% milk	240	13	39	3	33	6	4	170
Classic hot chocolate	sixteen w/ 2% milk	340	17	56	5	48	8	5	230
Classic hot chocolate	twelve w/ nonfat milk	220	15	42	3	36	1.5	1	210
Classic hot chocolate	sixteen w/ nonfat milk	320	21	60	5	51	2	1.5	280
Classic hot chocolate	twelve w/ soy milk	240	15	30	5	22	9	2	60
Classic hot chocolate	sixteen w/ soy milk	330	21	44	7	33	12	3	80
Five Fruit Frenzy™	original	340	2	82	6	63	1	0	30
Five Fruit Frenzy™	power	430	3	105	8	80	1.5	0	40
Five Fruit Frenzy™	sixteen	240	2	58	4	44	0.5	0	25
Flax & Fiber Boost	per serving	30	1	7	7		1.5		
Four Cheesy™	per serving	420	21	46	2	4	16	8	910
Fresh Banana Oatmeal	as Served	280	9	57	6	19	4	1	20
w/ brown sugar crumble	serving	40	0	8	0	7	1	0	0
w/ fruit	serving	50	1	13	2	7	0	0	0
Heavenly Green™	twelve w/ 2% milk	160	8	25	1	25	3	2	115
Heavenly Green™	sixteen w/ 2% milk	240	12	38	1	37	4.5	3	170
Heavenly Green™	twelve w/ nonfat milk	150	9	27	1	27	0	0	140
Heavenly Green™	sixteen w/ nonfat milk	220	14	41	1	40	0	0	210
Heavenly Green™	twelve w/ soy milk	150	9	27	1	27	0	0	140

JAMBA JUICE continued

Item	Serving Size	Calories	Protein	Carb	Fiber	Sugar	Total Fat	Sat Fat	Sodium
Heavenly Green™	sixteen w/ soy milk	220	14	41	1	40	0	0	210
Mango Mantra®	sixteen	150	6	31	2	27	0.5	0	190
Mango Mantra®	power	340	10	78	6	67	1	0	270
Mango Mantra®	original	250	8	56	4	48	1	0	230
Mango Peach Topper™	twelve	320	9	64	6	42	4.5	0.5	85
Mango Peach Topper™	sixteen	470	13	90	9	55	8	1	115
Mango-a-go-go®	original	400	3	94	3	85	1.5	0.5	45
Mango-a-go-go®	power	550	4	129	4	117	2.5	1	65
Mango-a-go-go®	sixteen	280	2	65	2	59	1	0	35
Matcha Energy Shot-Orange Juice	single shot	60	1	13	1	10	0	0	0
Matcha Energy Shot-Orange Juice	double shot	60	1	13	1	10	0	0	0
Matcha Energy Shot-Soymilk	single shot	70	3	14	0	12	0	0	45
Matcha Energy Shot-Soymilk	double shot	70	4	14	1	12	0	0	45
Matcha Green Tea Blast®	sixteen	290	8	62	1	55	0	0	160
Matcha Green Tea Blast®	power	590	14	127	2	114	0	0	320
Matcha Green Tea Blast®	original	420	10	90	1	80	0	0	230
MediterraneaYUM™	per serving	320	13	49	3	5	8	3.5	770
Mega Mango™	original	320	3 0	80	5	70	1	0	10
Mega Mango™	power	420	5 0	104	7	91	1	0	10
Mega Mango™	sixteen	230	2 0	57	4	50	0.5	0	5
Mocha Marvel™	twelve w/ 2% milk	250	13	41	2	33	5	3.5	170
Mocha Marvel™	sixteen w/ 2% milk	390	18	68	3	53	8	4.5	220
Mocha Marvel™	twelve w/ nonfat milk	240	15	44	2	36	1	0	210
Mocha Marvel™	sixteen w/ nonfat milk	370	21	72	3	57	1.5	1	280
Mocha Marvel™	twelve w/ soy milk	200	11	30	3	21	6	1	45
Mocha Marvel™	sixteen w/ soy milk	340	17	54	5	37	9	2	65

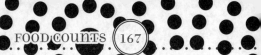

JAMBA JUICE continued

Item	Serving Size	Calories	Protein	Carb	Fiber	Sugar	Total Fat	Sat Fat	Sodium
Mocha Mojo	sixteen	350	9	73	1	62	1.5	1	220
Mocha Mojo	original	510	13	107	1	91	1.5	1	330
Mocha Mojo	power	680	18	142	2	122	3	1.5	430
Omega-3 chocolate brownie cookie	per serving	150	3	30	2	24	3.5	1	15
Omega-3 oatmeal cookie	per serving	150	2	26	3	15	6	1.5	85
Orange dark chocolate chip scone	per serving	380	6	57	2	27	15	3	65
Orange Dream Machine®	sixteen	350	8	75	1	68	1.5	1	150
Orange Dream Machine®	original	470	10	102	1	93	2	1	210
Orange juice	twelve	170	3	39	1	31	0.5	0	0
Orange juice	sixteen	220	3	52	1	42	1	0	0
Organic house blend	twelve	5	0	0	0	0	0	0	5
Organic house blend	sixteen	5	1	0	0	0	0	0	10
Organic house blend decaf	twelve	0	0	0	0	0	0	0	5
Organic house blend decaf	sixteen	0	0	0	0	0	0	0	10
Original Spiced Chai™	twelve w/ 2% milk	160	8	25	0	23	3	2	140
Original Spiced Chai™	sixteen w/ 2% milk	240	11	38	0	35	5	3	210
Original Spiced Chai™	twelve w/ nonfat milk	150	9	27	0	25	0	0	170
Original Spiced Chai™	sixteen w/ nonfat milk	220	14	41	0	38	0	0	250
Original Spiced Chai™	twelve w/ soy milk	160	9	19	1	16	5	1	65
Original Spiced Chai™	sixteen w/ soy milk	230	14	29	2	24	7	1	100
Passion Fruit Tea Infusion™	sixteen	150	1	37	1	32	0	0	20
Passion Fruit Tea Infusion™	power	300	2	72	1	63	0	0	35
Passion Fruit Tea Infusion™	original	230	1	54	1	48	0	0	30
Peach Perfection™	sixteen	210	1	53	4	42	0	0	20

JAMBA JUICE continued

Item	Serving Size	Calories	Protein	Carb	Fiber	Sugar	Total Fat	Sat Fat	Sodium
Peach Perfection™	power	400	3	99	7	80	0.5	0	35
Peach Perfection™	original	300	2	75	5	59	0.5	0	30
Peach Pleasure®	sixteen	260	2	61	3	51	1	0.5	35
Peach Pleasure®	power	490	4	114	5	96	2	1	65
Peach Pleasure®	original	370	3	88	4	73	1.5	1	50
Peanut Butter Moo'd®	sixteen	470	13	82	3	71	10	2.5	310
Peanut Butter Moo'd®	original	770	20	125	4	108	20	4.5	490
Perfectly Chocolate Chai™	twelve w/ 2% milk	190	9	32	2	27	4	2.5	140
Perfectly Chocolate Chai™	sixteen w/ 2% milk	280	13	48	3	41	6	3.5	210
Perfectly Chocolate Chai™	twelve w/ nonfat milk	170	10	34	2	29	1	0	170
Perfectly Chocolate Chai™	sixteen w/ nonfat milk	260	15	50	3	44	1.5	0.5	250
Perfectly Chocolate Chai™	twelve w/ soy milk	180	10	26	3	20	6	1.5	65
Perfectly Chocolate Chai™	sixteen w/ soy milk	270	15	39	5	30	9	2	100
Plain oatmeal with brown sugar	as Served	220	8	44	5	12	3.5	1	20
w/ brown sugar crumble	serving	40	0	8	0	7	1	0	0
Pomegranate Paradise™	sixteen	240	1	60	4	53	0.5	0	25
Pomegranate Paradise™	original	340	2	85	5	74	0.5	0	35
Pomegranate Paradise™	power	430	3	109	4	95	1	0	45
Pomegranate Pick-Me-Up™	sixteen	260	2	61	3	53	1	0	35
Pomegranate Pick-Me-Up™	original	370	3	88	4	75	2	0.5	50
Pomegranate Pick-Me-Up™	power	510	3	120	5	105	2.5	1	70
Pomegranate Tea Infusion™	sixteen	160	1	40	1	36	0	0	20
Pomegranate Tea Infusion™	original	240	1	59	1	53	0	0	30
Pomegranate Tea Infusion™	power	310	1	78	1	69	0	0	40
Prickly Pear Tea Infusion™	sixteen	150	1	38	1	33	0	0	20

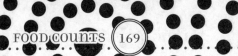

JAMBA JUICE continued

Item	Serving Size	Calories	Protein	Carb	Fiber	Sugar	Total Fat	Sat Fat	Sodium
Prickly Pear Tea Infusion™	original	230	1	56	2	49	0	0	30
Prickly Pear Tea Infusion™	power	300	1	74	2	64	0.5	0	35
Protein Berry Workout™	sixteen	280	17	52	3	42	0	0	115
Protein Berry Workout™	power	490	23	99	7	81	1	0	180
Protein Berry Workout™	original	370	20	72	4	59	0.5	0	150
Pumpkin Smash®	sixteen	390	10	83	1	75	0	0	320
Pumpkin Smash®	original	550	14	118	2	107	0.5	0	460
Razzmatazz®	sixteen	270	2	63	3	51	1	0.5	40
Razzmatazz®	original	390	3	91	4	74	1.5	1	55
Razzmatazz®	power	520	4	121	5	100	2.5	1	75
Reduced-fat blueberry lemon loaf	per serving	290	2	53	2	30	8	2	220
Reduced-fat cranberry orange loaf	per serving	310	6	52	4	31	9	2	200
Smokehouse Chicken	per serving	390	19	53	5	5	10	4	690
Sourdough Parmesan Pretzel	per serving	410	14	67	3	4	10	2	640
Soy Protein™ Boost	per serving	30	8	n/a	n/a	n/a	n/a	n/a	n/a
Strawberries Wild®	sixteen	250	3	60	2	52	0	0	95
Strawberries Wild®	original	370	5	87	3	77	0	0	140
Strawberries Wild®	power	510	7	118	5	104	0.5	0	210
Strawberry Energizer™	sixteen	280	2	67	5	58	1	0	20
Strawberry Energizer™	original	390	3	94	6	82	1.5	0.5	30
Strawberry Energizer™	power	540	4	128	7	113	2	1	35
Strawberry Nirvana®	sixteen	150	5	31	3	27	0	0	200
Strawberry Nirvana®	original	230	7	51	5	43	0.5	0	240
Strawberry Nirvana®	power	300	8	69	7	58	0.5	0	280
Strawberry Surf Rider™	sixteen	300	2	72	2	64	1	0	5
Strawberry Surf Rider™	original	430	3	103	3	93	1.5	0.5	10
Strawberry Surf Rider™	power	580	4	140	5	126	2	1	15
Strawberry Whirl™	sixteen	220	1	54	4	46	0	0	20
Strawberry Whirl™	original	300	2	75	6	64	0.5	0	25
Strawberry Whirl™	power	380	2	95	8	80	1	0	30
Tart cherry scone	per serving	360	6	58	1	23	12	1	60
The Coldbuster®	sixteen	240	3	65	3	49	1.5	0.5	20

JAMBA JUICE continued

Item	Serving Size	Calories	Protein	Carb	Fiber	Sugar	Total Fat	Sat Fat	Sodium
The Coldbuster®	original	350	4	81	4	70	2	1	30
The Coldbuster®	power	500	6	116	5	100	3	1.5	40
Vanilla Coffee Whirl™	twelve w/ 2% milk	250	12	40	0	34	4.5	3	200
Vanilla Coffee Whirl™	sixteen w/ 2% milk	360	16	60	0	50	6	4	270
Vanilla Coffee Whirl™	twelve w/ nonfat milk	230	14	43	0	27	0	0	240
Vanilla Coffee Whirl™	sixteen w/ nonfat milk	330	19	63	0	54	0	0	330
Vanilla Coffee Whirl™	twelve w/ soy milk	200	10	29	1	22	5	1	75
Vanilla Coffee Whirl™	sixteen w/ soy milk	300	14	46	2	34	7	1	115
Wheatgrass Detox Shot	1 fl oz	5	1	1	0	1	0		0
Wheatgrass Detox Shot	2 fl oz	15	1	2	0	1	0		10
Whey Protein™ Boost	per serving	50	10	1			0.5		25
Zucchini walnut loaf	per serving	270	5	43	4	26	9	1.5	250

JASON'S DELI

Item	Serving Size	Calories	Protein	Carb	Fiber	Sugar	Total Fat	Sat Fat	Sodium
POBOYS, PANINI, SANDWICHES, & WRAPS									
Amy's Turkey-O	each	648	33	71	7	11	27	11	2063
Beefeater poboy	each	794	64	41	1	1	38	15	2264
BLT	each	800	30	68	10	10	49	14	1850
California club	each	830	39	42	2	7	57	27	1660
Chicago club	each	776	46	46	7	2	50	15	2785
Chicken club Wrapini	each	648	43	41	4	3	35	11	1705
Chicken panini	each	717	43	49	2	3	38	10	2093
Club Light	each	475	41	49	7	10	15	5	1885
Club Royale	each	730	47	40	2	7	44	21	2230
Cranberry ciabatta sandwich	each	622	10	80	6	34	21	13	922
Deli club	each	827	57	67	11	11	41	14	2430
Grilled portobella Wrapini	each	672	24	45	7	5	47	16	925
JB's Bagelini	each	624	28	50	5	6	35	8	1652

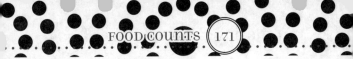

JASON'S DELI continued

Item	Serving Size	Calories	Protein	Carb	Fiber	Sugar	Total Fat	Sat Fat	Sodium
Meatball poboy	each	1065	52	62	3	6	65	26	2674
Mediterranean wrap	each	320	14	47	6	4	11	2	940
Pastrami melt poboy	each	1226	50	44	1	3	94	42	1631
Philly Chic wrap	each	609	47	52	5	8	25	9	1498
Pot roast melt poboy	each	766	67	47	4	2	32	13	1514
Ranchero wrap	each	891	57	62	14	7	49	17	3484
Reuben THE Great	each	860	75	56	9	6	35	15	4186
Santa Fe chicken sandwich	each	757	57	52	7	9	38	14	1909
Sergeant Pepper poboy	each	895	66	52	4	5	43	16	2271
Smokey Jack panini	each	671	44	50	3	8	33	9	2510
Spinach veggie wrap	each	359	16	40	6	3	17	8	607
The Big Joe Sandwich	each	829	28	54	6	4	55	10	1705
The New York Yankee, no dressing	each	1189	92	47	2	0	69	32	2270
Tuna melt	each	960	54	47	6	0	62	18	1310
Turkey Reuben	each	510	44	53	6	0	13	6	3047
Turkey wrap	each	359	22	40	5	3	14	4	920

FRUIT & SALADS

Item	Serving Size	Calories	Protein	Carb	Fiber	Sugar	Total Fat	Sat Fat	Sodium
Caesar salad, w/o chicken, w/o bread	each	703	30	33	4	7	51	20	1812
chicken Caesar salad, w/o bread	each	880	58	36	4	7	56	22	2900
Creamy fruit dip	each	144	1	18	3	16	7	4	74
Fresh fruit cup, w/ dip	each	234	3	41	3	34	8	5	77
Fresh fruit cup, w/o dip	each	89	1	23	3	18	0	0	2
Garlic olive oil focaccia bread for Caesar salad	2 pieces	220	4	19	1	1	16	2	205
Nutty Mixed Up Salad	each	920	38	90	9	63	45	8	2330
Nutty Mixed Up Salad, w/o chicken	each	740	10	87	9	63	40	7	1250
Nutty Mixed Up Salad, w/o chicken, w/o dressing	each	457	10	77	8	55	12	5	609
Nutty Mixed Up Salad, w/o dressing	each	636	41	80	8	55	18	6	1694
Taco salad w/ chili, w/o salsa	each	1972	55	189	27	11	111	27	1719
Taco salad w/ SW chicken chili, w/o salsa	each	1907	49	193	28	10	105	24	1723

JASON'S DELI continued

Item	Serving Size	Calories	Protein	Carb	Fiber	Sugar	Total Fat	Sat Fat	Sodium
The Big Chef Ssalad, w/o dressing	each	502	50	13	2	5	30	13	1656
POTATOES									
"Plain" Jane potato	each	2300	60	190	13	17	147	59	2423
Pollo Mexicano potato	each	1761	62	200	17	19	81	33	2558
Spud au broc	each	1535	68	203	17	17	56	28	3116
Texas style spud, beef	each	1812	58	192	13	18	84	29	1125
Texas style spud, pork	each	1553	48	191	13	19	68	26	1703
PASTA (all pastas listed w/o bread)									
Chicken pasta Alfredo	1 portion	793	48	31	1	3	53	29	2706
Chicken pasta primo	1 portion	589	39	30	3	7	35	15	2520
Garlic olive oil focaccia bread for pasta	2 pieces	220	4	19	1	1	16	2	205
Pasta Alfredo, w/o chicken	1 portion	614	21	28	1	3	47	28	1620
Pasta primo, w/o chicken	1 portion	397	11	27	3	7	27	13	1233
Penne pasta w/ meatballs	1 portion	703	33	36	2	8	46	18	2012
Portobello garden pasta w/ chicken	1 portion	714	46	39	10	2	42	15	2479
Portobello garden pasta w/ mushrooms	1 portion	541	19	37	10	2	36	13	1394
MUFFALETTAS									
Ham muffaletta	quarter	468	26	40	3	2	23	6	2274
Ham muffaletta	half	936	52	79	5	4	47	13	4548
Ham muffaletta	whole	1873	104	159	11	7	94	26	9097
Turkey muffaletta	quarter	422	25	39	3	3	18	5	230
Turkey muffaletta	half	843	51	79	5	6	36	10	4459
Turkey muffaletta	whole	1686	102	157	10	11	72	20	8918
Veggaletta muffaletta	quarter	258	11	39	3	3	7	3	590
Veggaletta muffaletta	half	517	23	77	6	6	14	6	1180
Veggaletta muffaletta	whole	1033	45	155	12	12	27	11	2360
SOUPS									
Beef stew	1 cup	181	15	25	5	6	3	1	660
Beef stew	1 bowl	318	27	44	9	10	5	2	1159

JASON'S DELI continued

Item	Serving Size	Calories	Protein	Carb	Fiber	Sugar	Total Fat	Sat Fat	Sodium
Broccoli cheese soup	1 cup	226	9	14	1	6	15	10	1018
Broccoli cheese soup	1 bowl	452	19	27	2	11	30	19	2035
Chicken noodle soup	1 cup	68	5	7	0	1	2	1	408
Chicken noodle soup	1 bowl	150	10	16	1	2	5	1	902
Creamy Irish potato	1 cup	221	4	16	1	2	16	8	526
Creamy Irish potato	1 bowl	463	8	33	2	5	33	17	1104
Fire roasted tortilla	1 cup	163	5	18	3	3	8	1	683
Fire roasted tortilla	1 bowl	317	9	35	5	6	16	2	1303
Seafood gumbo	1 cup	161	8	20	2	2	5	2	1001
Seafood gumbo	1 bowl	301	16	37	3	4	10	4	1902
SW chicken chili	1 cup	116	11	12	3	1	4	1	569
SW chicken chili	1 bowl	269	25	27	7	3	9	2	1324
Texas chili	1 cup	233	21	12	4	3	12	5	760
Texas chili	1 bowl	396	35	20	6	5	20	9	1292
Tomato basil	1 cup	171	2	12	2	6	13	7	600
Tomato basil	1 bowl	321	3	22	4	12	25	13	1123
Vegetarian French onion	1 cup	194	8	9	1	2	14	5	782
Vegetarian French onion	1 bowl	173	9	17	1	4	19	6	1113
Vegetarian vegetable	1 cup	76	2	13	2	4	2	0	485
Vegetarian vegetable	1 bowl	132	3	23	4	6	3	1	849
KIDS' MENUS									
Baked potato	each	796	23	70	5	6	48	28	694
Bowtie pasta & meatballs	each	500	22	55	3	7	21	7	880
Cheese pizza	each	470	20	53	4	3	20	7	820
Chicken pasta Alfredo	each	310	20	13	1	1	20	11	1137
Chic-N-Wrap	each	290	23	20	2	1	14	6	837
Grilled cheese, wheat	each	443	16	38	6	6	26	10	1054
Grilled cheese, white	each	483	14	42	1	8	27	10	1194
Ham & cheese Kidwich on organic wrap	each	241	20	19		1	10	5	991
Ham & cheese Kidwich, wheat	each	331	25	38	6	6	11	5	1201
Ham & cheese Kidwich, white	each	371	23	41	1	9	12	5	1384
Hot dog	each	271	13	28	1	3	11	5	678
Hot dog w/ chili	each	462	23	33	3	4	25	12	1163
Macaroni & cheese	each	420	17	37	2	4	23	14	820

JASON'S DELI continued

Item	Serving Size	Calories	Protein	Carb	Fiber	Sugar	Total Fat	Sat Fat	Sodium
Organic peanut butter & jelly, wheat	each	359	13	56	8	21	11	2	445
Organic peanut butter & jelly, white	each	375	10	56	2	22	12	2	540
Pasta Alfredo, no chicken	each	221	6	12	1	1	17	10	594
Pepperoni pizza	each	484	21	53	4	3	21	8	854
Turkey & cheese Kidwich on organic wrap	each	331	26	38	6	6	9	5	1215
Turkey & cheese Kidwich, wheat	each	241	21	19	2	1	9	5	1005
Turkey & cheese Kidwich, white	each	371	24	42	1	8	10	5	1355

SIDES & MORE

Item	Serving Size	Calories	Protein	Carb	Fiber	Sugar	Total Fat	Sat Fat	Sodium
American Potato Salad	1 container	350	5	28	3	3	25	4	500
Baked Lays	1 portion	120	2	23	2	2	2	0	180
Dill Pickle Spear	1 spear	5	0	1	1	0	0	0	410
Fresh Fruit Cup w/ dip	each	234	3	41		34	8	5	77
Fresh Fruit Cup w/o dip	each	89	1	23	3	18	0	0	2
Fresh Made Guacamole	1/4 cup	184	2	11	8	1	16	2	147
Fresh Made Salsa	1/4 cup	27	1	6	2	3	0	0	269
House Chips, Ruffled	1 portion	233	3	22	1	0	15	4	219
Individual Bag Chips, To Go	1 portion	150	2	15	1	0	10	3	150
Italian pasta Salad	1 container	300	8	33	2	0	17	3	880
Organic Blue Corn Tortilla Chips	1 portion	220	3	27	3	3	11	1	90
Roasted Red Pepper Hummus	1/4 cup	282	9	33	9	5	14	0	799
Steamed veggies	each	61	4	13	5	5	0	0	66
Three bean salad	1 container	360	20	37	11	6	12	1	500
Tuna pasta salad	1 container	250	10	19	2	2	16	3	480

DESSERTS

Item	Serving Size	Calories	Protein	Carb	Fiber	Sugar	Total Fat	Sat Fat	Sodium
Carrot cake	1 slice	530	7	57	4	40	33	11	420
Chocolate chip cookie	1 cookie	300	2	40	<1	28	15	6	135
Chocolate soft serve dessert	1 portion	170	5	25	0	24	5	3	79

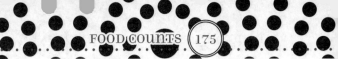

JASON'S DELI continued

Item	Serving Size	Calories	Protein	Carb	Fiber	Sugar	Total Fat	Sat Fat	Sodium
Chocolate topping for ice cream cone	1 portion	100	1	22	1	21	1	1	15
Classic plain cheese cake	1 slice	510	8	46	1	35	34	20	410
Classic strawberry shortcake	1 cake	625	5	74	3	45	36	18	553
Cranberry walnut cookie	1 cookie	300	55	36	3	20	16	4	170
Fruit topped cheese cake, strawberry	1 slice	520	8	49	2	37	34	20	410
Fudge nut brownie	1 brownie	420	6	51	3	40	24	12	25
Ice cream cone	1 cone	20	0	4	0	0	0	0	5
Macadamia white chip cookie	1 cookie	330	4	39	<1	25	18	6	150
Peanut butter cookie	1 cookie	330	5	41	0	27	16	7	160
Sugar free chocolate cheese cake	1 slice	340	6	39	6	0	23	13	320
Turtle cheese cake	1 slice	550	8	58	2	43	32	16	450
Vanilla soft serve dessert	1 portion	159	3	24	0	24	5	3	74

JIMMY JOHN'S

Item	Serving Size	Calories	Protein	Carb	Fiber	Sugar	Total Fat	Sat Fat	Sodium
Double Provolone Plain Slim®	each	545	29	65	0	n/a	16	9	991
Ham & cheese Plain Slim®	each	508	31	66	0	n/a	9.6	5	1244
Jimmy John's Big John®	each	533	26	49	1	n/a	24	4	1014
JJBLT® sandwich	each	634	25	49	1	n/a	35	9	1329
Pepe® sandwich	each	617	28	50	1	n/a	31	8	1262
Roast Beef Plain Slim®	each	424	29	64	0	n/a	2.8	1	966
Salami, capicola, & cheese Plain Slim®	each	599	33	66	0	n/a	19.8	8.8	1450
Totally Tuna® sandwich	each	548	33	54	3	n/a	31	4	1592
Tuna salad Plain Slim®	each	722	35	68	1	n/a	30.5	4	1746
Turkey breast Plain Slim®	each	401	27	65	0	n/a	0.6	0	1075
Turkey Tom® sandwich	each	515	24	50	1	n/a	22	3	1094
Vegetarian sandwich	each	578	19	53	2	n/a	30	7.6	873
Vito® sandwich	each	600	30	52	1	n/a	28	9	1377

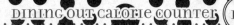

KFC

Item	Serving Size	Calories	Protein	Carb	Fiber	Sugar	Total Fat	Sat Fat	Sodium
CHICKEN (OR = Original Recipe EC= Extra Crispy)									
Boneless fiery Buffalo wings	1 wing	80	5	6	1	0	3.5	0.5	390
Boneless HBBQ wings	1 wing	80	5	7	1	2	3.5	0.5	340
Crispy strips	3 pieces	340	33	27	3	0	11	4	1280
Crispy strips	2 pieces	230	22	18	2	0	7	2.5	850
EC chicken, breast	each	510	39	16	0	1	33	7	1010
EC chicken, drumstick	each	150	12	5	0	0	10	2	360
EC chicken, thigh	each	340	20	10	0	0	24	5	780
EC chicken, whole Wing	each	190	12	6	0	0	13	2.5	410
Fiery Buffalo hot wings	1 wing	80	4	5	1	0	5	1	280
Fiery Buffalo wings	1 wing	80	4	4	1	0	5	1	230
Fiery grilled wings	1 wing	70	8	0	0	0	4	1	210
Grilled chicken, breast	each	210	34	0	0	0	8	2.5	460
Grilled chicken, drumstick	each	80	1	0	0	0	4	1	230
Grilled chicken, thigh	each	160	16	0	0	0	11	3	420
Grilled chicken, whole wing	each	80	9	1	0	0	5	1.5	250
HBBQ hot wings®	1 wing	90	4	7	0	2	5	1	260
HBBQ wings	1 wing	80	4	5	1	2	5	1	170
Hot wings®	1 wing	70	4	3	0	0	5	1	150
KFC® grilled fillet	each	140	26	1	0	1	3	1	560
KFC® OR fillet	each	170	23	4	1	0	7	1.5	360
OR chicken, breast	each	320	42	4	0	0	15	3.5	710
OR chicken, breast w/o skin or breading	each	150	31	0	0	0	2.5	0.5	430
OR chicken, drumstick	each	120	12	3	0	0	7	1.5	360
OR chicken, thigh	each	220	18	5	0	0	15	4	620
OR chicken, whole Wing	each	140	12	4	0	0	8	2	390
Popcorn chicken	kids	290	16	16	2	0	19	3.5	850
Popcorn chicken	individual	400	21	22	3	0	26	4.5	1160
Popcorn chicken	large	550	29	30	3	0	35	6	1600
Spicy crispy, breast	each	420	38	12	1	0	25	5	1250
Spicy crispy, drumstick	each	160	11	5	0	0	10	2	440
Spicy crispy, thigh	each	360	17	13	1	0	27	6	1010
Spicy crispy, whole Wing	each	170	11	6	0	0	12	2.5	470
SANDWICHES & WRAPS									
Crispy Twister® w/ crispy strip	each	560	29	59	4	5	23	6	1600

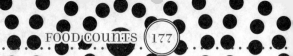

KFC continued

Item	Serving Size	Calories	Protein	Carb	Fiber	Sugar	Total Fat	Sat Fat	Sodium
Crispy Twister® w/ crispy strip w/o sauce	each	460	29	58	4	4	13	4.5	1480
Double Crunch sandwich w/ crispy strip	each	500	28	51	4	7	20	4.5	1150
Double Crunch sandwich w/ crispy strip w/o sauce	each	390	28	50	4	6	9	3	1020
Double Down w/ grilled fillet	each	480	60	4	0	2	25	9	1760
Double Down w/ OR fillet	each	540	53	11	1	1	32	10	1380
Doublicious w/ grilled fillet	each	380	35	35	2	9	11	4	950
Doublicious w/ OR fillet	each	480	33	36	2	7	23	6	990
Grilled fillet sandwich	each	400	32	33	2	7	16	3.5	850
Grilled fillet sandwich w/o sauce	each	290	32	32	2	6	4.5	1.5	720
Grilled Twister®	each	470	33	42	2	5	19	4.5	1300
Grilled Twister® w/o sauce	each	370	3	41	2	4	8	3	1180
Honey BBQ sandwich	each	320	24	47	3	21	3.5	1	770
KFC Snacker® with crispy strip	each	290	15	33	3	4	11	2.5	730
KFC Snacker® with crispy strip w/o sauce	each	240	15	33	2	4	6	1.5	600
KFC Snacker® with crispy strip, Buffalo	each	250	15	35	3	4	6	1.5	770
KFC Snacker® with crispy strip, ultimate cheese	each	270	16	34	2	4	8	2.5	750
KFC Snacker®, fish	each	320	16	31	2	5	14	3	640
KFC Snacker®, fish w/o sauce	each	290	16	29	1	4	12	2.5	550
KFC Snacker®, honey BBQ	each	210	13	32	2	12	3	1	470
Mini Melt	each	250	15	31	2	9	7	3	690
OR fillet sandwich	each	480	26	42	3	8	23	4	1160
OR fillet sandwich w/o sauce	each	370	25	41	3	7	12	2	1030
Toasted wrap w/ crispy strip	each	350	17	33	2	2	17	6	900
Toasted wrap w/ crispy strip w/o sauce	each	280	17	32	2	1	10	4.5	820
Toasted wrap w/ grilled fillet	each	310	20	24	1	2	15	5	760
Toasted wrap w/ grilled fillet w/o sauce	each	240	19	23	1	2	8	4	680

KFC continued

Item	Serving Size	Calories	Protein	Carb	Fiber	Sugar	Total Fat	Sat Fat	Sodium
Toasted wrap w/ tender roast fillet	each	310	21	24	1	2	15	5	700
Toasted wrap w/ tender roast fillet w/o sauce	each	240	20	23	1	2	8	3.5	630
POT PIE & BOWLS									
Chicken pot pie	each	690	27	57	3	14	40	31	1760
KFC® Famous Bowls, Mashed Potatoes w/ Gravy	each	700	26	77	6	8	32	8	2260
Snack-Size Bowl	each	320	12	34	3	1	15	4.5	990
SALADS & SIDES									
BBQ baked beans	each	200	8	39	9	18	1.5	0	680
Biscuit	each	180	4	23	1	2	8	6	530
Caesar salad w/o dressing & croutons	each	35	3	2	1	1	2	1	90
Cole slaw	each	180	1	19	2	14	11	1.5	160
Corn on the cob	3"	70	2	16	2	3	0.5	0	0
Corn on the cob	5.5"	140	5	33	4	5	1	0	5
Crispy chicken BLT salad w/o dressing	each	320	30	24	5	4	12	4	1210
Crispy chicken Caesar salad w/o dressing & croutons	each	300	28	22	4	2	11	5	1030
Green beans	each	20	1	3	1	1	0	0	290
Grilled chicken BLT salad w/o dressing	each	230	34	7	3	5	8	2.5	920
Grilled chicken Caesar salad w/o dressing & croutons	each	210	33	5	2	3	7	3.5	740
Heinz buttermilk ranch dressing	each	160	0	1	0	1	17	2	220
Hidden Valley® The Original Ranch® fat-free dressing	each	35	1	8	0	6	0	0	410
House Side salad w/o dressing	each	15	1	2	1	2	0	0	10
KFC® cornbread muffin	each	210	3	28	1	11	9	1.5	240
KFC® creamy Parmesan Caesar dressing	each	260	2	4	0	2	26	5	540
KFC® red beans w/ sausage & rice	each	160	24	26	4	0	2.5	0.5	340

KFC continued

Item	Serving Size	Calories	Protein	Carb	Fiber	Sugar	Total Fat	Sat Fat	Sodium
Macaroni & cheese	each	170	6	19	1	2	8	2.5	730
Macaroni salad	each	180	3	20	1	6	9	2	400
Marzetti light Italian dressing	each	10	0	2	0	1	0.5	0	510
Mashed potatoes w/ gravy	each	120	2	19	1	0	4	1	530
Mashed potatoes w/o gravy	each	90	2	15	1	0	3	0.5	320
Parmesan garlic croutons	each	70	2	8	1	1	3	0	140
Potato salad	each	200	2	24	3	5	10	2	540
Potato wedges	each	260	4	33	3	0	13	2.5	740
Sweet kernel Corn	each	110	4	23	2	4	0.5	0	0
Three bean salad	each	70	3	14	3	7	0	0	170

DESSERTS

Item	Serving Size	Calories	Protein	Carb	Fiber	Sugar	Total Fat	Sat Fat	Sodium
Apple turnover	each	260	2	35	1	14	13	3	170
Brownie tinis	1 pack	280	3	31	1	21	16	6	180
Café Valley Bakery chocolate chip cake	1 slice	280	3	47	1	21	9	3.5	160
Cookie dough pie	1 slice	240	3	31	1	21	12	7	190
Dutch apple pie	1 slice	320	2	27	1	24	14	6	300
Lemon meringue pie	1 slice	250	4	42	0	33	7	3.5	210
Lil' Bucket chocolate crème parfait cup	each	280	2	37	1	22	14	9	220
Lil' Bucket lemon crème parfait cup	each	390	7	60	0	47	14	8	220
Lil' Bucket strawberry shortcake crème parfait cup	each	230	2	39	1	20	8	4	220
Oreo cookies and crème pie	1 slice	290	3	34	1	23	16	10	210
Pecan pie	1 slice	410	4	52	1	22	21	6	220
Reese peanut butter pie	1 slice	310	5	31	1	22	19	10	200
Sara Lee sweet potato pie	1 slice	340	5	46	0	25	16	7	330
Strawberry cream cheese pie	1 slice	270	3	31	0	22	15	10	220
Sweet Life chocolate chip cookie	each	170	2	23	1	15	8	4	90
Sweet Life oatmeal raisin cookie	each	150	2	23	1	13	6	2.5	130

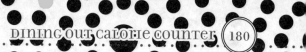

KFC continued

Item	Serving Size	Calories	Protein	Carb	Fiber	Sugar	Total Fat	Sat Fat	Sodium
Sweet Life sugar cookie	each	160	2	22	0	11	7	3	125

BEVERAGES

Capri Sun Roarin Waters	6 fl oz	30	0	8	0	8	0	0	15

LITTLE CAESARS

Item	Serving Size	Calories	Protein	Carb	Fiber	Sugar	Total Fat	Sat Fat	Sodium
PIZZAS									
3 Meat Treat®	1/8 pizza	350	17	30	1	3	18	8	730
Deep-dish cheese	1/8 pizza	320	14	38	1	3	13	5	490
Deep-dish pepperoni	1/8 pizza	360	16	38	1	4	16	6	610
Hula Hawaiian®	1/8 pizza	270	15	33	1	6	9	4.5	600
Just cheese	1/8 pizza	240	12	30	1	3	9	4.5	410
Meat and vegetable	1/8 pizza	350	17	30	1	3	18	8	730
Pepperoni	1/8 pizza	280	14	30	1	3	11	5	520
Thin crust, cheese	1/8 pizza	148	8	11	1	1	8	4	218
Ultimate Supreme	1/8 pizza	310	15	31	2	3	14	6	640
Vegetarian	1/8 pizza	270	13	32	2	4	10	4.5	530
SIDES & SAUCES									
Barbecue wings	1 piece	70	4	3	0	2	4	1	220
Buffalo dip	1 container	140	0	4	0	2	14	2	940
Buffalo ranch dip	1 container	230	0	3	0	2	24	3.5	520
Buttery garlic dip	1 container	380	0	0	0	0	42	9	420
Cheezy dip	1 container	210	1	3	0	2	21	4	450
Chipotle dip	1 container	220	0	2	0	0	4	3.5	560
Crazy Bread®	1 piece	100	3	15	1	1	3	0.5	150
Crazy Sauce®	1 container	45	2	10	1	8	0	0	260
Hot wings	1 piece	60	4	1	0	0	4.5	1	430
Little Caesars Italian Cheese Bread®	1 piece	130	6	13	1	1	7	2.5	230
Mild wings	1 piece	60	4	1	0	0	4	1	290
Oven-roasted wings	1 wing	50	4	0	0	0	3.5	1	150
Little Caesars Pepperoni Cheese Bread®	1 piece	150	7	13	0	1	8	3	280
Ranch dip	1 container	250	0	3	0	2	26	4	380

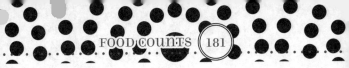

LONE STAR

Item	Serving Size	Calories	Protein	Carb	Fiber	Sugar	Total Fat	Sat Fat	Sodium
APPETIZERS									
Amarillo cheese fries	as served	2640.71	68.77	356.01	15.3	152.49	38.29	150.76	16887.52
Bavarian loaf	as served	150	n/a	28.5	1.8	2.9	0.91	0	264
Chicken tenders	as served	1093.82	35.33	91	7.06	65.55	12.12	100.7	1769.76
Chicken tenders, Buffalo style	as served	1197.43	37.18	92.32	6.95	77.42	15.6	119.04	4172.17
Lone Star® skins	as served	1310.52	53.23	134.38	8.41	62.46	21.75	112.99	1542.12
Lone Star® wings, mild	as served	953.65	83.35	15.25	2.77	62.02	8.19	322.89	841.56
Spinach artichoke dip	as served	491.49	18.53	13.98	3.25	40.31	24.12	129.47	1534.83
Texas Rose®	as served	1258.28	19.51	108.39	6.62	83.13	36.98	75.05	2704.19
Yeast rolls	1 roll	366.33	10.13	72.49	2.31	7.77	5.6	n/a	n/a
HOMEMADE SOUPS & CHILI									
Chili	10 oz bowl	345.71	30.56	13.5	3.82	17.69	6.59	88.52	878.12
Chili	4 oz cup	138.04	12.2	5.39	1.53	7.06	2.63	35.35	350.63
Steak soup	10 oz bowl	65.54	24.03	10.92	1.1	7.3	2.35	42.03	281.53
Steak soup	4 oz cup	26.17	9.59	4.36	0.44	2.92	0.94	16.78	112.41
FRESH GARDEN SALADS									
Caesar salad w/ grilled chicken	as served	479.25	46.18	19.34	5.22	23.59	5.21	114.38	2876.93
Dinner Caesar salad	as served	142.54	4.08	8.32	3.04	10.57	2.42	9.94	344.62
Dinner salad	as served	130.63	12.96	15.59	3.35	14.51	9.88	49.07	381.9
Signature lettuce wedge	as served	396.57	13.7	9.81	0.35	34.06	14.38	65.56	818.4
Steakhouse salad	as served	708.19	55.76	1.74	5.64	53.11	22.41	107.07	1328.28
HAND-CUT & MESQUITE-GRILLED STEAKS									
Cajun ribeye	12 oz	816.52	80.75	5.47	0	52.55	20.36	345.31	703.07
Chopped steak	10 oz	712.27	61.76	0	0	51.69	6.23	134.32	364.02
Five-star filet mignon, 6 oz	6 oz	332.9	41.92	1.84	0	17.57	6.83	160.64	241.54
Garlic lover's medallions & shrimp	8 oz	370.74	68.56	0	0	10.73	6.43	212.84	2242.57
New York strip	12 oz	524.74	68.87	0	0	27.6	15.55	194.45	617.49
Texas ribeye	as served	710.2	83.27	5.58	0.15	40.41	14.59	329.14	1339.19
SIDE ITEM SELECTIONS									
1/2 mushrooms & 1/2 onions	side	138.34	3.79	15.49	2.04	6.83	1.02	0.02	504.83

LONE STAR continued

Item	Serving Size	Calories	Protein	Carb	Fiber	Sugar	Total Fat	Sat Fat	Sodium
Baked potato, plain	each	226.2	6.13	50	5.36	0.3	0.06	0	32.65
Garlic mashed potatoes	1/2 cup	130	3	19	2	5	2.5	10	430
Jumbo baked sweet potato, plain	each	332.09	7.42	76.42	12.18	0.55	0.13	0	132.84
Sautéed mushrooms	side	140.38	4.5	10.79	0.21	8.84	1.29	0.05	419.22
Sautéed onions	side	85.68	1.73	14.23	3.01	2.41	0.4	0	400.23
Steak fries	8 oz	610.07	8.5	86.39	5.33	25.72	2.66	0	351.92
Texas rice	side	101.94	2.07	14	0.46	3.47	0.74	0.03	580.39

STEAK COMBOS
Item	Serving Size	Calories	Protein	Carb	Fiber	Sugar	Total Fat	Sat Fat	Sodium
Center cut sirloin	6 oz								
w/ 5 fried shrimp	as served	251.89	7.25	26.31	0.33	13.02	1.82	154.27	299.83
w/ 5 grilled shrimp	as served	44.2	9.45	0.58	0.28	0.43	0.19	60.26	1455.99

SEAFOOD
Item	Serving Size	Calories	Protein	Carb	Fiber	Sugar	Total Fat	Sat Fat	Sodium
Fried shrimp dinner	as served	865.68	21.76	96.94	0.99	39.57	5.46	462.82	1859.49
Mesquite-grilled shrimp dinner	as served	230.84	21.27	17.23	1.41	7.69	1.42	120.79	3665.71
Sweet bourbon salmon®	as served	309.88	36.48	0	0	18.22	4.87	111.44	538.9

MESQUITE-GRILLED SPECIALTIES
Item	Serving Size	Calories	Protein	Carb	Fiber	Sugar	Total Fat	Sat Fat	Sodium
Baby back ribs	full rack	972	58.8	0	0	80.4	32.4	264	252
Baby back ribs	1/2 rack	486	29.4	0	0	40.2	16.2	132	126
Grilled chicken	as served	169.15	32.68	0	0.1	4.24	0.34	58.86	1335.21
Grilled pork chops	as served	1432	85.22	0	0	32.62	9.3	257.9	6088.8
Texas trio	as served	1205.61	107.97	63.83	1.53	55.04	18.64	358.99	8386.36

GOURMET BURGERS & SANDWICHES
Item	Serving Size	Calories	Protein	Carb	Fiber	Sugar	Total Fat	Sat Fat	Sodium
Lone Star® cheeseburger	as served	893.96	70.22	49.77	2.5	45.35	20.18	243.68	2089.12
Swiss & mushroom burger	as served	843.65	69.19	52.52	2.56	37.88	16.62	209.77	1348.85

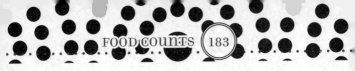

LONE STAR continued

Item	Serving Size	Calories	Protein	Carb	Fiber	Sugar	Total Fat	Sat Fat	Sodium
LUNCH MENU									
MAIN ENTRÉES									
Chicken tenders	as served	516.42	30.64	38.51	3.96	26.65	7.3	89.51	1241.13
Chopped steak	as served	712.27	61.76	0	0	51.69	6.23	134.32	364.02
Grilled chicken breast	as served	169.15	32.68	0	0.1	4.24	0.34	58.86	1335.21
Grilled pork chop	as served	317.47	42.61	0	0	16.31	4.65	128.95	3044.4
Grilled shrimp	as served	189.7	12.2	17.13	1.08	6.8	1.25	62.93	2362.67
Lunch cut steak	as served	389.91	36.46	0.61	0.23	26.9	7.19	100.21	1554.86
Sweet bourbon salmon	6 oz	240	33.6	0	0	10.8	1.8	96	678
SANDWICHES AND BURGERS									
Bacon bleu burger	as served	821.14	67.78	50.6	3.33	37.16	16.52	208.99	1641.32
Bubba burger	as served	1086.67	72.61	66.93	3.35	57.19	22.99	244.51	4268.22
Lone Star® burger	as served	639.96	60.22	47.77	2.5	27.35	10.19	183.68	1169.12
Lone Star® cheeseburger	as served	893.96	70.22	49.77	2.5	45.35	20.18	243.68	2089.12
Swiss & mushroom burger	as served	843.65	69.19	52.52	2.56	37.88	16.62	209.77	1348.85
The Perfect Chicken Sandwich™	as served	1047.08	49.92	135.03	8.45	34.17	4.02	73.86	4431.15
SALADS, SOUPS, SIDES									
Baked potato, plain	each	226.2	6.13	50	5.36	0.3	0.06	0	32.65
Chicken Caesar salad	as served	479.25	46.18	19.34	5.22	23.59	5.21	114.38	2876.93
Classic dinner salad	as served	130.63	12.96	15.59	3.35	14.51	9.88	49.07	381.9
Lone Star® chili	1 cup	138.04	12.2	5.39	1.53	7.06	2.63	35.35	350.63
Lone Star® steak soup	1 cup	26.17	9.59	4.36	0.44	2.92	0.94	16.78	112.41
Side Caesar salad	as served	142.54	4.08	8.32	3.04	10.57	2.42	9.94	344.62
Signature lettuce wedge	as served	396.57	13.7	9.81	0.35	34.06	14.38	65.56	818.4
Sweet potato, plain	each	332.09	7.42	76.42	12.18	0.55	0.13	0	132.84

LONG JOHN SILVER'S

Item	Serving Size	Calories	Protein	Carb	Fiber	Sugar	Total Fat	Sat Fat	Sodium
DOLLAR STRETCHER MENU									
Baja chicken taco	each	370	11	31	3	2	23	5	890
Baja fish taco	each	360	9	30	3	2	23	4.5	810
Chicken & fries	1 piece & 3 oz	370	11	42	4	0	18	4.5	820
Fish & fries	1 piece & 3 oz	490	14	50	4	0	26	6	1140
Fish sandwich	each	470	18	49	3	4	23	5	1180
Four battered shrimp	4 pieces	170	7	10	0	0	12	3	640
Popcorn shrimp	1 snack box	270	9	23	1	1	16	4	570
Six hushpuppies	6 pieces	360	9	56	4	5	19	4.5	1210
Small golden fries	3 oz	230	3	33	3	0	10	2.5	350
Three shrimp & Fries	3 pieces & 3 oz	360	8	41	3	1	19	5	830
Zesty chicken sandwich	each	380	14	39	3	2	19	4	880
FISH & SEAFOOD									
Battered Fish	1 piece	260	12	17	0	0	16	4	790
Battered Shrimp	3 pieces	130	5	8	0	0	9	2.5	480
Breaded clam strips	1 snack box	320	9	29	2	1	19	4.5	1190
Buttered Langostino lobster bites	1 snack box	230	13	24	2	0	9	3	520
Crispy breaded fish	1 piece	190	9	17	1	0	10	2.5	540
Grilled Pacific salmon	2 fillets	150	24	2	0	1	5	1	440
Grilled tilapia	1 fillet	110	22	1	0	1	2.5	1	250
Langostino lobster-stuffed crab cake	1 cake	170	6	16	1	0	9	2	390
Popcorn shrimp	1 snack box	270	9	23	1	1	16	4	570
Shrimp scampi	8 pieces	200	17	3	0	1	13	2.5	650
SANDWICHES, BOWLS, & MORE									
Chicken sandwich	each	360	14	40	3	4	15	3.5	900
Fish sandwich	each	470	18	49	3	4	23	5	1180
Freshside Grille® Smart Choice salmon	each	280	27	27	3	5	7	2	1010
Freshside Grille® Smart Choice shrimp scampi	each	330	20	29	3	5	15	3.5	1230
Freshside Grille® Smart Choice tilapia	each	250	25	27	3	4	4.5	2	820
Salmon bowl w/ sauce	each	460	30	65	4	22	8	2.5	1660
Salmon bowl w/o sauce	each	380	29	47	4	5	8	2	1270

LONG JOHN SILVER'S continued

Item	Serving Size	Calories	Protein	Carb	Fiber	Sugar	Total Fat	Sat Fat	Sodium
Shrimp bowl w/ sauce	each	390	22	65	4	21	5	1.5	1710
Shrimp bowl w/o sauce	each	310	21	47	4	5	4.5	1.5	1320
Ultimate fish sandwich®	each	530	21	50	3	4	27	8	1500
SAUCES & CONDIMENTS									
BBQ	1 portion	40	0	10	0	6	0	0	230
Cocktail	1 portion	25	0	6	0	5	0	0	250
Ginger Teriyaki sauce	1 portion	80	1	18	0	17	0	0	380
Honey mustard	1 portion	100	0	12	0	6	6	1.5	170
Ketchup	1 portion	10	0	2	0	2	0	0	100
Lemon juice	1 portion	0	0	0	0	0	0	0	0
Louisiana hot sauce	1 portion	0	0	0	0	0	0	0	140
Malt vinegar	1 portion	0	0	0	0	0	0	0	35
Marinara	1 portion	15	1	4	1	2	0	0	125
Ranch	1 portion	160	0	2	0	1	17	2.5	240
Sweet & sour	1 portion	45	0	12	0	7	0	0	120
Tartar sauce	1 portion	100	0	4	0	3	9	1.5	250
SIDES									
Breaded Mozzarella sticks	3 pieces	150	5	13	1	0	9	3.5	350
Breadstick	each	170	6	29	1	2	3.5	1	290
Broccoli cheese bites	5 pieces	230	5	25	2	2	12	4.5	550
Broccoli cheese soup	1 bowl	220	5	8	1	2	18	8	650
Cole slaw	4 oz	200	1	15	3	10	15	2.5	340
Corn cobbette w/ butter oil	1 cobbette	150	3	14	3	6	10	2	30
Corn cobbette w/o butter oil	1 cobbette	90	3	14	3	6	3	0.5	0
Crumblies®	1 oz	170	1	14	1	0	12	2.5	410
Fries	3 oz	230	3	34	3	0	10	2.5	350
Fries	4 oz	310	3	45	4	0	14	3.5	460
Hushpuppy	1 pup	60	1	9	1	1	2.5	0.5	200
Jalapeño Cheddar bites	5 pieces	240	6	23	2	2	14	5	730
Jalapeño peppers	1 pepper	15	1	2	0	1	0	0	190
Rice	5 oz	180	4	37	2	1	1	0.5	470
Vegetable medley	4 oz	50	1	8	3	3	2	0.5	360

LONG JOHN SILVER'S continued

Item	Serving Size	Calories	Protein	Carb	Fiber	Sugar	Total Fat	Sat Fat	Sodium
DESSERTS									
Chocolate cream pie	1 slice	280	3	28	1	19	17	10	230
Pineapple cream pie	1 slice	300	3	35	0	25	17	11	250
Turtle pie	1 slice	290	3	34	0	23	16	8	210

LONGHORN STEAKHOUSE

Item	Serving Size	Calories	Protein	Carb	Fiber	Sugar	Total Fat	Sat Fat	Sodium
STARTERS									
Boneless Buffalo wings	as served	990	n/a	40	n/a	n/a	63	11	4240
Crispy chicken trio	as served	730	n/a	32	n/a	n/a	39	9	1590
Firecracker chicken wraps	as served	640	n/a	52	n/a	n/a	36	13	2330
French onion soup	as served	320	n/a	20	n/a	n/a	21	9	1820
Housemade chips	as served	930	n/a	82	n/a	n/a	63	11	1470
Ranch House chili	as served	210	n/a	9	n/a	n/a	14	6	390
Shrimp & lobster chowder	as served	250	n/a	31	n/a	n/a	10	5	870
Shrimp & lobster dip	as served	1030	n/a	92	n/a	n/a	53	17	2080
Texas Tonian	as served	1130	n/a	116	n/a	n/a	68	12	2320
Western cheese fries	as served	1730	n/a	138	n/a	n/a	96	35	4940
Wild West shrimp	as served	760	n/a	43	n/a	n/a	49	13	4180
SALADS									
7-pepper sirloin salad	as served	670	n/a	32	n/a	n/a	36	12	1500
Grilled Caesar salmon salad	as served	730	n/a	29	n/a	n/a	50	10	1040
Grilled chicken strawberry salad	as served	950	n/a	58	n/a	n/a	60	10	860
Grilled salmon salad	as served	490	n/a	28	n/a	n/a	24	9	600
Sonoma chicken salad	as served	720	n/a	19	n/a	n/a	39	11	1770
DINNER ENTRÉES									
LEGENDARY STEAKS									
Bacon wrapped filet	9 oz	620	n/a	0	n/a	n/a	41	12	880
Chop steak	as served	980	n/a	45	n/a	n/a	67	20	3120
Crab stuffed filet	as served	490	n/a	5	n/a	n/a	26	11	900

LONGHORN STEAKHOUSE continued

Item	Serving Size	Calories	Protein	Carb	Fiber	Sugar	Total Fat	Sat Fat	Sodium
Fire-grilled T-bone	as served	830	n/a	1	n/a	n/a	57	22	1710
Flo's Filet	7 oz	450	n/a	0	n/a	n/a	30	9	800
Flo's Filet	9 oz	550	n/a	0	n/a	n/a	34	10	1700
Flo's Filet & grilled shrimp	as served	630	n/a	4	n/a	n/a	41	18	510
Flo's Filet & lobster tail	as served	550	n/a	0	n/a	n/a	30	8	630
Flo's Filet & Longhorn salmon	as served	740	n/a	3	n/a	n/a	43	11	1280
Flo's Filet & shrimp w/ crab	as served	750	n/a	6	n/a	n/a	44	16	1000
LongHorn Porterhouse	1	1200	n/a	1	n/a	n/a	85	31	2180
New York strip	11 oz	790	n/a	2	n/a	n/a	60	22	530
New York strip	14 oz	950	n/a	2	n/a	n/a	72	26	650
Outlaw ribeye	18 oz	1070	n/a	2	n/a	n/a	79	33	1640
Prime rib au jus	12 oz	745	n/a	0	n/a	n/a	46	21	1164
Prime rib au jus	16 oz	990	n/a	0	n/a	n/a	61	28	1304
Renegade top sirloin	6 oz	380	n/a	0	n/a	n/a	23	6	680
Renegade top sirloin	8 oz	470	n/a	0	n/a	n/a	26	7	990
Renegade top sirloin	12 oz	640	n/a	0	n/a	n/a	33	9	520
Ribeye	12 oz	910	n/a	0	n/a	n/a	69	25	1260
SEAFOOD									
Golden fried shrimp	as served	880	n/a	71	n/a	n/a	48	9	3180
Grilled fresh rainbow trout	as served	280	n/a	0	n/a	n/a	15	3	460
Grilled trout w/ shrimp	as served	490	n/a	5	n/a	n/a	29	8	1100
LongHorn salmon 7 oz	7 oz	290	n/a	3	n/a	n/a	13	2.5	300
LongHorn salmon 10 oz	10 oz	410	n/a	4	n/a	n/a	19	4	420
Redrock Grilled shrimp	as served	130	n/a	2	n/a	n/a	1.5	0.5	1690
CHICKEN									
Citrus grilled chicken	as served	520	n/a	35	n/a	n/a	18	5	1100
Fresh chicken tenders	as served	730	n/a	33	n/a	n/a	37	7	1450
Grilled chicken & portabella	as served	530	n/a	9	n/a	n/a	26	8	1550

LONGHORN STEAKHOUSE continued

Item	Serving Size	Calories	Protein	Carb	Fiber	Sugar	Total Fat	Sat Fat	Sodium
Parmesan crusted chicken	as served	1080	n/a	16	n/a	n/a	69	25	2440
Sierra chicken	as served	410	n/a	2	n/a	n/a	12	3	1240

RIBS, CHOPS, & MORE

Item	Serving Size	Calories	Protein	Carb	Fiber	Sugar	Total Fat	Sat Fat	Sodium
Baby back ribs	full rack	1090	n/a	4	n/a	n/a	74	25	1140
Baby back ribs	1/2 rack	550	n/a	2	n/a	n/a	37	13	570
Cowboy pork chops	as served	400	n/a	1	n/a	n/a	14	5	1600
LH churrasco steak	as served	1070	n/a	40	n/a	n/a	72	26	1090
LH steak tips	as served	650	n/a	26	n/a	n/a	29	9	2540

LUNCHTIME ENTRÉES & STEAKHOUSE SALADS

Item	Serving Size	Calories	Protein	Carb	Fiber	Sugar	Total Fat	Sat Fat	Sodium
7-pepper sirloin salad	as served	670	n/a	32	n/a	n/a	36	12	1500
Grilled Caesar chicken salad	as served	720	n/a	27	n/a	n/a	47	10	1190
Grilled Caesar salmon salad	as served	730	n/a	29	n/a	n/a	50	10	1040
Grilled chicken & strawberry	as served	950	n/a	58	n/a	n/a	60	10	860
Grilled chicken salad	as served	470	n/a	26	n/a	n/a	21	8	750
Grilled salmon salad	as served	490	n/a	28	n/a	n/a	24	9	600
Parmesan chicken salad	as served	770	n/a	48	n/a	n/a	38	11	1560
Sonoma chicken salad	as served	720	n/a	19	n/a	n/a	39	11	1770

HALF-POUND BURGERS & SANDWICHES

Item	Serving Size	Calories	Protein	Carb	Fiber	Sugar	Total Fat	Sat Fat	Sodium
Bacon & Cheddar	as served	920	n/a	53	n/a	n/a	52	22	1230
Black & bleu burger	as served	910	n/a	53	n/a	n/a	52	21	1190
Cheeseburger	as served	840	n/a	53	n/a	n/a	47	20	1180
Honey mustard chicken	as served	700	n/a	54	n/a	n/a	28	9	1320
Mushroom & Swiss	as served	871	n/a	55	n/a	n/a	49	18	1690
Parmesan Crusted Chicken	as served	770	n/a	48	n/a	n/a	38	11	1560
Shaved Prime Rib	as served	811	n/a	37	n/a	n/a	41	18	2250

LONGHORN STEAKS LUNCH ENTRÉES

Item	Serving Size	Calories	Protein	Carb	Fiber	Sugar	Total Fat	Sat Fat	Sodium
Chop Steak	as served	980	n/a	45	n/a	n/a	67	20	3120

LONGHORN STEAKHOUSE continued

Item	Serving Size	Calories	Protein	Carb	Fiber	Sugar	Total Fat	Sat Fat	Sodium
Flo's Filet	7 oz	450	n/a	0	n/a	n/a	30	6	510
NY /Kansas City Strip	11 oz	790	n/a	2	n/a	n/a	60	22	530
Renegade Top Sirloin	6 oz	380	n/a	0	n/a	n/a	23	6	520
Renegade Top Sirloin	8 oz	470	n/a	0	n/a	n/a	26	7	680
Renegade Top Sirloin	12 oz	640	n/a	0	n/a	n/a	33	9	990
Ribeye	12 oz	910	n/a	0	n/a	n/a	69	25	1260

SIGNATURE LUNCH
CHICKEN

Item	Serving Size	Calories	Protein	Carb	Fiber	Sugar	Total Fat	Sat Fat	Sodium
Citrus Grilled Chicken	as served	380	n/a	27	n/a	n/a	15	4.5	820
Fresh Chicken Tenders	as served	490	n/a	22	n/a	n/a	25	4.5	970
Grilled Chicken & Portabella	as served	430	n/a	9	n/a	n/a	23	7	1370
Parmesan crusted chicken	as served	630	n/a	5	n/a	n/a	37	14	1500
Sierra chicken	as served	310	n/a	2	n/a	n/a	9	2	930

SEAFOOD

Item	Serving Size	Calories	Protein	Carb	Fiber	Sugar	Total Fat	Sat Fat	Sodium
Golden fried shrimp	as served	620	n/a	50	n/a	n/a	34	6	2240
Grilled fresh rainbow trout	as served	280	n/a	0	n/a	n/a	15	3	460
Grilled trout w/ shrimp	as served	490	n/a	5	n/a	n/a	29	8	1100
LongHorn salmon	as served	290	n/a	3	n/a	n/a	13	2.5	300
Redrock grilled shrimp	as served	90	n/a	2	n/a	n/a	1	0	1120
Shrimp & crab gratin	as served	300	n/a	6	n/a	n/a	14	8	1190

RIBS, CHOPS, & MORE

Item	Serving Size	Calories	Protein	Carb	Fiber	Sugar	Total Fat	Sat Fat	Sodium
Baby Back Ribs	1/2 rack	550	n/a	2	n/a	n/a	37	13	570
Churrasco	as served	535	n/a	20	n/a	n/a	36	13	545
Cowboy pork chops	as served	200	n/a	0	n/a	n/a	7	2.5	800
Longhorn steak tips	as served	550	n/a	23	n/a	n/a	26	7	2260

LEGENDARY STEAKS

Item	Serving Size	Calories	Protein	Carb	Fiber	Sugar	Total Fat	Sat Fat	Sodium
Fire-grilled T-Bone	as served	830	n/a	1	n/a	n/a	57	22	1710
Flo's Filet	9 oz	550	n/a	0	n/a	n/a	34	10	630
Flo's Filet & lobster tail	as served	500	n/a	0	n/a	n/a	30	8	1000
Flo's Filet & Longhorn salmon	as served	740	n/a	3	n/a	n/a	43	11	800

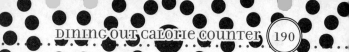

LONGHORN STEAKHOUSE continued

Item	Serving Size	Calories	Protein	Carb	Fiber	Sugar	Total Fat	Sat Fat	Sodium
Flo's Filet & shrimp crab	as served	750	n/a	6	n/a	n/a	44	16	1700
Longhorn Porterhouse	as served	1200	n/a	1	n/a	n/a	85	31	2180
NY/Kansas City strip	as served	950	n/a	2	n/a	n/a	72	26	650
Outlaw ribeye	18 oz	1070	n/a	0	n/a	n/a	79	33	1640

STEAK TOPPINGS & ADD-ONS

Item	Serving Size	Calories	Protein	Carb	Fiber	Sugar	Total Fat	Sat Fat	Sodium
Bleu cheese crusted topping	as served	180	n/a	9	n/a	n/a	14	5	350
Cedar grilled shrimp	as served	90	n/a	3	n/a	n/a	2.5	0.5	590
Grilled onions	as served	90	n/a	11	n/a	n/a	4	0.5	750
Grilled shrimp	as served	45	n/a	1	n/a	n/a	0.5	0	560
Lobster tail	as served	45	n/a	0	n/a	n/a	0	0	500
Parmesan crusted topping	as served	220	n/a	13	n/a	n/a	15	9	330
Sautéed mushroom	as served	90	n/a	5	n/a	n/a	5	1	530
Sautéed mushroom & onion	as served	90	n/a	8	n/a	n/a	4.5	1	640
Shrimp & crab gratin	as served	300	n/a	6	n/a	n/a	14	8	1190

SIDE DISHES

Item	Serving Size	Calories	Protein	Carb	Fiber	Sugar	Total Fat	Sat Fat	Sodium
Caesar side salad	as served	350	n/a	18	n/a	n/a	27	6	550
Fresh seasonal vegetables	as served	90	n/a	9	n/a	n/a	4	1	350
Fresh steamed asparagus	as served	80	n/a	5	n/a	n/a	4.5	1	55
Freshly baked bread (loaf)	as served	510	n/a	96	n/a	n/a	5	1	590
Loaded baked potato	as served	430	n/a	57	n/a	n/a	17	10	150
Mashed potatoes	as served	340	n/a	31	n/a	n/a	22	12	690
Mixed greens side salad	as served	110	n/a	12	n/a	n/a	4.5	2	200
Seasoned French fries	as served	290	n/a	38	n/a	n/a	13	2.5	370
Seasoned rice pilaf	as served	200	n/a	43	n/a	n/a	0.5	0	1600
Steakhouse BLT salad	as served	320	n/a	21	n/a	n/a	21	6	450
Steakhouse mac & cheese	as served	610	n/a	43	n/a	n/a	37	22	1210
Strawberry salad	as served	380	n/a	28	n/a	n/a	27	4.5	240

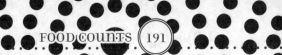

LONGHORN STEAKHOUSE continued

Item	Serving Size	Calories	Protein	Carb	Fiber	Sugar	Total Fat	Sat Fat	Sodium
Sweet potato w/ cinnamon	as served	270	n/a	57	n/a	n/a	1	0	0
DRESSINGS & DIPPING SAUCES									
Avocado-lime sauce	1.5 oz	160	n/a	3	n/a	n/a	16	2.5	350
Balsamic vinaigrette	1.5 oz	190	n/a	2	n/a	n/a	20	3	340
BBQ sauce	1.5 oz	45	n/a	10	n/a	n/a	0.5	0	540
Bleu cheese	1.5 oz	160	n/a	3	n/a	n/a	15	4	490
Caesar	1.5 oz	230	n/a	1	n/a	n/a	24	3.5	580
Chipotle ranch	1.5 oz	200	n/a	5	n/a	n/a	20	3	320
Creamy BBQ sauce	1.5 oz	121	n/a	8	n/a	n/a	10	1.5	500
Fat-free ranch	1.5 oz	45	n/a	12	n/a	n/a	0	0	540
Garlic butter	1.5 oz	170	n/a	1.5	n/a	n/a	18	9.5	200
Honey mustard	1.5 oz	240	n/a	7	n/a	n/a	23	3.5	240
Horseradish sauce	1.5 oz	70	n/a	4	n/a	n/a	6	3	200
Italian	1.5 oz	220	n/a	2	n/a	n/a	25	3.5	660
Oil & vinegar	1.5 oz	180	n/a	0	n/a	n/a	21	3	0
Ranch	1.5 oz	200	n/a	3	n/a	n/a	20	3.5	340
Rasberry vinaigrette	1.5 oz	210	n/a	13	n/a	n/a	18	3	105
Thousand Island	1.5 oz	190	n/a	5	n/a	n/a	17	2.5	400
Tonion sauce	1.5 oz	220	n/a	6	n/a	n/a	22	3.5	370
DESSERTS									
Caramel apple Goldrush	as served	1640	n/a	237	n/a	n/a	71	25	940
Chocolate stampede	serves 2	2180	n/a	229	n/a	n/a	131	73	760
Golden Nugget fried cheesecake	as served	930	n/a	94	n/a	n/a	56	26	510
Key lime pie	as served	630	n/a	102	n/a	n/a	20	9	270
LH Dessert Sampler	serves 2	1650	n/a	192	n/a	n/a	89	49	920
Mountain Top cheesecake	as served	1050	n/a	68	n/a	n/a	80	46	800
Ultimate brownie sundae	as served	1181	n/a	147	n/a	n/a	60	33	220
BEVERAGES, MARGARITAS, & SPECIALTY DRINKS									
1800 Texas Tornado	as served	240	n/a	37	n/a	n/a	0	0	790
Blackberry Firefly tea	as served	230	n/a	41	n/a	n/a	0	0	0
Blackberry mojito	as served	210	n/a	26	n/a	n/a	0	0	15

LONGHORN STEAKHOUSE continued

Item	Serving Size	Calories	Protein	Carb	Fiber	Sugar	Total Fat	Sat Fat	Sodium
Blazing berry sangria	as served	190	n/a	27	n/a	n/a	0	0	50
Desert pear margarita	as served	280	n/a	47	n/a	n/a	0	0	10
Frozen raspberry	as served	250	n/a	39	n/a	n/a	0	0	0
Frozen strawberry	as served	220	n/a	34	n/a	n/a	0	0	15
Goldrush martini	as served	130	n/a	4	n/a	n/a	0	0	4
Green apple martini	as served	160	n/a	11	n/a	n/a	0	0	0
LH Piña colada	as served	420	n/a	66	n/a	n/a	12	10	45
Mojito	as served	200	n/a	25	n/a	n/a	0	0	10
Pomegranate	as served	440	n/a	79	n/a	n/a	0	0	0
Raspberry Lynchburg lemonade	as served	160	n/a	23	n/a	n/a	0	0	10
Raspberry margarita	as served	220	n/a	39	n/a	n/a	0	0	10
Silver Lightening	as served	240	n/a	35	n/a	n/a	0	0	580
Strawberry-banana daiquiri	as served	250	n/a	49	n/a	n/a	0	0	5
Strawberry daiquiri	as served	200	n/a	36	n/a	n/a	0	0	0
Strawberry Goldrush	as served	190	n/a	27	n/a	n/a	0	0	20
Texas	as served	200	n/a	28	n/a	n/a	0	0	990
The Perfect	as served	260	n/a	41	n/a	n/a	0	0	990
Watermelon	as served	240	n/a	36	n/a	n/a	0	0	0
White peach sangria	as served	230	n/a	34	n/a	n/a	0	0	45

KIDS' MENU

Item	Serving Size	Calories	Protein	Carb	Fiber	Sugar	Total Fat	Sat Fat	Sodium
Banana berry smoothie	as served	230	n/a	56	n/a	n/a	0	0	0
Cheeseburger	as served	510	n/a	31	n/a	n/a	29	12.5	870
Chicken tenders	as served	340	n/a	15	n/a	n/a	18	3.5	450
Fresh fruit, cantaloupe	as served	53	n/a	13	n/a	n/a	0	0	25
Fresh fruit, oranges	as served	20	n/a	4	n/a	n/a	0	0	0
Fresh fruit, watermelon	as served	46	n/a	12	n/a	n/a	0	0	2
Grilled cheese sandwich	as served	350	n/a	29	n/a	n/a	20	11	1120
Grilled chicken salad	as served	270	n/a	5	n/a	n/a	9	3	190
Grilled chicken tenders	as served	140	n/a	0	n/a	n/a	2	0	150
Hot dog	as served	310	n/a	23	n/a	n/a	20	8	750

LONGHORN STEAKHOUSE continued

Item	Serving Size	Calories	Protein	Carb	Fiber	Sugar	Total Fat	Sat Fat	Sodium
Kids' fountain drink	as served	63	n/a	16	n/a	n/a	0	0	21
Kids' sirloin	as served	360	n/a	0	n/a	n/a	25	7	120
Kraft macaroni & cheese	as served	300	n/a	45	n/a	n/a	9	2.5	570
Peanut butter cup smoothie	as served	680	n/a	80	n/a	n/a	33	19	300
Rasberry dream smoothie	as served	320	n/a	51	n/a	n/a	12	8	65
Seasoned fries	as served	290	n/a	38	n/a	n/a	13	2.5	370

MCDONALD'S

Item	Serving Size	Calories	Protein	Carb	Fiber	Sugar	Total Fat	Sat Fat	Sodium
BEVERAGES									
Caramel frappe	small	450	6	62	0	56	20	13	130
Caramel frappe	medium	550	8	77	0	71	24	15	160
Caramel frappe	large	680	10	94	0	88	29	18	200
Caramel iced coffee	medium	190	2	27	0	27	8	5	115
Caramel iced coffee	large	270	2	41	0	41	11	7	160
Hazelnut iced coffee	medium	190	2	29	0	29	8	5	60
Hazelnut iced coffee	large	270	2	43	0	43	11	7	85
Mocha frappe	small	450	7	62	1	56	20	13	130
Mocha frappe	medium	560	8	78	1	70	24	15	160
Mocha frappe	large	680	1	96	1	87	28	18	200
Regular iced coffee	medium	200	2	30	0	30	8	5	60
Regular iced coffee	large	280	2	45	0	45	11	7	85
Strawberry banana smoothie w/ yogurt	small	210	2	49	2	44	0.5	0	35
Strawberry banana smoothie w/ yogurt	medium	260	2	60	3	54	1	0	40
Strawberry banana smoothie w/ yogurt	large	330	3	77	4	70	1	0.5	55
Sugar free vanilla iced coffee	medium	90	2	11	0	2	8	5	100
Sugar free vanilla iced coffee	large	120	2	16	0	2	11	7	140
Vanilla iced coffee	medium	190	2	29	0	28	8	5	60

MCDONALD'S continued

Item	Serving Size	Calories	Protein	Carb	Fiber	Sugar	Total Fat	Sat Fat	Sodium
Vanilla iced coffee	large	270	2	43	0	43	11	7	80
Wild berry smoothie w/ yogurt	small	210	2	48	3	44	0.5	0	30
Wild berry smoothie w/ yogurt	medium	260	3	60	4	55	1	0	35
Wild berry smoothie w/ yogurt	large	320	3	75	4	69	1	0.5	45

MCCAFE DRINKS MADE W/ NONFAT MILK

Item	Serving Size	Calories	Protein	Carb	Fiber	Sugar	Total Fat	Sat Fat	Sodium
Cappuccino	small	60	6	9	0	9	0	0	85
Cappuccino	medium	80	8	12	0	12	0	0	110
Cappuccino	large	90	9	13	0	13	0	0	130
Caramel cappuccino	small	150	5	33	0	32	0	0	120
Caramel cappuccino	medium	190	6	41	0	41	0	0	150
Caramel cappuccino	large	230	7	49	0	49	0	0	180
Caramel latte	small	170	7	36	0	36	0	0	150
Caramel latte	medium	220	9	45	0	45	0	0	180
Caramel latte	large	260	10	53	0	53	0	0	220
Hazelnut cappuccino	small	150	5	34	0	34	0	0	70
Hazelnut cappuccino	medium	190	6	43	0	43	0	0	90
Hazelnut cappuccino	large	230	7	51	0	51	0	0	100
Hazelnut latte	small	180	7	37	0	37	0	0	95
Hazelnut latte	medium	220	9	46	0	46	0	0	115
Hazelnut latte	large	260	10	55	0	55	0	0	135
Hot chocolate	small	250	8	43	0	37	5	3	140
Hot chocolate	medium	310	11	55	0	47	6	3.5	190
Hot chocolate	large	390	16	68	0	59	6	3.5	250
Iced caramel latte	small	140	3	30	0	30	0	0	105
Iced caramel latte	medium	150	5	32	0	32	0	0	120
Iced caramel latte	large	190	6	40	0	40	0	0	150
Iced hazelnut latte	small	140	3	32	0	32	0	0	50
Iced hazelnut latte	medium	150	5	33	0	33	0	0	70
Iced hazelnut latte	large	190	6	42	0	42	0	0	80
Iced latte	small	50	5	7	0	7	0	0	70
Iced latte	medium	60	6	9	0	9	0	0	90
Iced latte	large	70	7	11	0	11	0	0	105
Iced mocha	small	230	6	35	0	29	7	4.5	115

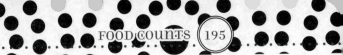
MCDONALD'S continued

Item	Serving Size	Calories	Protein	Carb	Fiber	Sugar	Total Fat	Sat Fat	Sodium
Iced mocha	medium	27	7	43	0	35	8	4.5	140
Iced mocha	large	340	8	58	0	48	8	5	180
Iced sugar free vanilla latte	small	40	4	13	0	5	0	0	85
Iced sugar free vanilla latte	medium	50	5	14	0	6	0	0	100
Iced sugar free vanilla latte	large	110	11	21	0	15	0	0	190
Iced vanilla latte	small	140	3	31	0	31	0	0	50
Iced vanilla latte	medium	150	5	33	0	33	0	0	70
Iced vanilla latte	large	190	6	41	0	41	0	0	85
Latte	small	90	9	13	0	13	0	0	115
Latte	medium	110	10	15	0	15	0	0	140
Latte	large	120	12	18	0	18	0	0	160
Mocha	small	240	7	41	0	34	5	3	130
Mocha	medium	280	8	50	0	42	6	3.5	160
Mocha	large	330	10	58	0	50	6	3.5	190
Sugar free vanilla cappuccino	small	50	5	15	0	8	0	0	100
Sugar free vanilla cappuccino	medium	70	7	19	0	10	0	0	130
Sugar free vanilla cappuccino	large	80	8	22	0	11	0	0	150
Sugar free vanilla latte	small	80	7	18	0	11	0	0	130
Sugar free vanilla latte	medium	9	9	22	0	13	0	0	160
Sugar free vanilla latte	large	110	11	27	0	15	0	0	190
Vanilla cappuccino	small	150	5	34	0	34	0	0	70
Vanilla cappuccino	medium	190	6	42	0	42	0	0	90
Vanilla cappuccino	large	230	7	51	0	51	0	0	100
Vanilla latte	small	180	7	37	0	37	0	0	95
Vanilla latte	medium	220	9	46	0	46	0	0	115
Vanilla latte	large	260	10	55	0	55	0	0	135

MCCAFE DRINKS MADE W/ WHOLE MILK

Item	Serving Size	Calories	Protein	Carb	Fiber	Sugar	Total Fat	Sat Fat	Sodium
Cappuccino	small	120	6	9	0	9	7	4	85
Cappuccino	medium	140	8	11	0	11	8	4.5	90
Cappuccino	large	180	9	1	0	13	10	6	130
Caramel cappuccino	small	20	5	32	0	32	5	3	125

MCDONALD'S continued

Item	Serving Size	Calories	Protein	Carb	Fiber	Sugar	Total Fat	Sat Fat	Sodium
Caramel cappuccino	medium	240	6	41	0	40	6	3.5	150
Caramel cappuccino	large	290	8	49	0	49	8	4.5	190
Caramel latte	small	230	7	35	0	35	7	4	140
Caramel latte	medium	280	8	43	0	43	8	4.5	170
Caramel latte	large	330	9	52	0	51	9	5	210
Hazelnut cappuccino	small	200	5	34	0	34	5	3	70
Hazelnut cappuccino	medium	240	6	42	0	42	6	3.5	85
Hazelnut cappuccino	large	290	7	51	0	51	8	4.5	105
Hazelnut latte	small	230	7	36	0	36	7	4	90
Hazelnut latte	medium	280	8	45	0	45	8	4.5	110
Hazelnut latte	large	330	9	53	0	53	9	5	130
Hot chocolate	small	300	8	41	0	35	12	7	135
Hot chocolate	medium	340	10	53	0	45	15	9	170
Hot chocolate	Large	460	13	63	0	54	18	10	220
Iced caramel latte	large	160	3	29	0	29	3	1.5	100
Iced caramel latte	medium	180	4	31	0	31	4.5	2.5	120
Iced caramel latte	large	230	6	40	0	40	6	3.5	150
Iced hazelnut latte	small	160	3	31	0	31	3	1.5	45
Iced hazelnut latte	medium	180	4	33	0	33	4.5	2.5	65
Iced hazelnut latte	large	230	6	41	0	41	6	3.5	85
Iced latte	small	80	4	6	0	6	4.5	2.5	65
Iced latte	medium	100	6	8	0	8	6	3.5	80
Iced latte	large	140	7	10	0	10	8	4.5	105
Iced mocha	small	260	5	34	0	28	12	7	115
Iced mocha	medium	310	7	42	0	35	13	8	140
Iced mocha	large	390	7	57	0	47	14	9	170
Iced sugar free vanilla latte	small	60	3	12	0	4	3	2	80
Iced sugar free vanilla latte	medium	90	5	14	0	6	5	3	105
Iced sugar free vanilla latte	large	180	10	25	0	13	10	6	180
Iced vanilla latte	small	160	3	31	0	31	3	1.5	45
Iced vanilla latte	medium	190	5	33	0	33	4.5	2.5	70
Iced vanilla latte	large	230	6	41	0	41	6	3.5	85
Latte	small	150	8	11	0	11	8	4.5	105
Latte	medium	180	10	13	0	13	10	6	130

MCDONALD'S continued

Item	Serving Size	Calories	Protein	Carb	Fiber	Sugar	Total Fat	Sat Fat	Sodium
Latte	large	210	11	16	0	16	11	7	150
Mocha	small	280	6	40	0	33	11	6	125
Mocha	medium	330	7	48	0	41	12	7	150
Mocha	large	400	10	58	0	49	14	8	190
Sugar free vanilla cappuccino	small	100	5	15	0	7	5	3	105
Sugar free vanilla cappuccino	medium	120	6	18	0	9	6	3.5	130
Sugar free vanilla cappuccino	large	150	8	22	0	11	8	4.5	160
Sugar free vanilla latte	small	130	7	17	0	10	7	4	125
Sugar free vanilla latte	medium	160	8	21	0	11	8	5	150
Sugar free vanilla latte	large	180	10	25	0	13	10	6	180
Vanilla cappuccino	small	200	5	34	0	34	5	3	70
Vanilla cappuccino	medium	240	6	42	0	42	6	3.5	85
Vanilla cappuccino	large	290	7	51	0	51	8	4.5	105
Vanilla latte	small	230	7	36	0	36	7	4	90
Vanilla latte	medium	280	8	44	0	44	8	4.5	110
Vanilla latte	large	330	9	53	0	53	9	5	130

SANDWICHES & WRAPS

Item	Serving Size	Calories	Protein	Carb	Fiber	Sugar	Total Fat	Sat Fat	Sodium
Angus bacon & cheese Snack Wrap®	each	790	45	63	4	13	39	17	2070
Angus deluxe Snack Wrap®	each	750	40	61	4	11	39	17	1700
Angus mushroom & Swiss Snack Wrap®	each	770	44	59	4	8	40	17	1170
Big Mac®	each	540	25	45	3	9	29	10	1040
Big N' Tasty®	each	460	24	37	3	8	24	8	720
Big N' Tasty® w/ cheese	each	510	27	38	3	8	28	11	960
Cheeseburger	each	300	15	33	2	6	12	6	750
Chicken McNuggets®	each	190	10	11	0	0	12	2	400
Chicken McNuggets®	each	280	14	16	0	0	17	3	600
Chicken McNuggets®	each	460	24	27	0	0	29	5	1000
Chicken Selects®	3 pieces	400	23	23	0	0	24	3.5	1010
Chicken Selects®	5 pieces	660	38	39	0	0	40	6	1680
Chipotle Snack Wrap®, crispy	each	330	14	35	1	4	15	4.5	810

MCDONALD'S continued

Item	Serving Size	Calories	Protein	Carb	Fiber	Sugar	Total Fat	Sat Fat	Sodium
Chipotle Snack Wrap®, grilled	each	260	18	28	1	5	9	3.5	830
Double cheeseburger	each	440	25	34	2	7	23	11	1150
Double Quarter Pounder® w/ cheese	each	740	48	40	3	9	42	19	1380
Filet-O-Fish®	each	380	15	38	2	5	18	3.5	640
Hamburger	each	250	12	31	2	6	9	3.5	520
Honey Mustard Snack Wrap®, crispy	each	330	14	34	1	4	16	4.5	780
Honey Mustard Snack Wrap®, grilled	each	260	18	27	1	4	9	3.5	800
Mac Snack Wrap®	each	330	15	26	1	3	19	7	690
McChicken®	each	360	14	40	2	5	16	3	830
McDouble®	each	390	22	33	2	7	19	8	920
Premium Chicken Classic Sandwich, crispy	each	530	28	59	3	12	20	3.5	1150
Premium Chicken Classic Sandwich, grilled	each	420	32	51	3	11	10	2	1190
Premium Chicken Club Sandwich, crispy	each	630	35	60	4	13	28	7	1360
Premium Chicken Club Sandwich, grilled	each	530	39	52	4	12	18	6	1410
Premium Chicken Ranch BLT Sandwich, crispy	each	580	31	62	3	13	23	4.5	1400
Premium Chicken Ranch BLT Sandwich, grilled	each	470	36	53	3	13	12	3	1440
Quarter Pounder®	each	410	24	37	2	8	19	7	730
Quarter Pounder® w/ cheese	each	510	29	40	3	9	26	12	1190
Ranch Snack Wrap®, crispy	each	340	14	33	1	2	17	4.5	810
Ranch Snack Wrap®, grilled	each	270	18	26	1	2	10	4	830
Southern Style Chicken Sandwich	each	400	24	39	1	6	17	3	1030
FRENCH FRIES									
French fries	small	230	3	29	3	0	11	1.5	160
French fries	medium	380	4	48	5	0	19	2.5	270
French fries	large	500	6	63	6	0	25	3.5	350

MCDONALD'S continued

Item	Serving Size	Calories	Protein	Carb	Fiber	Sugar	Total Fat	Sat Fat	Sodium
CONDIMENTS, DRESSINGS, & SAUCES									
Barbecue sauce	1 pkg	50	0	12	0	10	0	0	260
Butter garlic croutons	1 pkg	60	0	10	1	0	1.5	0	140
Creamy ranch sauce	1 pkg	170	0	2	0	1	18	3	270
Grape jam	1 pkg	35	9	9	0	9	0	0	0
Honey	1 pkg	50	0	12	0	11	0	0	0
Hot mustard sauce	1 pkg	60	1	9	2	6	2.5	0	250
Hotcake syrup	1 pkg	180	33	45	0	33	0	0	20
Ketchup	1 pkg	15	0	3	0	2	0	0	110
Low fat caramel dip	1 pkg	70	9	15	0	9	0.5	0	35
Margarine	1 pat	40	0	0	0	0	4.5	1.5	55
Newman's Own creamy Caesar dressing	1 pkg	190	2	4	0	2	18	3.5	500
Newman's Own creamy Southwest dressing	1 pkg	100	3	11	0	3	6	1	340
Newman's Own low-fat balsamic vinaigrette	1 pkg	40	3	4	0	3	3	0	730
Newman's Own low-fat Family Recipe Italian dressing	1 pkg	60	1	8	0	1	2.5	0	730
Newman's Own ranch dressing	1 pkg	170	4	9	0	4	15	2.5	530
Picante sauce, hot	1 pkg	5	0	1	0	0	0	0	140
Picante sauce, mild	1 pkg	5	0	1	0	0	0	0	120
Southwestern chipotle barbecue sauce	1 pkg	60	0	15	1	11	0	0	210
Spicy Buffalo sauce	1 pkg	60	0	1	1	0	6	1	800
Strawberry preserves	1 pkg	35	9	9	0	9	0	0	0
Sweet n' sour sauce	1 pkg	50	0	12	0	10	0	0	150
Tangy honey mustard sauce	1 pkg	60	0	10	0	8	2	0	140
SALADS									
Premium bacon ranch salad w/ crispy chicken	each	370	29	20	3	6	20	6	970
Premium bacon ranch salad w/ grilled chicken	each	260	33	12	3	5	9	4	1010
Premium bacon ranch salad w/out chicken	each	140	9	10	3	4	7	3.5	300

MCDONALD'S continued

Item	Serving Size	Calories	Protein	Carb	Fiber	Sugar	Total Fat	Sat Fat	Sodium
Premium Caesar salad w/ crispy chicken	each	330	26	20	3	6	17	4.5	840
Premium Caesar salad w/ grilled chicken	each	220	30	12	3	5	6	3	890
Premium Caesar salad w/out chicken	each	90	7	9	3	44	4	2.5	180
Premium Southwest salad w/ crispy chicken	each	430	26	38	6	12	20	4	920
Premium Southwest salad w/ grilled chicken	each	320	30	30	6	11	9	3	960
Premium Southwest salad w/out chicken	each	140	6	20	6	6	4.5	2	150
Side salad	each	20	2	4	1	2	0	0	10
Snack Size Fruit & Walnut Salad	each	210	25	31	2	25	8	1.5	60

BREAKFAST

Item	Serving Size	Calories	Protein	Carb	Fiber	Sugar	Total Fat	Sat Fat	Sodium
Bacon, egg, & cheese bagel	each	560	7	56	3	7	27	9	1300
Bacon, egg, & cheese biscuit	regular	420	3	37	n/a	3	23	12	1160
Bacon, egg, & cheese biscuit	large	480	4	43	3	4	27	12	1270
Bacon, egg, & cheese McGriddles®	each	420	15	48	2	15	18	8	1110
Bagel, plain	each	26	6	49	2	6	3	0	520
Big Breakfast®	regular	740	3	51	3	3	48	17	1560
Big Breakfast®	large	800	3	56	4	3	52	18	1680
Big Breakfast® w/ hotcakes	regular	1090	17	111	6	17	56	19	2150
Big Breakfast® w/ hotcakes	large	1150	17	116	7	17	60	20	2260
Egg McMuffin®	each	300	3	30	2	3	12	5	820
Hash browns	each	150	0	15	2	0	9	1.5	310
Hotcakes & sausage w/o syrup or margarine	as served	520	14	61	3	14	24	7	930
Hotcakes w/o syrup or margarine	as served	350	14	60	3	14	9	2	590

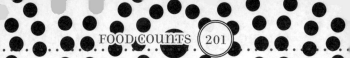

MCDONALD'S continued

Item	Serving Size	Calories	Protein	Carb	Fiber	Sugar	Total Fat	Sat Fat	Sodium
McSkillet™ Burrito w/ Sausage	each	610	4	44	3	4	36	14	1390
Sausage biscuit	regular	430	2	34	2	2	27	12	1080
Sausage biscuit	large	480	3	39	3	3	31	13	1190
Sausage biscuit w/ egg	regular	510	2	36	2	2	33	14	1170
Sausage biscuit w/ egg	large	570	3	42	3	3	37	15	1280
Sausage burrito	each	300	2	26	1	2	16	7	830
Sausage McGriddles®	each	420	15	44	2	15	22	8	1030
Sausage McMuffin®	each	370	2	29	2	2	22	8	850
Sausage McMuffin® w/ egg	each	450	2	30	2	2	27	10	920
Sausage, egg & cheese McGriddles	each	560	15	48	2	15	32	12	1360
Southern style chicken biscuit	regular	410	3	41	2	3	20	8	1180
Southern style chicken biscuit	large	470	4	46	3	4	24	9	1290
Scrambled eggs	2 eggs	170	0	1	0	0	11	4	180

DESSERT

Item	Serving Size	Calories	Protein	Carb	Fiber	Sugar	Total Fat	Sat Fat	Sodium
Apple dippers	1 pkg	35	6	8	0	6	0	0	0
Baked hot apple pie	each	250	13	32	4	13	13	7	170
Caramel sundae	each	340	44	60	1	44	8	5	160
Chocolate chip cookie	each	160	15	21	1	15	8	3.5	90
Chocolate McCafé® shake w/ whipped cream & cherry	small	580	77	94	1	77	17	10	240
Chocolate McCafé® shake w/ whipped cream & cherry	medium	720	98	119	1	98	20	12	300
Chocolate McCafé® shake w/ whipped cream & cherry	large	880	121	147	1	121	24	15	370
Cinnamon melts	each	460	32	66	3	32	19	9	370
Fruit 'n yogurt parfait w/ granola	each	160	21	31	1	21	2	1	85
Fruit 'n yogurt parfait w/o granola	each	130	19	25	0	19	2	1	55
Hot fudge sundae	each	330	48	54	2	48	10	7	180

MCDONALD'S continued

Item	Serving Size	Calories	Protein	Carb	Fiber	Sugar	Total Fat	Sat Fat	Sodium
McDonaldland® cookies	1 bag	250	13	42	1	13	8	2	280
McFlurry® w/ M&M'S	small	430	59	64	2	59	16	10	130
McFlurry® w/ M&M'S	medium	710	97	105	4	97	25	16	220
McFlurry® w/ M&M'S	large	930	128	137	5	128	33	21	280
McFlurry® w/ Oreo cookies	small	340	43	53	2	43	12	6	200
McFlurry® w/ Oreo cookies	medium	580	73	89	3	73	19	10	320
McFlurry® w/ Oreo cookies	large	750	95	116	4	95	25	13	430
Oatmeal raisin cookie	each	150	13	22	1	13	6	2.5	135
Peanuts, for sundaes	1 pkg	45	0	2	1	0	3.5	0.5	0
Strawberry McCafé® shake w/ whipped cream & cherry	small	570	79	92	0	79	17	10	170
Strawberry McCafé® shake w/ whipped cream & cherry	medium	710	100	116	0	100	20	12	210
Strawberry McCafé® shake w/ whipped cream & cherry	large	860	124	144	0	124	24	15	260
Strawberry sundae	each	280	45	49	1	45	6	4	95
Sugar cookie	each	160	11	21	0	11	7	3	120
Vanilla McCafé® shake w/ whipped cream & cherry	small	540	64	88	0	64	16	10	170
Vanilla McCafé® shake w/ whipped cream & cherry	medium	680	82	111	0	82	20	12	220
Vanilla McCafé® shake w/ whipped cream & cherry	large	830	103	138	0	103	24	14	270
Vanilla reduced-fat ice cream cone	each	150	18	24	0	18	3.5	2	60

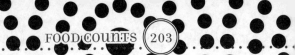

MRS. FIELDS

Item	Serving Size	Calories	Protein	Carb	Fiber	Sugar	Total Fat	Sat Fat	Sodium
MRS. FIELDS® COOKIES									
Butter	each	200	2	29	<1	15	8	3.5	180
Cut Out	each	400	2	56	0	32	19	7	230
Debra's special	each	200	3	28	1	16	9	3	160
Macadamia	each	230	3	27	1	18	12	5	150
Peanut butter	each	210	4	24	1	12	12	4	190
Semi-sweet chocolate	each	210	2	29	1	19	10	5	170
Semi-sweet chocolate w/ walnuts	each	220	2	29	2	18	11	4.5	140
Triple chocolate	each	210	2	28	2	18	11	5	140
White chunk macadamia	each	230	3	27	1	18	12	5	150
BITE-SIZE NIBBLER® COOKIES									
Cinnamon sugar	3 cookies	180	2	25	0	12	8	2.5	210
Debra's Special Nibbler	3 cookies	160	2	22	1	13	7	2	160
Peanut butter	3 cookies	170	3	19	1	10	9	2.5	180
Semi-sweet chocolate	3 cookies	170	2	23	1	14	8	3.5	140
Triple chocolate	3 cookies	160	2	22	1	15	8	4	150
White chunk macadamia	3 cookies	180	2	22	0	15	9	4	140
BROWNIE BITES									
Butterscotch blondie	3 bites	200	n/a	29	0	22	8	5	15
Double fudge	3 bites	200	2	27	1	21	10	5	75
Toffee fudge	3 bites	200	n/a	26	1	21	11	5	85
BROWNIES									
Butterscotch blondie	each	260	3	38	0	28	10	6	20
Double fudge	each	260	3	34	1	27	13	8	95
Pecan fudge	each	270	3	32	2	25	15	7	95
Special walnut fudge & blondie	each	260	3	35	1	27	13	7	55
Toffee fudge	each	260	3	34	1	27	14	7	110
Walnut fudge	each	270	3	32	2	25	15	7	95
COFFEE CAKE									
Chocolate chip	large	250	3	32	1	16	12	3.5	340
Chocolate chip	small	240	3	30	1	16	11	3.5	320

MRS. FIELDS continued

Item	Serving Size	Calories	Protein	Carb	Fiber	Sugar	Total Fat	Sat Fat	Sodium
ENROBED COOKIES									
Peanut butter	each	340	5	37	1	26	19	10	230
Semi-sweet	each	380	5	40	1	37	23	15	65
White chunk macadamia	each	330	3	39	1	29	19	10	170
MRS. FIELDS® CAKES									
Chocolate chip	each	350	4	45	-1	27	17	8	330
MRS. FIELDS® MUFFINS									
Blueberry	each	190	3	24	1	12	9	2.5	280
Chocolate chip	each	200	3	26	1	14	10	3	270
Raspberry	each	190	3	24	1	12	9	2.5	280

NOODLES & COMPANY

Item	Serving Size	Calories	Protein	Carb	Fiber	Sugar	Total Fat	Sat Fat	Sodium
ASIAN BOWLS									
Bangkok curry	as served	490	9	85	7	n/a	13	9	860
Chinese chop salad	as served	310	6	40	6	n/a	15	1.5	370
Indonesian peanut sauté	as served	950	22	165	13	n/a	23	4	2110
Japanese pan noodles	as served	690	19	133	10	n/a	9	1.5	2160
Pad Thai	as served	700	11	117	5	n/a	20	3	1840
Thai curry soup	as served	480	0	70	3	n/a	19	15	1580
MEDITERRANEAN BOWLS									
Pasta fresca	as served	780	27	111	6	n/a	22	6	770
Penne rosa	as served	810	24	119	15	n/a	26	13	1100
Pesto cavatappi	as served	910	36	124	8	n/a	30	12	1240
The Med Salad	as served	310	10	39	4	n/a	13	4.5	960
Tomato bisque	as served	420	0	45	13	n/a	23	12	3530
Whole grain Tuscan linguine	as served	770	26	108	20	n/a	26	8	1370
AMERICAN BOWLS									
Buttered noodles	as served	620	33	84	7	n/a	16	3.5	1590
Caesar salad	as served	320	11	11	2	n/a	28	7	780
Chicken noodle soup	as served	300	20	44	10	n/a	4	1	2290

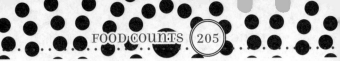

NOODLES & COMPANY continued

Item	Serving Size	Calories	Protein	Carb	Fiber	Sugar	Total Fat	Sat Fat	Sodium
Mushroom Stroganoff	as served	780	28	100	10	n/a	31	17	980
Spaghetti	as served	670	26	101	9	n/a	18	6	1170
Spaghetti & meatballs	as served	900	43	104	9	n/a	35	12	1790
Wisconsin mac & cheese	as served	900	36	119	13	n/a	31	18	1100

PROTEINS

Item	Serving Size	Calories	Protein	Carb	Fiber	Sugar	Total Fat	Sat Fat	Sodium
Braised beef	as served	190	28	0	0	n/a	10	3.5	370
Chicken breast	as served	130	22	0	0	n/a	2.5	0.5	720
Meatballs	as served	230	17	3	0	n/a	17	6	620
Organic tofu	as served	180	16	4	0	n/a	11	1.5	220
Parmesan-crusted chicken	as served	190	17	1	0	n/a	8	1.5	620
Sautéed beef	as served	210	25	1	0	n/a	12	4	480
Sautéed shrimp	as served	35	8	0	0	n/a	0	0	190

SANDWICHES

Item	Serving Size	Calories	Protein	Carb	Fiber	Sugar	Total Fat	Sat Fat	Sodium
Caesar dressing	side	180	1	1	0	n/a	19	3	440
Mmmeatball	as served	620	36	60	4	n/a	26	10	2040
Spicy chicken Caesar	as served	320	24	40	2	n/a	8	2	920
The Med	as served	340	23	40	2	n/a	11	3	1110
Veggie Med	as served	300	45	10	3	n/a	11	3	890
Wisconsin cheesesteak	as served	610	41	52	4	n/a	27	12	1560
Wisconsin cheesesteak on flatbread	as served	580	38	42	2	n/a	30	12	1470

EXTRAS & DESSERTS

Item	Serving Size	Calories	Protein	Carb	Fiber	Sugar	Total Fat	Sat Fat	Sodium
Chocolate chunk cookie	each	360	6	65	2	n/a	8	2.5	135
Ciabatta roll	as served	160	6	31	2	n/a	1.5	0	430
Cucumber tomato salad	as served	80	2	18	2	n/a	0	0	190
Flat bread	as served	210	7	37	2	n/a	3.5	0.5	370
Potstickers	as served	340	16	49	3	n/a	9	1.5	1630
Rice Crispy Treat	each	530	4	90	0	n/a	19	12	640
Snoodledoodle cookie	each	350	6	65	2	n/a	7	3.5	350
Tossed green salad	as served	60	1	3	1	n/a	6	0.5	140
Tossed green salad w/ fat free Asian	as served	30	1	7	1	n/a	0	0	50

NOTHING BUT NOODLES

Item	Serving Size	Calories	Protein	Carb	Fiber	Sugar	Total Fat	Sat Fat	Sodium
ENTRÉES									
Basil pesto	1 serving	574	14	36	3	1	42	18	334
Beef Stroganoff	1 serving	508	26	33	2	3	31	14	1499
Buttery noodles	1 serving	651	19	46	2	1	44	26	1538
Cappelini primavera	1 serving	500	10	56	4	18	28	5	333
Cheesy chicken & vegetables	1 serving	318	29	6	2	2	21	12	970
Chicken pomodoro	1 serving	452	28	7	2	2	34	19	1040
Eggplant Parmesan	1 serving	725	19	79	6.5	8	37	8	746
Fettuccini Alfredo	1 serving	723	20	36	2	1	56	35	1053
General Tso's chicken	1 serving	760	24	69	1	12	44	5	1538
Kung Pao chicken	1 serving	935	31	89	5	23	51	6	460
Lobster ravioli	1 serving	637	24	21	3.5	2	80.5	38.5	1189
Margherita pasta	1 serving	474	9	36	3	3	31	5	2153
Marinara pasta	1 serving	487	23	77	8	4	11	5	1075
Pad Thai noodles	1 serving	602	14	118	4	39	10	2	2817
Primavera chicken & vegetable wrap	1 serving	318	22	26	2	16	15	3	722
Santa Fe pasta	1 serving	705	18	40	3	4	54	29	1714
Sesame lo mein	1 serving	411	5	64	4	8	11	2	1737
Shrimp pesto Florentine	1 serving	308	16	5	2	1	25	12	357
Southwest chipotle	1 serving	713	11	41	4	3	58	32	1822
Spicy cajun pasta	1 serving	660	9	44	4	6	50	29	1517
Spicy Japanese noodles	1 serving	419	10	74	4	13	8	1	1453
Stuffed shells	1 serving	701	27	28	3	3	57	33.5	1238
Thai curry beef & vegetables	1 serving	443	32	16	4	7	30	13	899
Thai peanut	1 serving	568	11	89	5	12	20	5	1638
Thai peanut stir fry	1 serving	595	29	59	3	12	27	5	885
Three-cheese macaroni	1 serving	446	20	45	2	2	21	12	392
ADD-ONS									
Beef	1 serving	110	17	0	0	0	4	1	227
Chicken	1 serving	100	18	0	0	0	3	1	487
Shrimp	1 serving	53	10	1	0	0	1	0	74

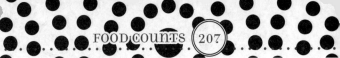

NOTHING BUT NOODLES continued

Item	Serving Size	Calories	Protein	Carb	Fiber	Sugar	Total Fat	Sat Fat	Sodium
Tofu	1 serving	60	7	1	0	0	4	1	7
SALADS									
BBQ chicken salad	1 serving	205	9	11	3	3	15	3	225
Caesar salad	1 serving	247	7	14	2	3	19	4	677
Chopped salad	1 serving	229	7	10	3	3	15	4	480
Cranberry spinich salad	1 serving	154	3	18	3	10	10	2	92
Cucumber side salad	1 serving	193	2	13	1	6	16	1	653
Garden fresh salad	1 serving	110	5	12	2	2	5	2	249
Greek salad	1 serving	409	9	26	3	2	31	8	661
Hunk of lettuce	1 serving	229	6	7	2	2	21	6	706
Mandarin orange salad	1 serving	205	2	13	2	10	14	2	245
Oriental salad	1 serving	187	4	20	4	5	11	2	151
Pear & balsamic spinach salad	1 serving	395	7	38	3	24	28	5	249
Spicy cucumber & chicken salad	1 serving	284	28	10	3	4	15	5	911
Steak salad	1 serving	135	11	7	2	2	19	5	220
Sun-dried tomato salad	1 serving	271	11	32	4	5	12	2	773
DRESSING									
Buttermilk ranch	1 portion	55	0	1	0	1	6	1	140
Creamy balsamic	1 portion	151	0	20	0	14	10	1	12
Golden Italian	1 portion	55	0	2	0	2	6	1	150
Oriental salad dressing	1 portion	135	0	12	1	10	10	1	132
Poppy seed	1 portion	70	0	5	0	4	6	1	175
Roasted garlic balsamic vinaigrette	1 portion	30	0	2	0	2	3	1	155
Tuscan Caesar	1 portion	70	1	1	0	0	7	1	8
KIDS'									
Alfredo	kid's portion	719	19	39	2	1	55	34	949
Buttery noodles	kid's portion	723	21	51	2	1	49	29	1709
Macaroni & cheese	kid's portion	454	18	38	2	2	26	16	748
Spaghetti	kid's portion	290	13	47	5	2	6	3	611

NOTHING BUT NOODLES continued

Item	Serving Size	Calories	Protein	Carb	Fiber	Sugar	Total Fat	Sat Fat	Sodium
STARTERS									
Fresh mozzarella	per serving	767	20	134	1	88	27	10	488
Garlic breadsticks	per serving	106	2	28	1	1	4	1	214
Mozzarella cheese bread	per serving	633	33	86	3	5	17	8	1314
Potstickers	per serving	479	11	39	5	10	33	3	2163
Thai lettuce wraps	per serving	361	24	15	2	7	23	6	1241
SOUP									
Tomato bisque	as served	253	2	9	1	2	23	0	434
DESSERTS									
Cannoli	per serving	374	10	44	1	34	17	7	88
Cotton candy	per serving	65	0	17	0	18	0	0	7
Key lime pie	per serving	590	11	67	1	50	33	19	290
New York cheesecake	per serving	710	15	59	0	49	53	32	0
Triple chocolate Cake	per serving	710	6	106	4	61	33	9	620

O'CHARLEY'S

Item	Serving Size	Calories	Protein	Carb	Fiber	Sugar	Total Fat	Sat Fat	Sodium
BREAKFAST, BRUNCH, LUNCH, & DINNER									
12-spice chicken pasta	as served	1390	64	103	7	15	77	35	1760
12-spice chicken pasta	Lunch Combo	710	33	52	3	7	39	18	910
Authentic spinach & artichoke dip	as served	780	14	86	6	2	44	13	1530
Baked penne Italiano	as served	1700	54	142	7	10	99	41	3350
Barbacoa quesadilla	as served	1170	62	64	4	8	73	31	2810
Bayou shrimp pasta	as served	1640	59	155	8	17	87	32	3420
Better Cheddar bacon burger	as served	990	59	55	3	8	57	23	1710
Better with bacon patty melt	as served	1110	64	63	3	3	64	25	1740
Boneless Buffalo O'Tenders	as served	880	46	27	2	4	66	12	3500

O'CHARLEY'S continued

Item	Serving Size	Calories	Protein	Carb	Fiber	Sugar	Total Fat	Sat Fat	Sodium
Broccoli, à la carte	as served	140	5	11	5	4	10	2	1130
Broccoli cheese casserole, à La carte	as served	270	10	20	4	5	16	5	830
Brunch quesadilla	as served	1220	53	65	4	7	82	33	2490
Brunch quesadilla w/ chopped Applewood bacon	as served	1370	62	65	4	7	95	38	3020
Brunch toast w/ Jelly	as served	260	5	38	1	15	10	2	320
Buffalo kickin' sandwich	as served	1180	46	79	4	8	74	13	4010
Build Your Own Waffle	as served	460	10	57	1	1	20	11	950
Build Your Own Waffle, w/ side of chocolate chips semi sweet	as served	210	3	27	0	26	12	0	40
Build Your Own Waffle, w/ side of chopped pecans	as served	210	3	4	2	1	21	2	0
Build Your Own Waffle, w/ side of fresh strawberries	as served	10	0	3	1	2	0	0	0
Build Your Own Waffle, w/ side of Reeses peanut butter cups	as served	160	4	18	1	15	10	3.5	125
Catfish platter	as served	1430	38	46	23	4	121	20	2800
Cedar-planked salmon	as served	530	57	2	1	1	32	6	940
Cedar-planked tilapia	as served	280	42	2	1	1	11	3	410
Chicken Parmesan pasta	as served	1500	65	138	7	15	77	18	3980
Chicken tenders	appetizer	800	44	29	1	6	57	11	1520
Chicken tenders & Naked Twisted chips w/o sauces	as served	1150	55	110	9	6	60	11	3170
Chicken tenders w/ Buffalo sauce	as served	810	51	31	2	1	53	11	2260
Chicken Tenders w/ chipotle BBQ sauce	appetizer	1040	61	119	4	39	37	8	4230
Chicken tenders w/ honey mustard w/o side	5 Tenders	1090	59	82	4	6	61	10	3680
Classic burger	as served	740	44	54	3	8	37	12	1180
Classic burger w/ Cheddar	as served	900	53	55	3	8	50	20	1440

O'CHARLEY'S continued

Item	Serving Size	Calories	Protein	Carb	Fiber	Sugar	Total Fat	Sat Fat	Sodium
Classic club sandwich	as served	990	41	82	5	20	58	14	2620
Classic Combos, panko-crusted shrimp & hand-battered cod	as served	1170	69	55	3	2	75	14	2370
Classic Combos, steak & chicken tenders	as served	1200	78	53	3	6	75	16	3220
Classic Combos, steak & grilled Atlantic salmon	as served	800	81	3	1	1	50	13	1110
Classic Combos, steak & 1/2-rack baby back ribs	as served	1170	81	38	2	26	75	26	3550
Classic Combos, steak & panko-crusted shrimp	as served	920	71	28	1	1	57	14	1970
Classic Combos, steak & shrimp Scampi	as served	750	58	9	1	1	54	21	1740
Cowboy sirloin	as served	890	51	38	4	4	55	17	980
Eggs (2) & bacon (3)	as served	420	22	2	0	0	36	10	730
Eggs (2) & sausage (2)	as served	500	25	2	0	0	42	12	690
Filet mignon	as served	450	47	0	0	0	28	9	910
French fries, à La carte	as served	390	4	40	3	0	24	4.5	760
Fried shrimp dinner	as served	740	44	35	1	1	47	8	1280
Grilled Atlantic salmon	6 oz	370	38	2	1	1	22	4.5	190
Grilled Atlantic salmon	9 oz	540	57	2	1	1	33	7	240
Grilled Atlantic salmon w/chipotle	6 oz	430	38	17	1	14	22	4.5	450
Grilled Atlantic salmon w/ Chipotle	9 oz	610	57	17	1	14	33	7	500
Grilled Baja chicken	as served	1010	64	103	11	10	36	8	3620
Grilled shrimp dinner	as served	290	22	32	1	2	7	1.5	1220
Grilled top sirloin	7 oz	430	43	1	0	0	28	9	920
Grilled turkey burger	as served	890	47	54	3	8	54	14	1710
Half club sandwich, Lunch Combo	as served	620	21	45	2	13	42	9	1410
Half white Cheddar grilled cheese	as served	410	19	29	1	0	23	12	750

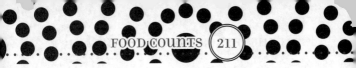

O'CHARLEY'S continued

Item	Serving Size	Calories	Protein	Carb	Fiber	Sugar	Total Fat	Sat Fat	Sodium
Half white Cheddar grilled cheese w/bacon & tomato	as served	500	24	30	1	1	31	15	1070
Half club sandwich, Lunch	as served	510	22	42	2	10	30	8	1330
Ham & cheese omelette	as served	1210	49	76	4	13	76	22	2510
Hand battered fish n' chips	as served	1140	52	43	3	3	85	16	2040
Loaded baked potato	as served	480	12	54	6	8	29	10	570
Louisiana sirloin	as served	680	74	3	1	0	40	14	1220
O'Charley's baby back ribs	full rack	1480	77	76	3	52	96	34	5260
O'Charley's baby back ribs	1/2 rack	740	39	38	2	26	48	17	2630
O'Charley's Butchers Cut Premium USDA Choice steak	5 oz	260	30	0	0	0	14	5	170
O'Charley's Grillers	as served	1260	56	112	5	15	64	21	2400
O'Charley's Overloaded Brunch Platter	as served	1690	68	116	4	47	103	28	2080
Overloaded potato skins	as served	1260	56	43	0	4	98	43	1980
Pancakes (3) with syrup	as served	520	5	84	1	46	18	4	680
Philly burger	as served	1230	61	71	4	11	77	22	2580
Prime rib omelette w/o sides	as served	1420	61	78	5	14	91	28	2580
Prime rib pasta	as served	1530	63	90	5	12	101	38	2580
Prime rib Philly sandwich	as served	980	41	82	5	20	56	14	2540
Prime Time prime rib	10 oz	670	44	3	0	1	43	23	1790
Prime Time prime rib	16 oz	1060	70	4	1	1	68	36	2470
Ranch-hand burger	as served	930	53	63	3	13	50	19	1800
Rice Pilaf à la carte	as served	190	4	30	1	1	5	1	790
Roast beef sandwich	as served	880	42	74	4	4	47	14	2660
Sausage patty	1 patty	110	5	0	0	0	9	3	220
Seasoned brunch potatoes	as served	430	4	40	4	0	27	5	220

O'CHARLEY'S continued

Item	Serving Size	Calories	Protein	Carb	Fiber	Sugar	Total Fat	Sat Fat	Sodium
Sicilian meatballs & linguini	as served	1250	56	103	6	10	69	25	3390
Smashed potatoes, à la carte	as served	400	4	47	5	5	14	6	810
Southwestern cheese dip & chips	as served	820	24	84	4	6	45	18	1630
Southwestern chicken quesadilla	as served	1060	63	64	4	7	60	28	2690
Southwestern twisted chips	as served	1280	31	111	12	18	89	26	2140
Spicy Jack cheese wedges	7 wedges	880	29	55	0	2	60	25	2540
Spinach mushroom omelette w/o sides	as served	1110	42	80	6	14	67	18	1930
Sweet potato fries, à la carte	as served	470	4	46	6	18	31	3.5	500
Sweet potato fries	side	470	4	46	6	18	31	4.5	500
Teriyaki sesame chicken	as served	1030	46	151	5	82	25	4.5	3740
Teriyaki sesame tilapia	as served	850	53	102	3	41	24	5	2690
Three cheese shrimp dip	as served	870	32	86	10	0	49	16	1540
Top Shelf Combo Appetizer	as served	1880	80	105	3	8	130	43	4690
Two eggs (w/o sides)	as served	290	14	2	0	0	24	6	250
Ultimate open-faced Omelette	as served	1230	49	85	6	17	75	22	2420
Wild West burger	as served	1210	53	67	4	10	79	23	1860
Your Favorite ribeye steak	as served	810	72	0	0	0	55	20	960

KIDS' MENU

Item	Serving Size	Calories	Protein	Carb	Fiber	Sugar	Total Fat	Sat Fat	Sodium
Brunch, eggs only	as served	200	7	1	0	0	19	4	390
Brunch, fries	as served	330	3	31	3	0	21	5	200
Brunch, plate	as served	800	15	70	4	15	50	11	910
Cheeseburger	as served	650	31	57	3	8	33	12	3790
Corn dogs	as served	500	11	32	3	8	38	12	770
French toast	as served	1040	8	117	2	33	50	7	720

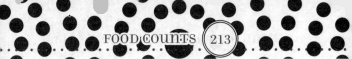

O'CHARLEY'S continued

Item	Serving Size	Calories	Protein	Carb	Fiber	Sugar	Total Fat	Sat Fat	Sodium
Fruit cup, peaches	as served	70	0	18	1	17	0	n/a	15
Fruit cup, pears	as served	70	0	18	0	17	n/a	n/a	70
Grilled chicken	as served	240	32	0	0	0	11	2	320
Hamburger	as served	540	23	57	3	8	24	7	3600
Macaroni & cheese	as served	360	14	27	0	5	23	9	1560
Pancakes	as served	670	5	121	1	80	18	4	760
Pasta	as served	260	8	46	2	5	4.5	0	660
Pizza	as served	440	18	45	2	4	21	11	980
Shrimp	as served	310	12	25	1	3	18	6	210
Waffle	as served	1070	11	146	1	82	48	28	1250

DRESSINGS, DIPS, & TOPPINGS

Item	Serving Size	Calories	Protein	Carb	Fiber	Sugar	Total Fat	Sat Fat	Sodium
Bacon topping for baked potato	as served	15	1	0	0	0	1	0	45
Balsamic vinaigrette dressing	2 oz	240	0	18	0	8	18	3	100
Bleu cheese dressing	2 oz	280	2	2	0	2	30	4	560
Brunch jelly	as served	50	0	13	0	12	0	0	0
Cheese, shredded for baked potato	as served	110	7	1	0	0	9	5	180
Cranberry orange vinaigrette	1.5 oz	130	0	15	1	14	10	1.5	640
Greek feta vinaigrette	2 oz	620	4	7	2	5	64	11	1590
Honey mustard dressing	2 oz	350	0	12	0	8	34	6	260
Honey mustard light	1.5 oz	100	0	16	0	7	3	0	250
Margarine for baked potato	0.88 oz	170	0	0	0	0	20	5	200
Pico de gallo	1/4 Cup	10	0	2	0	1	0	0	180
Ranch dressing	2 oz	200	1	4	0	0	20	4	400
Ranch dressing, light	2 oz	70	1	8	0	4	4.5	1	500
Sour cream for baked potato	0.88 oz	50	2	2	0	2	4.5	3	40
Southwestern ranch dressing	2 oz	100	2	5	0	3	9	1	90
Thousand Island dressing	2 oz	210	0	8	0	0	19	4	530

O'CHARLEY'S continued

Item	Serving Size	Calories	Protein	Carb	Fiber	Sugar	Total Fat	Sat Fat	Sodium
SOUP & SALADS									
Black & Bleu Caesar salad	as served	1050	61	22	5	8	79	25	2270
Broccoli & three cheese soup, bowl	1 bowl	340	11	14	2	3	26	11	1700
Broccoli & three cheese soup, cup	1 cup	200	7	9	1	2	15	7	1020
Caesar salad	Lunch Combo	280	7	10	1	3	24	5	520
Caesar salad, à la carte	as served	270	7	13	2	4	22	5	600
California chicken salad w/o dressing	as served	700	45	48	8	25	37	9	760
California shrimp salad w/o dressing	as served	700	33	53	9	27	42	9	1520
Chicken harvest soup	1 bowl	270	15	19	1	2	13	3.5	1530
Chicken harvest soup	1 cup	160	9	12	1	1	8	2	920
Chicken tortilla soup	1 bowl	260	9	21	2	6	15	3	1600
Chicken tortilla soup	1 cup	150	5	12	1	3	9	2	960
Chili	1 Bowl	250	13	31	6	9	9	2.5	1630
Chili	1 cup	150	8	19	3	5	5	1.5	980
Clam chowder	1 bowl	340	14	23	0	3	20	7	1220
Clam chowder	1 cup	200	9	14	0	2	12	4.5	730
Classic Caesar salad	as served	450	9	16	3	5	39	8	960
House salad w/o dressing	Lunch Combo	120	6	12	1	1	6	2.5	270
House salad w/o dressing, à la carte	as served	140	6	16	2	2	6	2.5	300
Original Southern fried chicken salad w/o dressing	as served	900	60	74	6	3	42	12	3130
Overloaded potato soup, bowl	as served	280	8	27	1	4	17	6	1920
Overloaded potato soup, cup	as served	160	5	16	1	2	9	3	1130
Pecan chicken tender salad w/o dressing	as served	1020	46	81	10	25	60	11	2020
Pepper steak soup	1 bowl	210	8	13	1	2	13	5	1210
Pepper steak soup	1 cup	130	5	8	1	1	8	3	730
Roasted tomato basil soup	1bowl	260	6	20	2	9	17	7	1020

O'CHARLEY'S continued

Item	Serving Size	Calories	Protein	Carb	Fiber	Sugar	Total Fat	Sat Fat	Sodium
Roasted tomato basil soup	1 cup	130	3	10	1	4	9	3.5	510
Southwestern steak soup	1 bowl	200	6	20	2	6	10	3	1390
Southwestern steak soup	1 cup	100	3	10	1	3	5	1.5	690
Tortilla chicken salad w/o dressing	as served	610	47	41	5	6	27	9	1590
Wild mushroom cream soup	1 bowl	260	6	11	0	3	23	9	1190
Wild mushroom cream soup	1 cup	150	3	7	0	2	14	5	710

SIDE ITEMS & ADD-ONS

Item	Serving Size	Calories	Protein	Carb	Fiber	Sugar	Total Fat	Sat Fat	Sodium
Applewood smoked bacon	1 slice	45	3	0	0	0	4	1.5	160
Baked potato (plain)	side	240	8	50	6	6	5	1	720
Beer battered onion rings	side	380	3	32	1	7	26	5	660
Broccoli	side	140	5	10	5	3	10	2	500
Broccoli cheese casserole	side	230	8	17	3	4	14	4	710
Caesar salad	side	290	8	12	2	4	24	5	520
Chips & salsa	as served	520	12	82	4	4	18	3	1160
French fries	as served	390	4	40	3	0	24	5	760
Fresh asparagus	as served	80	2	4	2	2	6	1.5	380
House salad	side	210	10	15	2	2	11	5	310
Onions, sautéed	add-on	280	1	8	1	3	28	6	230
Smashed potatoes	side	370	2	47	5	5	12	4.5	720
Toast	side	220	5	28	1	0	9	2	400
Whipped potatoes	side	110	2	13	2	1	2	2.5	350
Yeast roll w/ margarine	side	180	4	25	0	6	7	1.5	170
Yeast roll w/o Margarine	side	130	4	25	0	6	1.5	0	11

DESSERTS

Item	Serving Size	Calories	Protein	Carb	Fiber	Sugar	Total Fat	Sat Fat	Sodium
Cinnamon sugar donuts	1 donut	1130	11	139	1	76	54	10	1160
Ooey gooey caramel pie	1 slice	730	12	106	0	87	28	15	210
Ultimate chocolate chocolate cake	1 slice	1080	12	151	6	114	59	12	770

OLIVE GARDEN

Item	Serving Size	Calories	Protein	Carb	Fiber	Sugar	Total Fat	Sat Fat	Sodium
ANTIPASTI (APPETIZERS)									
Breadstick	1 order	150	n/a	28	2	n/a	2	0	400
Bruschetta	1 order	610	n/a	100	10	n/a	13	2.5	1760
Calamari	as served	440	n/a	32	0	n/a	27	2.5	1160
Calamari	as served	890	n/a	64	2	n/a	54	5	2340
Caprese flatbread	1 order	600	n/a	46	5	n/a	36	11	1520
Chicken fingers	as served	330	n/a	22	0	n/a	16	1.5	930
Fried mozzarella	as served	370	n/a	26	2	n/a	22	9	800
Fried Zucchini	as served	370	n/a	42	4	n/a	20	1.5	630
Grilled chicken flatbread	1 order	760	n/a	47	5	n/a	44	15	1500
Hot artichoke-spinach dip	1 order	650	n/a	68	6	n/a	31	15	1430
Lasagna fritta	1 order	1030	n/a	82	9	n/a	63	21	1590
Marinara dipping sauce	1 order	70	n/a	10	3	n/a	2.5	0	540
Mussels di Napoli	1 order	180	n/a	13	0	n/a	8	4	1770
Sicilian scampi	1 order	500	n/a	43	7	n/a	22	10	1850
Smoked mozzarella fonduta	1 order	940	n/a	72	7	n/a	48	28	1940
Stuffed mushrooms	as served	280	n/a	15	3	n/a	19	5	720
Stuffed mushrooms	1 order	280	n/a	15	3	n/a	19	5	720
Toasted beef & pork ravioli	as served	360	n/a	39	2	n/a	16	2.5	780
ZUPPE E INSALATA (SOUPS & SALADS)									
Chicken & gnocchi	1 order	250	n/a	29	2	n/a	8	3	1180
Garden-fresh salad	1/2 order	120	n/a	17	3	n/a	3.5	0.5	550
Garden-fresh salad	1 order	350	n/a	22	3	n/a	26	4.5	1930
Grilled chicken Caesar	1 order	850	n/a	14	4	n/a	64	13	1880
Minestrone	1 order	100	n/a	18	3	n/a	1	0	1020
Pasta e fagioli	1 order	130	n/a	17	6	n/a	2.5	1	680
Zuppa toscana	1 order	170	n/a	24	2	n/a	4	2	960
PIZZA									
Chicken Alfredo pizza	1 order	1180	n/a	144	11	n/a	40	17	3330
Create Your Own pizza, cheese & sauce Only	1 order	910	n/a	129	8	n/a	28	12	2970
w/ bell peppers	as served	10	n/a	2	1	n/a	0	0	0
w/ black olives	as served	45	n/a	3	1	n/a	4	0.5	350

OLIVE GARDEN continued

Item	Serving Size	Calories	Protein	Carb	Fiber	Sugar	Total Fat	Sat Fat	Sodium
w/ Italian sausage	as served	130	n/a	1	0	n/a	11	4	360
w/ mushrooms	as served	5	n/a	1	0	n/a	0	0	0
w/ onions	as served	15	n/a	4	1	n/a	0	0	0
w/ pepperoni	as served	120	n/a	0	0	n/a	11	4	460
w/ roma tomatoes	as served	10	n/a	2	1	n/a	0	0	0

CUCINA CLASSICA (CLASSIC RECIPES)

Item	Serving Size	Calories	Protein	Carb	Fiber	Sugar	Total Fat	Sat Fat	Sodium
Chianti-braised short ribs	1 order	1060	n/a	71	17	n/a	58	26	2970
Chicken & shrimp carbonara	1 order	1440	n/a	80	9	n/a	88	38	3000
Chicken Alfredo	1 order	1440	n/a	103	5	n/a	82	48	2070
Chicken Marsala	1 order	770	n/a	59	16	n/a	37	5	1800
Chicken Parmigiana	1 order	1090	n/a	79	27	n/a	49	18	3380
Chicken scampi	1 order	1070	n/a	88	8	n/a	53	20	2220
Eggplant Parmigiana	1 order	850	n/a	98	19	n/a	35	10	1900
Fettuccine Alfredo	1 order	1220	n/a	99	5	n/a	75	47	1350
Five-cheese ziti al forno	1 order	1050	n/a	112	9	n/a	48	26	2370
Garlic n' herb chicken con broccoli	1 order	960	n/a	90	12	n/a	41	18	2180
Grilled shrimp caprese	1 order	900	n/a	82	0	n/a	40	17	3490
Herb-grilled salmon	1 order	510	n/a	5	2	n/a	26	6	760
Lasagna classico	1 order	850	n/a	39	19	n/a	47	25	2830
Lasagna rollata al forno	1 order	1170	n/a	90	11	n/a	68	39	2510
Mixed grill	1 order	830	n/a	72	10	n/a	28	5	1840
Parmesan-crusted bistecca	1 order	690	n/a	40	7	n/a	35	19	1480
Parmesan-crusted tilapia	1 order	590	n/a	42	6	n/a	25	10	910
Pork Milanese	1 order	1510	n/a	118	11	n/a	87	37	3100
Ravioli di portobello	1 order	670	n/a	74	15	n/a	30	17	1400
Seafood Alfredo	1 order	1020	n/a	88	9	n/a	52	31	2430
Seafood brodetto	1 order	480	n/a	35	7	n/a	16	3	2250
Seafood Portofino	1 order	800	n/a	85	16	n/a	33	14	1880
Shrimp & crab tortelli Romana	1 order	840	n/a	67	4	n/a	42	24	1710
Shrimp primavera	1 order	730	n/a	110	14	n/a	12	2	1620
Spaghetti & Italian sausage	1 order	1270	n/a	97	15	n/a	67	24	3090

OLIVE GARDEN continued

Item	Serving Size	Calories	Protein	Carb	Fiber	Sugar	Total Fat	Sat Fat	Sodium
Spaghetti & meatballs	1 order	1110	n/a	103	9	n/a	50	20	2180
Spaghetti w/ seat sauce	1 order	710	n/a	94	9	n/a	22	8	1340
Steak Gorgonzola-Alfredo	1 order	1310	n/a	82	9	n/a	73	41	2190
Steak Toscano	1 order	810	n/a	62	11	n/a	35	8	1690
Stuffed chicken Marsala	1 order	800	n/a	40	6	n/a	36	16	2830
Tour of Italy	1 order	1450	n/a	97	10	n/a	74	33	3830
Venetian apricot chicken	1 order	380	n/a	32	8	n/a	4	1.5	1420

LUNCH ENTRÉES
CUCINA CLASSICA (CLASSIC RECIPES)

Item	Serving Size	Calories	Protein	Carb	Fiber	Sugar	Total Fat	Sat Fat	Sodium
Capellini pomodoro	as served	480	n/a	78	11	n/a	11	2	970
Chicken Parmigiana	as served	570	n/a	67	18	n/a	18	5	1720
Eggplant Parmigiana	as served	620	n/a	70	11	n/a	26	8	1540
Fettuccine Alfredo	as served	800	n/a	69	4	n/a	48	30	810
Five-cheese ziti al forno	as served	770	n/a	89	5	n/a	32	17	1450
Lasagna classico	as served	580	n/a	35	7	n/a	32	0	1930
Spaghetti & meatballs	as served	820	n/a	66	6	n/a	40	16	1600
Spaghetti Italian sausage	as served	830	n/a	61	9	n/a	44	16	1920
Spaghetti w/ meat sauce	as served	550	n/a	59	6	n/a	21	8	1040
Tour of Italy	as served	1450	n/a	97	10	n/a	74	33	3830

CHICKEN & SEAFOOD

Item	Serving Size	Calories	Protein	Carb	Fiber	Sugar	Total Fat	Sat Fat	Sodium
Chicken Alfredo	as served	910	n/a	71	4	n/a	52	30	1150
Chicken scampi	as served	740	n/a	57	7	n/a	38	14	1350
Grilled Chicken Spiedini	as served	460	n/a	26	7	n/a	13	2.5	1180
Grilled shrimp caprese	as served	820	n/a	81	0	n/a	39	17	2800
Seafood Alfredo	as served	670	n/a	59	5	n/a	36	21	1320
Shrimp primavera	as served	510	n/a	79	12	n/a	9	1.5	1130
Venetian Apricot Chicken	as served	280	n/a	32	8	n/a	3	1	1180

FILLED PASTAS

Item	Serving Size	Calories	Protein	Carb	Fiber	Sugar	Total Fat	Sat Fat	Sodium
Braised beef & tortelloni	as served	740	n/a	60	5	n/a	41	17	1280
Cheese ravioli w/ marinara	as served	430	n/a	64	6	n/a	18	9	1160

OLIVE GARDEN continued

Item	Serving Size	Calories	Protein	Carb	Fiber	Sugar	Total Fat	Sat Fat	Sodium
Cheese ravioli w/ meat sauce	as served	600	n/a	65	8	n/a	22	12	1210
Lasagna rollata al forno	as served	840	n/a	65	8	n/a	49	28	1830
Ravioli di portobello	as served	450	n/a	53	8	n/a	19	11	960
KIDS' MENU									
Broccoli	side	25	n/a	4	2	n/a	0	0	10
Cheese pizza	as served	470	n/a	66	4	n/a	14	6	1170
Cheese ravioli	as served	300	n/a	43	4	n/a	8	4	440
Chicken fingers	as served	330	n/a	22	0	n/a	16	1.5	930
Fettuccine Alfredo	as served	800	n/a	69	4	n/a	48	30	810
Fries	side	400	n/a	47	4	n/a	21	2	880
Grilled chicken w/ pasta	as served	310	n/a	33	6	n/a	5	1	680
Macaroni & cheese	as served	340	n/a	58	3	n/a	6	2.5	1000
Spaghetti w/ tomato sauce	as served	250	n/a	45	4	n/a	3	0.5	370
DESSERTS									
Amaretto tiramisu	each	240	n/a	16	0	n/a	17	9	50
Black Tie Mousse Cake	each	700	n/a	73	6	n/a	41	20	390
Cheesecake	each	610	n/a	69	2	n/a	35	16	430
Chocolate milk shake	each	520	n/a	72	7	n/a	22	14	230
Chocolate mousse w/ dark chcoclate cookie crust	each	290	n/a	23	2	n/a	21	10	120
Dark chocolate cake w/ chocolate mousse & caramel	each	270	n/a	25	0	n/a	18	8	140
Lemon cream cake	each	760	n/a	70	8	n/a	48	27	270
Limoncello mousse	each	230	n/a	28	0	n/a	13	8	70
Strawberry & white chocolate cream cake	each	210	n/a	27	0	n/a	11	6	70
Strawberry milk shake	each	500	n/a	62	10	n/a	24	15	160
Sundae	each	180	n/a	21	0	n/a	9	6	45
Tiramisu	each	510	n/a	48	2	n/a	32	19	75
Triple chocolate strata	each	920	n/a	73	4	n/a	41	3.5	590
Vanilla milk shake	each	530	n/a	73	16	n/a	23	14	170

OLIVE GARDEN continued

Item	Serving Size	Calories	Protein	Carb	Fiber	Sugar	Total Fat	Sat Fat	Sodium
Warm apple crostata	each	730	n/a	104	6	n/a	32	15	240
White chocolate raspberry	each	890	n/a	70	6	n/a	62	36	490
Zeppoli	each	210	n/a	131	4	n/a	35	3.5	75

SIGNATURE COCKTAILS

Item	Serving Size	Calories	Protein	Carb	Fiber	Sugar	Total Fat	Sat Fat	Sodium
Berry sangria	Glass	230	n/a	35		n/a	0	0	15
Berry sangria	Pitcher	910	n/a	138		n/a	0	0	50
Chocolate martini	each	260	n/a	36		n/a	3.5	2	45
Italian margarita	each	240	n/a	32		n/a	0	0	10
Mango martini	each	180	n/a	31		n/a	0	0	0
Peach sangria	Glass	250	n/a	40		n/a	0	0	50
Peach sangria	Pitcher	1010	n/a	158		n/a	0	0	200
Pomegranate margarita martini	each	290	n/a	44		n/a	0	0	5
Strawberry fresco	each	230	n/a	31		n/a	0	0	5
Strawberry-limoncello martini	each	300	n/a	42		n/a	0	0	15
Tropical sangria	Glass	220	n/a	31		n/a	0	0	10
Tropical sangria	Pitcher	870	n/a	126		n/a	0	0	45
Venetian Sunset	each	190	n/a	38		n/a	0	0	10

DRINK SPECIALTIES & FROZEN SPECIALTIES

Item	Serving Size	Calories	Protein	Carb	Fiber	Sugar	Total Fat	Sat Fat	Sodium
Bella limonata	each	190	n/a	48		n/a	0	0	35
Berry acqua fresca	each	390	n/a	94		n/a	1.5	1	40
Cream sodas	each	190	n/a	35		n/a	5	3	40
Italian sodas	each	120	n/a	29		n/a	0	0	5
Limoncello lemonade	each	260	n/a	42		n/a	0	0	5
Mango daiquiri	each	240	n/a	43		n/a	0	0	10
Peach Bellini	each	170	n/a	33		n/a	0	0	0
Peach daiquiri	each	270	n/a	51		n/a	0	0	10
Strawberry Bellini	each	220	n/a	46		n/a	0	0	0
Strawberry daiquiri	each	250	n/a	47		n/a	0	0	15
Strawberry-mango limonata	each	200	n/a	50		n/a	0	0	30
Strawberry mango margarita	each	350	n/a	68		n/a	0	0	20
Strawberry margarita	each	340	n/a	67		n/a	0	0	25
Wild Berry Bellini	each	160	n/a	31		n/a	0	0	10

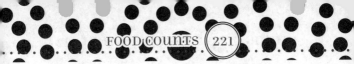

OLIVE GARDEN continued

Item	Serving Size	Calories	Protein	Carb	Fiber	Sugar	Total Fat	Sat Fat	Sodium
Wild Berry daiquiri	each	270	n/a	49	n/a		0	0	5
Wild Berry margarita	each	290	n/a	55	n/a		0	0	20

COFFEE & HOT TEAS

Caffe la Toscana Coffee	each	0	n/a	0	n/a		0	0	5
Caffe latte	each	130	n/a	15	n/a		4	2	85
Caffe mocha	each	180	n/a	30	n/a		4	2.5	75
Cappuccino	each	150	n/a	14	n/a		8	4	65
Caramel hazelnut macchiato	each	220	n/a	43	n/a		4.5	2.5	40
Frozen cappuccino	each	320	n/a	52	n/a		10	6	60
Herbal teas	each	0	n/a	0	n/a		0	0	0
Lavazza espresso	each	0	n/a	0	n/a		0	0	10

ON THE BORDER

Item	Serving Size	Calories	Protein	Carb	Fiber	Sugar	Total Fat	Sat Fat	Sodium
APPETIZER									
Border Sampler	as served	2050	94	100	14		144	54	4000
Chicken flautas w/ original queso	4 each	1160	48	62	8		80	20	1920
Chips and salsa	basket	430	5	52	5		22	4	460
Empanadas, chicken w/ original queso	5 each	1300	38	75	4		95	31	1310
Empanadas, ground beef w/ original queso	5 each	1340	37	75	5		99	32	1380
Fajita quesadillas, chicken	as served	1220	56	54	5		87	35	2460
Fajita quesadillas, steak	as served	1240	50	54	7		93	40	1960
Firecracker stuffed jalapenos w/ original queso	as served	1930	63	124	5		136	39	6180
Grande fajitas nacho, chicken	as served	1470	99	82	16		86	42	4090
Grande fajitas nachos, steak	as served	1520	86	82	20		98	52	3070
Guacamole w/o chips	as served	260	6	16	13		23	5	480
Guacamole Live! w/o chips	as served	570	11	34	31		50	10	2330

ON THE BORDER continued

Item	Serving Size	Calories	Protein	Carb	Fiber	Sugar	Total Fat	Sat Fat	Sodium
Original queso w/o chips	1 bowl	430	21	15	1		31	19	2090
Original queso w/o chips	1 cup	270	13	9	1		19	12	1310
Original queso carne style w/o chips	1 bowl	510	28	17	2		36	21	2410
Original queso carne style w/o chips	1 cup	350	20	11	2		2	14	1590
OTB dip trio w/o chips	as served	480	17	26	7		35	14	1740
Ultimate loaded queso w/o chips	as served	780	43	34	11		54	28	2410

SOUPS & SALADS

Item	Serving Size	Calories	Protein	Carb	Fiber	Sugar	Total Fat	Sat Fat	Sodium
Chicken tortilla Soup	side	330	17	26	4	n/a	18	7	960
Chicken tortilla Soup	regular	510	25	50	6	n/a	25	8	1950
Citrus chipotle chicken salad w/ mango w/ citrus vinaigrette	as served	290	25	42	11	n/a	4	2	840
Grande taco salad w/ chicken w/ dressing	as served	1290	53	83	12	n/a	85	28	2110
Grande taco salad w/ ground beef w/ dressing	as served	1380	53	83	14	n/a	95	33	2200
House salad w/o dressing	as served	200	6	20	4	n/a	12	4	260
Sizzling chicken fajita salad w/o dressing	as served	710	52	25	7	n/a	46	20	1930
Sizzling steak fajita salad w/o dressing	as served	830	56	24	8	n/a	58	29	2090

MAIN ENTRÉES

Item	Serving Size	Calories	Protein	Carb	Fiber	Sugar	Total Fat	Sat Fat	Sodium
Cheese onion enchiladas w/ chili con carne	as served	360	17	20	2	n/a	24	12	930
Cheese stuffed chile relleno w/ ranchero sauce	as served	680	31	28	6	n/a	57	5	1190
Chicken empanadas w/ chili con queso	as served	540	20	33	1	n/a	37	14	780
Chicken enchiladas w/ sour cream sauce	as served	210	12	18	1	n/a	11	5	490
Chicken flautas w/ chili con queso	as served	330	17	19	2	n/a	21	7	790

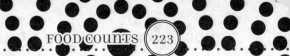

ON THE BORDER continued

Item	Serving Size	Calories	Protein	Carb	Fiber	Sugar	Total Fat	Sat Fat	Sodium
Chicken soft taco	as served	240	19	24	2	n/a	11	4	830
Chicken tortilla soup	as served	330	17	26	4	n/a	18	7	960
Crispy beef taco	as served	320	18	19	4	n/a	19	7	600
Crispy chicken taco	as served	260	18	19	3	n/a	12	4	530
Ground beef empanadas w/ chili con queso	as served	550	19	33	2	n/a	39	15	810
Ground beef enchiladas w/ chili con carne	as served	260	14	19	2	n/a	15	6	650
Ground beef soft taco	as served	310	19	24	3	n/a	18	8	900
Pork tamale w/ chili con carne	as served	290	13	14	3	n/a	20	7	960
Tostadas, chicken	as served	90	9	6	2	n/a	3	1	330
Tostadas, ground beef	as served	120	9	6	2	n/a	7	3	370
Tostadas, guacamole	as served	140	4	10	7	n/a	10	3	290

SIDES

Item	Serving Size	Calories	Protein	Carb	Fiber	Sugar	Total Fat	Sat Fat	Sodium
Black beans w/ cheese	side	130	8	20	6	n/a	3	1	630
Cilantro lime rice	side	390	8	83	1		330	3	0
Grilled vegetables	side	70	2	16	3	n/a	0	0	20
Guacamole	side	50	1	3	3	n/a	5	1	90
House vegetables	side	180	2	13	3	n/a	14	3	190
Mexican rice	side	290	6	54	0	n/a	5	1	620
Pico de gallo	side	10	0	1	0	n/a	1	0	55
Refried beans w/ cheese	side	230	10	24	7	n/a	10	4	730

FRESH GRILL

Item	Serving Size	Calories	Protein	Carb	Fiber	Sugar	Total Fat	Sat Fat	Sodium
Bacon wrapped shrimp skewer	as served	560	22	3	0		53	15	990
Carne asada	as served	970	51	105	5		38	15	1830
Chicken salad fresca	as served	520	50	60	12		9	3	2410
Jalapeño-BBQ salmon	as served	590	54	45	24		21	6	1220
Queso chicken	as served	1080	65	111	8		41	14	2300
Tomatillo chicken	as served	890	58	109	7		25	6	2070

OTB TACO STAND (LIST W/O RICE OR BEANS)

Item	Serving Size	Calories	Protein	Carb	Fiber	Sugar	Total Fat	Sat Fat	Sodium
Brisket tacos w/ jalapeño BBQ sauce	as served	1370	58	157	4		56	21	4780
Dos XX fish tacos w/ creamy red chile sauce	as served	2280	63	163	4		154	33	3920

ON THE BORDER continued

Item	Serving Size	Calories	Protein	Carb	Fiber	Sugar	Total Fat	Sat Fat	Sodium
Grilled mahi mahi tacos w/ creamy red chile sauce	as served	1130	41	116	9		58	13	2150
Loaded carne asada tacos w/ creamy red chile sauce	as served	1410	52	94	5		94	25	2250
Southwest chicken tacos w/ creamy red chile sauce	as served	1580	62	135	4		87	22	3360
Street-style mini tacos, carnitas	as served	950	43	91	10		49	16	2380
Street-style mini tacos, chicken	as served	910	47	89	9		41	13	2020
Street-style mini tacos, steak	as served	990	47	87	9		52	21	1540
Taco melt, beef, crispy	as served	870	34	79	7		46	18	1820
Taco melt, beef, soft	as served	1010	40	110	5		46	20	2670
Taco melt, chicken, crispy		770	34	79	5		36	13	1720
Taco melt, chicken, soft	as served	920	40	110	3		35	14	2570
Tacos al carbon, chicken w/o condiments	as served	920	59	124	3		20	5	2740
Tacos al carbon, steak w/o condiments	as served	970	47	121	4		32	14	2670

FAJITA GRILL (LIST W/O RICE OR BEANS, TORTILLAS, & CONIDMENTS)

Item	Serving Size	Calories	Protein	Carb	Fiber	Sugar	Total Fat	Sat Fat	Sodium
Baja Blend veggies	as served	210	3	16	4		15	3	530
Chili con queso	as served	80	4	3	0		6	4	390
Classic veggies	as served	90	2	11	3		5	1	510
El Diablo veggies	as served	50	1	8	1		2	0	5
Grilled vegetables w/ portobello mushrooms	as served	230	4	25	4		15	1	360
Guacamole	side	50	1	3	3		5	1	90
Guajillo steak sauce	as served	45	1	6	0		3	1	420
Homemade flour tortillas	side	360	9	57	0		11	3	900
Mesquite-grilled chicken		350	43	5	0		16	1	910
Mesquite-grilled steak	as served	390	32	1	0		28	10	830

ON THE BORDER continued

Item	Serving Size	Calories	Protein	Carb	Fiber	Sugar	Total Fat	Sat Fat	Sodium
Mexican rice	side	280	5	55	1		5	1	630
Mixed Cheeses	side	110	7	0	0		9	6	160
Monterey ranch chicken	as served	700	62	13	1		44	14	2190
Pico de gallo	side	15	0	1	0		1	0	55
Pulled pork (carnitas)	as served	770	35	2	2		70	13	1220
Red chilé-tomatillo salsa	as served	15	0	3	1		0	0	140
Seasoned, sautéed shrimp	as served	390	22	2	0		33	6	900
Sour cream	side	60	1	2	0		5	3	50
The Ultimate Fajita	as served	1090	49	26	6		90	21	2640

BURRITOS & CHIMIS (LISTED W/ RICE & W/O BEANS)

Item	Serving Size	Calories	Protein	Carb	Fiber	Sugar	Total Fat	Sat Fat	Sodium
Big chicken bordurrito w/ side salad w/o dressing	as served	1760	74	173	16		87	20	4550
Big steak bordurrito w/ side salad w/o dressing	as served	1810	61	174	21		98	30	3540
Chili con carne for chimi/burrito	side	100	6	8	2		5	1	550
Classic chicken burrito w/o sauce	as served	920	47	105	5		35	16	2320
Classic chimichanga chicken w/o sauce	as served	1300	47	105	5		78	23	2320
Classic chimichanga ground beef w/o sauce	as served	1410	47	105	6		89	29	2440
Classic shredded beef burrito w/o sauce	as served	1020	58	102	3		41	19	2010
Fresh sour cream for chimi/burrito	side	80	1	5	0		6	4	290
Queso for chimi/burrito	side	160	8	6	0		12	7	790
Ranchero sauce for chimi/burrito	side	50	1	7	1		3	0	430
Three sauce fajita chicken burrito	as served	1190	68	117	5		49	18	4460
Three sauce fajita steak burrito	as served	1240	55	118	9		61	27	3450

ON THE BORDER continued

Item	Serving Size	Calories	Protein	Carb	Fiber	Sugar	Total Fat	Sat Fat	Sodium
KIDS' MENU LISTED W/O SIDES									
Black beans	side	180	12	29	10		3	1	830
Cheeseburger	as served	530	22	17	0		42	15	300
Chicken tenders	as served	520	22	40	2		35	6	1530
Corn dog	as served	280	5	25	2		17	4	650
Dessert, sundae w/ chocolate syrup	as served	370	4	51	1		18	13	95
Dessert, sundae w/ strawberry puree	as served	330	3	41	1		17	13	55
French fries	side	250	3	36	4		10	2	350
Grilled chicken	as served	110	22	2	0		1	0	450
Grilled chicken sandwich	as served	330	23	19	0		18	3	550
Hamburger	as served	420	15	16	0		33	9	135
House salad w/o dressing	side	10	1	2	1		0	0	5
Mexican rice	side	280	5	55	1		5	1	630
Mexican Plate, cheese enchiladas	as served	340	17	17	2		23	13	890
Mexican Plate, crispy chicken taco	as served	260	18	19	3		12	4	530
Mexican Plate, crispy ground beef taco	as served	320	18	19	4		20	8	590
Mexican Plate, soft chicken taco	as served	270	20	24	1		11	5	820
Mexican Plate, soft ground beef taco	as served	340	20	24	2		18	8	880
Mixed vegetables	side	180	2	12	3		14	33	10
Nachos, bean & cheese	as served	770	42	57	11		45	25	1440
Nachos, cheese	as served	560	32	28	3		37	23	720
Quesadilla, cheese	as served	890	33	36	1		69	30	1170
Refried beans	side	220	10	25	6		9	4	660
BORDER LUNCH (LISTED W/ RICE & W/O BEANS UNLESS INDICATED)									
Border's Best Lunch chicken fajitas	as served	470	37	46	3		15	2	1580
Border's Best Lunch steak fajitas	as served	580	38	43	3		28	11	1610
Brisket tacos	as served	1040	41	129	4		39	14	3600
Chili con carne for chimi/burrito	side	100	6	8	2		5	1	550

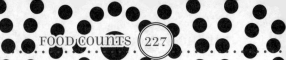

ON THE BORDER continued

Item	Serving Size	Calories	Protein	Carb	Fiber	Sugar	Total Fat	Sat Fat	Sodium
Dos XX fish tacos	as served	1690	44	127	3	n/a	112	23	2930
Fresh sour cream for chimi/burrito	side	80	1	5	0	n/a	6	4	290
Little bordurrito, chicken w/ salad, no dressing	as served	1050	38	92	10	n/a	60	13	2310
Little bordurrito, steak w/ salad, no dressing	as served	1070	31	92	12	n/a	65	18	1800
Lunch beef burrito w/o sauce	as served	790	40	93	3	n/a	27	12	1610
Lunch chicken burrito w/o sauce	as served	720	32	94	4	n/a	24	10	1820
Lunch chimichanga, chicken w/o sauce	as served	950	32	94	4	n/a	50	14	1820
Lunch chimichanga, ground beef w/o sauce	as served	1080	32	94	5	n/a	64	19	1900
Queso for chimi/burrito	side	160	8	6	0	n/a	12	7	790
Ranchero sauce for chimi/burrito	side	50	1	7	1	n/a	3	0	430

BORDER LUNCH CREATE YOUR OWN (LISTED W/O RICE OR BEANS)

Item	Serving Size	Calories	Protein	Carb	Fiber	Sugar	Total Fat	Sat Fat	Sodium
Black beans	side	180	12	29	10	n/a	3	1	830
Cheese stuffed chili relleno w/ ranchero sauce	as served	670	31	26	6	n/a	57	5	1180
Chicken flautas w/ chile con queso	as served	370	16	18	2	n/a	26	8	840
Chicken tortilla soup	as served	300	16	24	3	n/a	16	7	910
Crispy taco, chicken	as served	260	18	19	3	n/a	12	4	530
Crispy taco, ground beef	as served	320	18	19	4	n/a	20	8	590
Empanadas, beef w/ chili con queso	as served	590	18	31	2	n/a	44	16	840
Empanadas, chicken w/ chili con queso	as served	580	18	31	1	n/a	42	15	810
Enchiladas, cheese & onion w/ chili con queso	as served	360	18	20	2	n/a	24	12	900
Enchiladas, chicken w/ sour cream sauce	as served	210	12	16	1	n/a	11	5	460

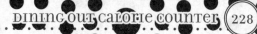

ON THE BORDER continued

Item	Serving Size	Calories	Protein	Carb	Fiber	Sugar	Total Fat	Sat Fat	Sodium
Enchiladas, ground beef w/ chili con carne	as served	260	14	18	3	n/a	14	6	630
House salad w/o dressing	side	200	6	20	4	n/a	12	4	260
Mexican rice	side	280	5	55	1	n/a	5	1	630
Pork tamale w/ chili con carne	as served	290	13	14	3	n/a	19	6	960
Refried beans	side	220	10	25	6	n/a	9	4	660
Soft taco, chicken	as served	270	20	24	1	n/a	11	5	820
Soft taco, ground beef	as served	340	20	24	2	n/a	18	8	880

DESSERTS

Item	Serving Size	Calories	Protein	Carb	Fiber	Sugar	Total Fat	Sat Fat	Sodium
Border brownie sundae w/ vanilla ice cream	as served	1310	16	161	7	n/a	72	34	420
Chocolate turtle empanadas	as served	1710	15	175	6	n/a	109	35	200
Kahlúa ice cream pie	as served	950	11	111	6	n/a	50	24	500
Sizzling apple crisp	as served	1120	10	177	6	n/a	44	22	460
Sopapillas	5 pieces	1350	14	236	7	n/a	43	8	1100
Sopapillas, two w/ chocolate syrup	2 pieces	540	7	92	4	n/a	18	4	490
Sopapillas, two w/ honey	2 pieces	630	5	119	2	n/a	17	3	410

OUTBACK STEAKHOUSE

Item	Serving Size	Calories	Protein	Carb	Fiber	Sugar	Total Fat	Sat Fat	Sodium
ENTRÉES									
Alice Springs Chicken® w/o sides	as served	1297	84	30	2	n/a	93	40	2292
Atlantic salmon	as served	582	39	2	1	0	45	17	708
Baby back ribs w/o sides	full rack	2013	109	24	1	n/a	160	59	2600
Bloomin' Burger®	sandwich	1221	56	76	7	n/a	77	30	2831
Chicken & Swiss grilled sandwich	1 sandwich	750	48	50	3	0	39	13	1371
Chicken grilled on the Barbie	as served	587	54	32	4	0	26	13	1533

OUTBACK STEAKHOUSE continued

Item	Serving Size	Calories	Protein	Carb	Fiber	Sugar	Total Fat	Sat Fat	Sodium
Chicken grilled on the Barbie w/o sides	as served	444	52	21	1	n/a	15	7.3	1256
Filet w/ wild mushroom sauce w/o sides	as served	344	36	7	1	n/a	18	10	1193
New York strip steak	8 oz	407	49	0.7	0.2	n/a	22	11.1	594
New Zealand rack of lamb w/o sides	as served	1303	61	5	1	n/a	112	58	1473
No Rules Parmesan pasta	as served	909	20	89	4	n/a	53	31	1075
Outbacker burger	1 burger	759	43	43	4	0	45	17	1250
Prime rib	8 oz	537	29	2	0	n/a	45	18.6	888
Ribs, w/ fries	1/2 rack	1403	59	66	6	0	99	39	1727
Sweet-glazed roasted pork tenderloin w/o sides	as served	385	37	32	1	n/a	12	6	462
Victoria's Filet® w/o sides	9 oz	725	50	1	0	n/a	57	25.5	593

SIDES, SALADS, & APPETIZERS

Item	Serving Size	Calories	Protein	Carb	Fiber	Sugar	Total Fat	Sat Fat	Sodium
Aussie fries	side	354	4	43	5	n/a	19	9.3	110
Baked potato, dressed	1 potato	520	8	65	7	0	26	13	2456
Bleu cheese pecan chopped salad	as served	523	13	35	6	n/a	36	9	892
Bloomin' Onion®	1/6 order	259	4.6	31	4	n/a	13.8	5.3	918
Chicken Caesar salad	1 salad	1044	68	27	6	0	73	24	2101
Fresh seasonal vegetables	1 order	143	3	11	4	0	11	6	277
Gold Coast coconut shrimp	1/4 order	142	7	17	2	n/a	5.4	4.2	187.5
Kookaburra Wings®	1/4 order	344	22	7	1	n/a	25	7.8	955
Potato boats	side	165	4	32.4	3.5	n/a	2.2	0.2	1149
Potato wedges	side	277	4	35.5	3.5	n/a	15	6.4	1255
Queensland salad without dressing	as served	839	54	53	5	n/a	59	22.5	1322

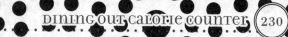
P. F. CHANG'S

Item	Serving Size	Calories	Protein	Carb	Fiber	Sugar	Total Fat	Sat Fat	Sodium
STARTERS/SMALL PLATES									
Crab wontons	6 wontons	163	5	13	0		10	4	303
Chang's chicken lettuce wraps	5 oz	160	8	17	2		7	1	650
Chang's spare ribs	4 oz	344	26	7	1		24	7	336
Chang's vegetarian lettuce wraps	5 oz	140	6	11	2		7	1	530
Crispy green beans	4 oz	260	2	21	2		18	3	140
Crispy wontons	1 oz	45	2	4	0		3	0	60
Dynamite shrimp	4 oz	290	5	6	0		12	2	285
Egg rolls	3 oz	174	5	22	3		8	1	673
Northern style spare ribs	4 oz	343	31	11	0		19	2	985
Pork dumplings, pan-fried	1 oz	70	4	6	0		4	1	125
Pork dumplings, steamed	1 oz	60	4	6	0		2	1	125
Salt & pepper calamari	2 oz	160	6	11	0		10	2	208
Seared Ahi tuna	4 oz	160	10	7	1		11	2	860
Shrimp dumplings, pan-fried	1 oz	60	4	6	0		2	0	170
Shrimp dumplings, steamed	1 oz	45	4	6	0		0	0	170
Sichuan chicken flatbread	3 oz	195	15	12	1		10	5	523
Spring rolls	2 rolls	156	4	17	2		8	1	271
Vegetable dumplings, pan-fried	1 oz	60	2	8	0		2	0	80
Vegetable dumplings, steamed	1 oz	45	2	8	0		0	0	80
DRESSINGS & SAUCES									
Citrus dressing	2 oz	200	0	6	0		20	3	140
Crab wontons' Spicy plum sauce	2 oz	200	0	50	0		0	0	1460
Crispy green beans' sauce	2 oz	310	0	2	0		32	5	520
Potsticker sauce	2 oz	50	1	7	0		2	0	610
Salt & pepper calamari sauce	2 oz	50	1	7	0		2	0	610
Shrimp dumpling sauce	2 oz	15	2	2	0		0	0	1250
Sichuan chicken flatbread sauce	2 oz	310	0	2	0		32	5	520

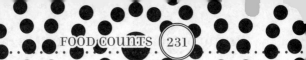

P. F. CHANG'S continued

Item	Serving Size	Calories	Protein	Carb	Fiber	Sugar	Total Fat	Sat Fat	Sodium
Sweet & sour mustard sauce	2 oz	90	1	17	1	n/a	2	0	140
Sweet & sour sauce	2 oz.	80	0	21	0	n/a	0	0	210
SOUPS, SALADS, & SIDES									
Asian shrimp salad	9 oz	225	14	16	3	n/a	13	2	635
Asian slaw	3 oz	170	1	3	1	n/a	17	3	280
Asian slaw	5 oz	237	2	7	2	n/a	22	3	360
Brown rice, steamed	6 oz	190	4	40	3	n/a	2	0	0
Chang's chicken noodle soup	7 oz	120	6	15	1	n/a	4	1	510
Chicken chopped salad with ginger dressing	8 oz	365	23	13	2	n/a	24	4	640
Egg drop soup	7 oz	60	1	8	0	n/a	3	0	640
Garlic snap peas	3 oz	64	2	7	2	n/a	2	0	107
Green tea noodles	4 oz	284	6	37	2	n/a	12	2	163
Hot and sour soup	7 oz	80	5	9	0	n/a	3	1	1000
Shanghai cucumbers	4 oz	40	2	3	1	n/a	2	0	743
Sichuan-style asparagus	5 oz	100	3	10	2	n/a	6	1	730
Spicy green beans	5 oz	110	3	13	4	n/a	6	1	720
Spinach stir-fried with garlic	5 oz.	53	4	5	3	n/a	3	1	300
White rice, steamed	6 oz	220	4	49	1	n/a	0	0	0
Wok-seared mushrooms	4 oz	115	4	6	0	n/a	9	4	645
Wonton soup	7 oz	92	7	9	0	n/a	3	1	482
LUNCH BOWLS									
Almond & cashew chicken on brown rice	14 oz	535	25	59	5	n/a	22	4	2085
Almond & cashew chicken on white rice	14 oz	560	25	66	3	n/a	21	3	2085
Asian grilled salmon on brown rice	9 oz	320	22	44	3	n/a	6	1	575
Asian grilled salmon on white rice	9 oz	345	22	50	1	n/a	5	1	570
Beef with broccoli on brown rice	11 oz	420	23	52	4	n/a	13	3	1760
Beef with broccoli on white rice	11 oz	440	23	58	3	n/a	12	3	1760

P. F. CHANG'S continued

Item	Serving Size	Calories	Protein	Carb	Fiber	Sugar	Total Fat	Sat Fat	Sodium
Buddha's feast, steamed on brown rice	9 oz	210	10	39	5	n/a	2	0	80
Buddha's feast, steamed on white rice	9 oz	235	10	45	3	n/a	1	0	575
Buddha's feast, stir-fried on brown rice	11 oz	290	11	48	5	n/a	6	1	1050
Buddha's feast, stir-fried on white rice	11 oz	310	11	54	3	n/a	5	1	1050
Crispy honey chicken on brown rice	11 oz	655	15	92	3	n/a	24	4	710
Crispy honey chicken on white rice	11 oz	680	15	99	1	n/a	23	4	705
Moo goo gai pan on brown rice	13 oz	380	21	43	3	n/a	13	2	1000
Moo goo gai pan on white rice	13 oz	390	24	47	1	n/a	11	2	1035
Pepper steak on brown rice	12 oz	395	22	47	3	n/a	13	3	1225
Pepper steak on white rice	12 oz	415	22	54	2	n/a	12	3	1225
Sesame chicken on brown rice	14 oz	510	24	69	5	n/a	16	3	1320
Sesame chicken on white rice	14 oz	535	24	76	3	n/a	15	2	1320
Shrimp w/ lobster sauce on white rice	12 oz	340	16	45	1	n/a	10	2	1120
Shrimp w/ lobster sauce on brown rice	12 oz	315	16	39	1	n/a	11	2	1120
CHICKEN & DUCK									
Almond & cashew chicken	10 oz	373	29	24	2	n/a	18	3	1960
Chang's spicy chicken	6 oz	323	28	23	0	n/a	13	2	550
Chicken w/ black bean sauce	7 oz	300	29	14	0	n/a	16	2	1850
Crispy honey chicken	6 oz	477	16	49	0	n/a	23	4	510
Dali chicken	6 oz	283	27	15	1	n/a	13	2	707
Ginger chicken w/ broccoli	9 oz	273	28	18	2	n/a	11	2	1457
Ground chicken & eggplant	7 oz	288	8	17	2	n/a	20	3	1233
Kung pao chicken	5 oz	383	33	14	2	n/a	23	4	940
Mandarin chicken	10 oz	360	33	29	3	n/a	15	2	1715
Moo goo gai pan	9 oz	247	18	13	1	n/a	13	2	823

P. F. CHANG'S continued

Item	Serving Size	Calories	Protein	Carb	Fiber	Sugar	Total Fat	Sat Fat	Sodium
Mu shu chicken	10 oz	285	26	16	3	n/a	13	3	1540
w/ Hoisin sauce	2 oz	210	2	23	0	n/a	12	0	1150
w/ Mu shu pancake	1 pancake	90	2	14	0	n/a	2	0	30
Orange peel chicken	5 oz	333	29	20	1	n/a	15	3	770
Philip's Better Lemon chicken	7 oz	343	26	30	1	n/a	14	2	187
Sesame chicken	8 oz	343	30	25	2	n/a	14	2	1020
Sweet & sour chicken	5 oz	370	12	38	0	n/a	19	3	367
VIP duck	12 oz	650	52	55	1	n/a	29	8	1880
BEEF									
Asian marinated New York strip	8 oz	370	33	17	0	n/a	20	9	933
Beef à la Sichuan	7 oz	303	22	25	1	n/a	12	3	1084
Beef with broccoli	7 oz	290	24	21	2	n/a	12	3	1573
Hong Kong beef w/ snow peas	9 oz	310	24	24	3	n/a	14	3	926
Mongolian beef	6 oz	337	29	20	1	n/a	15	4	1340
Orange peel beef	5 oz	283	12	21	1	n/a	13	3	833
Pepper steak	8 oz	297	24	19	1	n/a	13	3	1300
Wok-charred beef	8 oz	317	25	16	1	n/a	17	5	1157
PORK & LAMB									
Chengdu spiced lamb	5 oz	237	23	11	1	n/a	12	3	740
Crispy honey shrimp	6 oz	460	10	55	1	n/a	22	4	805
Hunan pork	9 oz	395	16	38	2	n/a	19	1	1850
Mu shu pork	10 oz	320	21	16	3	n/a	19	7	2275
w/ Hoisin sauce	2 oz	210	2	23	0	n/a	12	0	1150
w/ Mu shu pancake	1 pancake	90	2	14	0	n/a	2	0	30
Sweet & sour pork	10 oz	460	14	72	2	n/a	14	7	950
Wok-seared lamb	7 oz	283	25	9	1	n/a	16	3	1410
SEAFOOD									
Asian grilled salmon w/ rice	9 oz	345	32	38	1	n/a	6	2	715
Calamari	5 oz	348	12	28	1	n/a	21	4	538
Cantonese scallops	7 oz	245	15	17	2	n/a	14	2	1000
Cantonese shrimp	7 oz	215	21	10	2	n/a	10	2	950

P. F. CHANG'S continued

Item	Serving Size	Calories	Protein	Carb	Fiber	Sugar	Total Fat	Sat Fat	Sodium
Chang's lemon scallops	6 oz	243	11	28	1	n/a	10	2	540
Combo	4 oz	215	12	14	0	n/a	12	2	553
Hot fish	8 oz	340	16	21	1	n/a	22	3	1043
Kung pao scallops	5 oz	307	16	17	2	n/a	20	3	1126
Kung pao shrimp	5 oz	280	21	12	2	n/a	17	3	1083
Lemon pepper shrimp	9 oz	235	21	19	3	n/a	10	2	1080
Lemongrass prawns w/ garlic noodles	10 oz	485	24	32	2	n/a	30	10	935
Mahi-mahi	10 oz	420	25	42	2	n/a	17	8	605
Oolong marinated sea bass	9 oz	315	24	15	2	n/a	19	5	1550
Orange peel shrimp	5 oz	187	15	14	1	n/a	14	1	937
Salmon steamed w/ ginger	10 oz	330	31	12	3	n/a	19	3	605
Salt & pepper prawns	6 oz	197	21	8	2	n/a	11	2	1070
Scallops	7 oz	295	16	26	1	n/a	15	3	1230
Shanghai shrimp w/ garlic sauce	9 oz	195	17	10	3	n/a	20	2	1050
Shrimp	5 oz	173	16	10	0	n/a	7	1	747
Shrimp w/ candied walnuts	7 oz	377	16	25	1	n/a	24	4	654
Shrimp w/ lobster sauce	10 oz	250	23	11	1	n/a	14	2	1745

NOODLES & RICE

Item	Serving Size	Calories	Protein	Carb	Fiber	Sugar	Total Fat	Sat Fat	Sodium
Cantonese chow fun w/ beef	14 oz	745	27	94	5	n/a	20	4	903
Cantonese chow fun w/ chicken	14 oz	790	32	88	5	n/a	20	4	1615
Dan Dan noodles	9 oz	270	13	30	2	n/a	7	1	1388
Double pan-fried noodles w/ beef	8 oz	395	15	44	2	n/a	17	1	1665
Double pan-fried noodles w/ chicken	8 oz	393	16	43	2	n/a	17	1	1608
Double pan-fried noodles w/ combo	9 oz	455	16	44	1	n/a	21	2	1923
Double pan-fried noodles w/ pork	8 oz	413	13	42	2	n/a	21	3	1975
Double pan-fried noodles w/ shrimp	8 oz	363	12	42	2	n/a	16	0	1698
garlic noodles	5 oz	178	5	31	1	n/a	4	1	360
Lo mein w/ beef	7 oz	270	15	33	2	n/a	9	2	1070
Lo mein w/ chicken	7 oz	267	17	30	2	n/a	9	2	997

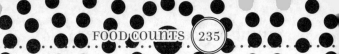

P. F. CHANG'S continued

Item	Serving Size	Calories	Protein	Carb	Fiber	Sugar	Total Fat	Sat Fat	Sodium
Lo mein w/ combo	9 oz	347	23	23	2	n/a	14	0	1413
Lo mein w/ pork	7 oz	290	13	30	2	n/a	13	4	1483
Lo mein w/ shrimp	7 oz	227	12	30	2	n/a	6	1	1113
P. F. Chang's fried rice w/ beef	7 oz	303	13	41	1	n/a	9	2	803
P. F. Chang's fried rice w/ chicken	7 oz	303	15	39	1	n/a	9	2	748
P. F. Chang's fried rice w/ combo	8 oz	363	19	41	1	n/a	13	3	1063
P. F. Chang's fried rice w/ pork	7 oz	320	12	39	1	n/a	13	4	1115
P. F. Chang's fried rice w/ shrimp	7 oz	273	11	39	1	n/a	8	1	838
Singapore street noodles	6 oz	300	11	42	3	n/a	6	1	1157

VEGETARIAN

Item	Serving Size	Calories	Protein	Carb	Fiber	Sugar	Total Fat	Sat Fat	Sodium
Buddha's Feast, steamed	6 oz	55	4	11	4	n/a	0	0	40
Buddha's Feast, stir-fried	11 oz	220	14	29	5	n/a	6	1	1620
Canton chicken & mushrooms	17 oz	550	38	48	3	n/a	23	4	1410
Coconut curry vegetables	13 oz	510	22	26	5	n/a	36	12	650
Ma po tofu	10 oz	350	20	17	2	n/a	23	5	1060
Stir-fried eggplant	6 oz	270	2	14	2	n/a	22	3	760
Vegetable chow fun	7 oz	250	2	46	3	n/a	2	0	750
Vegetarian fried rice	7 oz	190	5	38	2	n/a	2	0	230

DESSERTS

Item	Serving Size	Calories	Protein	Carb	Fiber	Sugar	Total Fat	Sat Fat	Sodium
Banana spring rolls	4 oz	235	4	34	1	n/a	10	4	128
Flourless chocolate dome	3 oz	235	5	55	3	n/a	4	2	85
Mini apple pie	1 serving	150	1	29	0	n/a	4	1	85
Mini carrot cake	1 serving	130	1	19	0	n/a	6	2	85
Mini cheesecake	1 serving	220	2	15	1	n/a	18	10	80
Mini Great Wall	1 serving	100	1	18	0	n/a	4	1	115
Mini Lemon Dream	1 serving	190	4	30	0	n/a	4	2	30
Mini red velvet cake	1 serving	130	1	18	0	n/a	7	2	85
Mini tiramisu	1 serving	100	2	10	0	n/a	11	5	50
Mini triple chocolate mousse	1 serving	300	3	25	1	n/a	22	14	50
New York-style cheesecake	6 oz	460	9	46	1	n/a	28	18	310

P. F. CHANG'S continued

Item	Serving Size	Calories	Protein	Carb	Fiber	Sugar	Total Fat	Sat Fat	Sodium
The Great Wall of Chocolate™	5 oz	383	4	61	3	n/a	18	6	355
GLUTEN-FREE MENU									
Buddha's Feast, steamed	6 oz	55	4	11	4	n/a	0	0	40
Buddha's Feast, steamed lunch bowl	8 oz	210	10	39	5	n/a	2	0	80
Egg drop soup cup	7 oz	60	1	8	0	n/a	3	0	640
Beef a la Sichuan	7 oz	293	23	26	1	n/a	11	3	910
Beef w/ broccoli	6 oz	290	24	21	2	n/a	12	3	1300
Beef w/ broccoli lunch bowl	11 oz	420	24	52	5	n/a	13	3	1435
Cantonese scallops	7 oz	245	15	17	2	n/a	14	2	1000
Cantonese Shrimp	7 oz	215	21	10	2	n/a	10	2	950
Chang's chicken lettuce wraps	5 oz	158	9	15	2	n/a	7	1	670
Chang's lemon scallops	6 oz	233	11	27	1	n/a	10	3	540
Chang's spicy chicken	6 oz	323	28	23	0	n/a	13	2	550
Dali chicken	6 oz	280	27	16	1	n/a	12	2	370
Garlic snap Peas	3 oz	63	2	7	2	n/a	2	0	107
Ginger chicken w/ broccoli	8 oz	270	28	17	2	n/a	11	2	990
Hong Kong beef w/ snow peas	9 oz	335	25	28	3	n/a	14	3	1480
Mongolian beef	6 oz	337	30	21	1	n/a	15	4	1123
Moo goo gai pan	8 oz	223	23	9	2	n/a	10	2	987
Moo goo gai pan lunch bowl	13 oz	365	24	41	3	n/a	12	2	1035
P. F. Chang's fried rice w/ chicken	7 oz	293	14	39	1	n/a	9	2	585
P. F. Chang's fried rice w/ beef	7 oz	293	13	41	1	n/a	9	2	640
P. F. Chang's fried rice w/ Combo	8 oz	353	19	40	1	n/a	13	3	900
P. F. Chang's fried rice w/ Pork	7 oz	320	12	39	1	n/a	13	4	953
P. F. Chang's fried rice w/ Shrimp	7 oz	260	10	38	1	n/a	7	0	675
Pepper steak	8 oz	300	25	19	1	n/a	13	3	1197
Pepper steak lunch bowl	12 oz	400	22	48	3	n/a	13	3	1045

P. F. CHANG'S continued

Item	Serving Size	Calories	Protein	Carb	Fiber	Sugar	Total Fat	Sat Fat	Sodium
Philip's better lemon chicken	7 oz	350	29	31	1	n/a	13	2	207
Salmon, steamed w/ ginger	10 oz	220	32	13	2	n/a	3	1	1160
Shrimp w/ lobster sauce	10 oz	255	23	13	1	n/a	14	2	1745
Shrimp w/ lobster sauce lunch bowl	6 oz	315	16	39	3	n/a	11	2	1120
Singapore street noodles	7 oz	300	11	41	3	n/a	7	1	980
Spinach, stir-fried w/ garlic	4 oz	40	2	3	1	n/a	2	0	743
Spinach, stir-fried w/ garlic	5 oz	53	4	5	2	n/a	3	1	300

KIDS' MENU

Item	Serving Size	Calories	Protein	Carb	Fiber	Sugar	Total Fat	Sat Fat	Sodium
Baby Buddha's Feast, stir-fried	5 oz	90	3	12	2	n/a	4	1	760
Baby Buddha's Feast, steamed	3 oz	30	2	6	3	n/a	0	0	25
Chicken honey sauce	2 oz	140	0	33	0	n/a	0	0	360
Chicken sweet & sour sauce	2 oz	90	0	23	0	n/a	0	0	210
Fried rice w/ chicken	6 oz	290	15	37	1	n/a	9	2	755
Lo mein	4 oz	195	9	21	1	n/a	8	1	720

PANDA EXPRESS

Item	Serving Size	Calories	Protein	Carb	Fiber	Sugar	Total Fat	Sat Fat	Sodium
BEEF & PORK									
BBQ pork	4.6 oz	360	34	13	1	12	19	8	1310
Broccoli beef	5.4 oz	150	11	12	3	2	6	1.5	720
Mongolian beef	6.9 oz	230	17	17	3	6	11	2.5	1040
Sweet & sour pork	5.6 oz	400	13	36	2	15	23	4.5	360
CHICKEN									
Broccoli chicken	5.5 oz	180	13	11	3	2	9	2	630
Kung pao chicken	6.1 oz	300	19	13	2	4	19	3.5	880
Mushroom chicken	5.9 oz	220	17	9	2	3	13	3	780
Orange chicken	5.4 oz	400	15	42	0	18	20	3.5	640
Pineapple chicken breast	6 oz	220	17	20	1	14	8	1.5	640
String bean chicken breast	5.1 oz	190	12	11	2	4	10	2	720

PANDA EXPRESS continued

Item	Serving Size	Calories	Protein	Carb	Fiber	Sugar	Total Fat	Sat Fat	Sodium
String bean chicken breast	5.6 oz	170	15	13	2	5	7	1.5	720
Sweet & sour chicken	5.5 oz	400	15	46	1	23	17	3	370
Thai cashew chicken breast	6.3 oz	280	23	21	2	6	19	3.5	980

SHRIMP

Item	Serving Size	Calories	Protein	Carb	Fiber	Sugar	Total Fat	Sat Fat	Sodium
Crispy shrimp	6 pieces	260	9	26	1	2	13	2.5	810
Honey walnut shrimp	3.7 oz	370	14	27	2	9	23	4	470
Kung pao shrimp	6.4 oz	250	14	14	2	4	15	2.5	880
Tangy shrimp	6.4 oz	190	13	19	2	14	7	1.5	820

SOUPS & SIDES

Item	Serving Size	Calories	Protein	Carb	Fiber	Sugar	Total Fat	Sat Fat	Sodium
Chicken egg roll	each	200	8	16	2	2	12	4	390
Chicken potstickers	3 pieces	220	7	23	1	2	11	2.5	280
Chow mein	8.3 oz	400	12	61	8	10	12	2	1060
Eggplant and tofu	6.1 oz	310	7	19	3	13	24	3	680
Fortune cookie	each	32	1	7	0	3	0	0	8
Fried rice	10 oz	570	16	85	8	0	18	4	900
Hot and sour soup	10.6 oz	90	4	12	1	3	3.5	0.5	970
Mixed veggies	8.6 oz	70	4	13	5	4	0.5	0	530
Veggie spring rolls	2 rolls	160	4	22	4	2	7	1	540

PANERA BREAD

Item	Serving Size	Calories	Protein	Carb	Fiber	Sugar	Total Fat	Sat Fat	Sodium

BAGELS

Item	Serving Size	Calories	Protein	Carb	Fiber	Sugar	Total Fat	Sat Fat	Sodium
Asiago cheese	each	330	13	55	2	3	6	3.5	570
Blueberry	each	330	10	67	2	9	1.5	0	490
Chocolate chip	each	370	10	69	2	14	6	4	480
Cinnamon crunch	each	430	9	81	3	30	8	5	430
Cinnamon swirl and raisin	each	320	10	65	3	11	2.5	1	460
Everything	each	300	10	59	2	4	2.5	0	630
French toast	each	350	9	67	2	15	5	2	610
Jalapeño & cheddar	each	310	12	56	2	3	3	1.5	740
Plain	each	290	10	59	2	3	1.5	0	450
Sesame	each	310	10	59	2	3	3	0	450

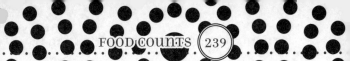

PANERA BREAD continued

Item	Serving Size	Calories	Protein	Carb	Fiber	Sugar	Total Fat	Sat Fat	Sodium
Sweet onion poppy seed	each	400	14	72	4	7	7	1	510
Whole grain	each	370	13	70	6	5	3.5	0	420
Asiago cheese, demi	each	160	7	22	1	0	4	2.5	320

BREADS

Item	Serving Size	Calories	Protein	Carb	Fiber	Sugar	Total Fat	Sat Fat	Sodium
Ciabatta	6.25 oz	460	16	84	3	3	6	1	760
Cinnamon raisin loaf	2 oz	180	5	34	1	11	3	1.5	135
Focaccia	2 oz	180	5	28	1	1	4.5	0.5	320
Focaccia w/ Asiago cheese	2 oz	160	5	23	1	1	5	1.5	230
French baguette	2 oz	150	5	30	1	0	1	0	370
Honey wheat loaf	2 oz	170	5	30	2	4	3	1.5	240
Sesame semolina loaf	2 oz	140	4	29	1	1	0.5	0	350
Sourdough round loaf	2 oz	140	5	28	1	0	0.5	0	290
Sourdough soup bowl	8 oz	590	21	118	4	1	2.5	0	1210
Stone-milled rye loaf	2 oz	140	5	28	2	0	0.5	0	380
Three-cheese demi	2 oz	160	6	29	1	1	2	1	320
Three-Seed demi	2 oz	160	6	27	2	0	3.5	0	300
Tomato basil loaf	2 oz	140	5	27	1	1	0.5	0	330
White whole-grain loaf	2 oz	140	5	26	2	1	2.5	1	310
Whole-grain loaf	2 oz	140	6	27	3	2	1	0	300

PASTRIES, COOKIES, & CAKES

Item	Serving Size	Calories	Protein	Carb	Fiber	Sugar	Total Fat	Sat Fat	Sodium
Apple crunch muffin	5 oz	450	7	80	2	49	12	3	340
Carrot walnut muffin	5 oz	500	8	72	3	37	21	4.5	580
Cheese pastry	3.75 oz	400	8	42	1	15	22	14	340
Cherry pastry	5 oz	500	7	77	2	45	18	11	320
Chocolate Chip Muffie	2.5 oz	280	4	40	1	24	12	3.5	180
Chocolate Chipper	3.25 oz	440	5	59	2	33	23	14	250
Chocolate Duet w/ walnuts	3.25 oz	450	6	55	3	36	24	13	150
Chocolate fudge brownie	3.5 oz	410	5	64	2	33	14	8	260
Chocolate pastry	3.5 oz	410	8	46	2	18	24	14	260
Cinnamon coffee crumb cake	4.25 oz	470	6	54	1	30	25	9	310
Macadamia nut blondie	3.5 oz	460	4	62	1	25	21	11	200
Oatmeal raisin	3.25 oz	370	5	57	2	28	14	8	310
Pecan braid	4.25 oz	470	8	52	2	23	26	12	270
Pumpkin Muffie	3 oz	290	3	45	1	26	11	2	240

PANERA BREAD continued

Item	Serving Size	Calories	Protein	Carb	Fiber	Sugar	Total Fat	Sat Fat	Sodium
Pumpkin muffin	6 oz	580	7	89	2	51	22	4	470
Shortbread	2.5 oz	350	3	36	1	11	21	12	160
Wild blueberry muffin	4.5 oz	440	6	66	2	39	17	3	330
SANDWICHES & PANINI									
Asiago roast beef on asiago cheese	1/2 sandwich	350	24	32	1	2	13	7	630
Bacon Turkey Bravo® on tomato basil	1/2 sandwich	420	26	44	2	6	14	5	1500
Chicken Caesar on three-cheese	1/2 sandwich	360	21	33	2	2	16	4.5	730
Chipotle chicken on artisan French	1/2 sandwich	500	26	34	2	3	28	8	1180
Cuban chicken panini	1/2 panini	430	23	43	2	5	19	5	950
Frontega Chicken® on focaccia	1/2 panini	430	23	40	2	3	20	4.5	1080
Italian combo on ciabatta	1/2 sandwich	520	31	47	2	3	23	9	1510
Mediterranean veggie on tomato basil	1/2 sandwich	300	11	50	5	3	7	1.5	730
Napa almond chicken salad on sesame semolina	1/2 sandwich	340	15	44	2	6	13	2	660
Sierra Turkey on focaccia w/ asiago cheese	1/2 sandwich	480	19	40	2	3	27	6	990
Smoked ham and swiss on stone-milled rye	1/2 sandwich	350	23	33	3	2	14	5	1180
Smoked turkey breast on country	1/2 sandwich	280	16	34	2	2	9	1.5	980
Smokehouse Turkey® on three-cheese	1/2 panini	360	25	33	2	3	14	6	1230
Tomato and mozzarella on ciabatta	1/2 panini	380	15	48	3	5	15	5	650
Tuna salad on honey wheat	1/2 sandwich	380	10	32	3	6	23	4.5	570
Turkey artichoke on focaccia	1/2 panini	370	20	44	3	5	13	3.5	1170

PANERA BREAD continued

Item	Serving Size	Calories	Protein	Carb	Fiber	Sugar	Total Fat	Sat Fat	Sodium
SALADS									
Asian sesame chicken	full salad	400	31	31	3	6	20	3.5	810
Asian sesame chicken	half salad	200	15	15	2	3	10	2	410
BBQ chopped chicken	full salad	500	31	50	6	15	22	3	770
BBQ chopped chicken	half salad	250	16	25	3	8	11	1.5	380
Caesar	full salad	390	12	25	3	2	27	8	610
Caesar	half salad	200	6	13	1	1	14	4	310
Chopped chicken cobb	full salad	500	38	11	3	3	36	9	1120
Chopped chicken cobb	half salad	250	19	6	1	1	18	4.5	560
Classic café	full salad	170	2	18	4	12	11	1.5	270
Classic café	half salad	80	1	9	2	6	5	1	135
Fruit cup	full salad	60	1	16	1	12	0	0	15
Fuji apple with chicken	full salad	520	32	36	5	21	31	7	830
Fuji apple with chicken	half salad	260	16	18	2	11	15	3.5	410
Greek	full salad	380	8	14	5	4	34	8	1670
Greek	half salad	190	4	7	2	2	17	4	840
Grilled chicken Caesar salad	Full salad	510	37	29	3	2	29	9	820
Grilled chicken Caesar salad	half salad	260	18	14	1	1	15	4.5	410
Orchard harvest chicken	full salad	550	34	34	5	21	34	7	940
Orchard harvest chicken	half salad	270	17	17	2	10	17	4	470
SOUPS & SIDES									
Baked potato	12 oz	340	7	29	0	2	22	11	850
Baked potato w/ You Pick Two®	8 oz	210	5	18	0	1	14	7	1180
Broccoli cheddar soup	12 oz	290	12	24	7	0	16	9	1540
Cream of chicken & wild rice soup	12 oz	320	10	33	0	3	17	7	1270

PANERA BREAD continued

Item	Serving Size	Calories	Protein	Carb	Fiber	Sugar	Total Fat	Sat Fat	Sodium
French onion soup	13.25 oz	240	9	24	1	7	12	5	2210
Low fat chicken noodle soup	12 oz	110	8	10	0	2	4	1.5	1360
Low fat chicken tortilla soup	12.75 oz	190	10	24	1	1	6	1.5	1110
Low fat garden vegetable w/ pesto soup	12 oz	160	5	28	6	8	3.5	0	1240
Low fat vegetarian black bean soup	12 oz	170	10	29	5	4	4	1.5	1590
New England clam chowder	12 oz	450	8	29	3	0	34	20	1190
Signature macaroni & cheese	15.5 oz	980	33	75	3	14	61	26	2030
Signature macaroni & cheese	7.75 oz	490	17	37	1	7	30	13	1020
CREAM CHEESE									
Plain	1 oz	100	2	1	0	1	10	6	110
Plain	2 oz	180	3	2	0	1	18	11	210
Reduced fat hazelnut	1 oz	80	2	3	0	3	6	3.5	110
Reduced fat hazelnut	2 oz	140	5	6	1	6	11	6	210
Reduced fat honey walnut	1 oz	80	2	4	0	4	6	3.5	105
Reduced fat honey walnut	2 oz	150	5	8	1	7	11	6	200
Reduced fat plain	1 oz	70	3	1	0	1	6	4	120
Reduced fat plain	2 oz	130	5	2	1	1	12	7	230
Reduced fat raspberry	1 oz	70	2	4	1	3	5	3	105
Reduced fat raspberry	2 oz	130	4	7	1	6	10	6	200
Reduced fat sun-dried tomato	1 oz	70	3	2	1	1	6	3.5	115
Reduced fat sun-dried tomato	2 oz	130	5	4	1	2	11	7	220
Reduced fat veggie	1 oz	60	2	1	1	1	5	3	110
Reduced fat veggie	2 oz	120	5	3	1	2	10	6	210
GRILLED BREAKFAST SANDWICHES									
Asiago cheese bagel breakfast sandwich w/ bacon	1 sandwich	610	33	55	2	4	27	13	1250

PANERA BREAD continued

Item	Serving Size	Calories	Protein	Carb	Fiber	Sugar	Total Fat	Sat Fat	Sodium
Asiago cheese bagel breakfast sandwich w/ egg & cheese	1 sandwich	480	23	54	2	3	18	9	800
Asiago cheese bagel breakfast sandwich w/ sausage	1 sandwich	640	31	56	2	4	31	14	1130
Bacon, egg & cheese on ciabatta	1 sandwich	510	28	44	2	2	24	10	1060
Breakfast power sandwich	1 sandwich	330	22	31	4	3	14	6	830
Egg & cheese on ciabatta	1 sandwich	380	18	43	2	1	14	6	620
French toast bagel breakfast sandwich w/ sausage	1 sandwich	660	27	69	2	15	30	13	1190
Jalapeno & cheddar bagel w/ bacon	1 sandwich	590	32	58	3	4	25	11	1430
Jalapeno & cheddar bagel w/ egg & cheese	1 sandwich	460	22	57	3	3	12	7	990
Jalapeno & cheddar bagel w/ sausage	1 sandwich	620	31	59	3	3	28	12	1320
Jalapeno & cheddar bagel w/ smoked ham	1 sandwich	490	27	58	3	4	16	8	1290
Sausage, egg & cheese on ciabatta	1 sandwich	540	26	44	2	2	28	11	950
FROZEN DRINKS									
Caramel	16 fl oz	600	5	97	0	85	22	15	170
Low fat black cherry smoothie	16 fl oz	290	6	63	2	53	1.5	1	90
Low fat mango smoothie	16 fl oz	230	6	51	2	48	1.5	1	90
Low fat strawberry smoothie with ginseng	16 fl oz	260	6	59	2	53	1.5	1	90
Mango	16 fl oz	330	2	61	2	56	10	7	20
Mocha	16 fl oz	570	7	92	2	77	21	14	140
Peppermint mocha	16 fl oz	710	7	133	3	107	19	12	160

PANERA BREAD continued

Item	Serving Size	Calories	Protein	Carb	Fiber	Sugar	Total Fat	Sat Fat	Sodium
ICED DRINKS									
Iced chai tea latte	16 fl oz	160	6	26	0	25	3.5	2	75
Iced green tea	16 fl oz	90	0	23	0	23	0	0	10
Lemonade	16 fl oz	90	0	22	0	22	0	0	10
HOT DRINKS									
Caffe latte	8.5 fl oz	120	8	11	0	11	4.5	3	95
Caffe mocha	11.5 fl oz	380	11	49	2	41	17	11	160
Cappuccino	8.5 fl oz	120	8	11	0	11	4.5	3	95
Caramel latte	11.5 fl oz	420	10	53	0	49	18	12	190
Chai tea latte	10 fl oz	200	7	32	0	32	4.5	2.5	85
Hot chocolate	11 fl oz	380	11	48	2	41	17	11	160
Peppermint hot chocolate	13.5 fl oz	510	12	88	3	70	14	9	190
Peppermint mocha latte	13.5 fl oz	520	13	86	3	69	14	10	190

PAPA JOHN'S

Item	Serving Size	Calories	Protein	Carb	Fiber	Sugar	Total Fat	Sat Fat	Sodium
PIZZAS, 14"									
BBQ Chicken & Bacon	1/8 pizza	350	15	44	2	7	12	5	1020
Cheese	1/8 pizza	290	11	37	2	4	10	4.5	720
Garden Fresh	1/8 pizza	280	11	39	2	5	9	4	700
Hawaiian BBQ Chicken	1/8 pizza	290	11	37	2	4	10	4.5	720
Pepperoni	1/8 pizza	330	13	37	2	4	14	6	870
Sausage	1/8 pizza	330	12	37	2	4	15	6	830
Spicy Italian	1/8 pizza	380	14	38	2	4	18	7	980
Spinach Alfredo	1/8 pizza	290	10	36	1	4	11	6	640
The Meats	1/8 pizza	370	15	38	2	5	19	7	1050
The Works	1/8 pizza	330	13	39	2	5	14	6	930
Tuscan six-cheese	1/8 pizza	320	14	38	2	4	13	6	800

PAPA MURPHY'S

Item	Serving Size	Calories	Protein	Carb	Fiber	Sugar	Total Fat	Sat Fat	Sodium
PIZZAS									
50/50	1/8 pizza	330	16	29	<1	6	17	8	850
5-meat	1/8 pizza	370	18	39	0	7	16	7	910
All-meat	1/8 pizza	320	17	28	0	5	16	8	790
Awesome Foursome	1/8 pizza	320	116	34	<1	9	15	8	800
Barbecue chicken	1/8 pizza	310	17	35	0	11	11	6	680
Big Murphy	1/8 pizza	370	17	40	<1	7	16	7	890
Cheese	1/8 pizza	250	12	27	0	5	10	6	500
Chicago-style	1/8 pizza	370	17	40	<1	7	16	7	850
Chicken & bacon	1/8 pizza	370	20	39	0	6	15	7	820
Chicken Florentine	1/8 pizza	460	26	46	1	7	19	9	1040
Combo	1/8 pizza	450	21	46	<1	8	21	11	1030
Cowboy	1/8 pizza	320	16	29	<1	5	16	8	810
Forty-Niner	1/8 pizza	370	18	31	<1	6	19	9	880
Gourmet chicken garlic	1/8 pizza	290	17	27	0	4	13	6	560
Gourmet classic Italian	1/8 pizza	350	17	31	<1	5	18	8	790
Gourmet supreme	1/8 pizza	280	13	30	2	6	12	6	600
Gourmet vegetarian	1/8 pizza	300	14	31	1	5	14	7	700
Hawaiian	1/8 pizza	270	13	30	<1	8	10	6	600
Herb chicken Mediterranean	1/8 pizza	340	17	35	3	7	14	7	630
Italian	1/8 pizza	450	22	46	<1	8	20	10	1090
Meat sampler	1/8 pizza	280–340	15–17	31–32	<1	6	11–16.0	6–8	670–840
Murphy's combo	1/8 pizza	330	16	29	<1	6	17	8	850
Papa's Favorite	1/8 pizza	330	16	29	<1	6	17	8	820
Papa-Roni	1/8 pizza	300	14	28	0	5	15	8	690
Pepperoni	1/8 pizza	290	13	27	0	5	14	7	640
Perfect	1/8 pizza	290–320	15	30–34	<1	6–9	11–15	6–8	670–710
Rancher	1/8 pizza	300	16	28	0	6	14	7	700
Specialty of the House	1/8 pizza	320	16	32	<1	6	15	7	800
Taco grande	1/8 pizza	310	16	30	1	5	14	6	760
Vegetarian combo	1/8 pizza	270	13	30	<1	6	11	6	610
Veggie Mediterranean	1/8 pizza	280	12	31	2	6	12	6	540

PAPA MURPHY'S continued

Item	Serving Size	Calories	Protein	Carb	Fiber	Sugar	Total Fat	Sat Fat	Sodium
SIDES & DESSERT									
Apple dessert pizza	1 slice	240	4	46	<1	19	4.5	1	340
Caesar salad	each	50	4	4	2	2	2	1	120
Caesar salad dressing	1 oz	140	1	2	0	1	14	1	170
Cheesy bread w/o sauce	each	220	7	31	0	5	7	3	480
Cherry dessert pizza	1/8 pizza	240	4	44	<1	16	4.5	1	330
Chicken Caesar salad	each	140	18	5	3	2	5	2.5	320
Cinnamon wheel	2 slices	250	5	42	0	13	7	2	410
Club salad	1/2 salad	140	13	6	3	2	8	4	480
Cookie dough w/ Hershey's chocolate chips	1 oz	120	1	17	0	10	6	2	115
Garden salad	each	100	6	8	3	2	6	3	260
Italian salad	each	140	7	7	3	1	10	4	400
Lasagna	each	330	17	26	2	9	18	9	760
Low-calorie Italian salad dressing	1 oz	10	0	1	0	0	0.5	0	280

PIZZA HUT

Item	Serving Size	Calories	Protein	Carb	Fiber	Sugar	Total Fat	Sat Fat	Sodium
PIZZAS (MEDIUM PAN UNLESS OTHERWISE SPECIFIED)									
Cheese	1/8 pizza	240	11	27	1	2	11	4.5	530
Chicken supreme	1/8 pizza	270	13	28	1	3	12	4	580
Italian sausage	1/8 pizza	270	11	28	1	3	13	4.5	560
Meat Lover's®	1/8 pizza	330	14	27	1	2	18	7	830
Pepperoni Lover's ®	1/8 pizza	250	11	26	1	2	12	4.5	590
Sausage Lover's ®	1/8 pizza	330	13	29	2	2	20	7	830
Super supreme	1/8 pizza	340	14	30	2	7	18	6	760
Supreme	1/8 pizza	240	11	26	2	3	12	5	690
Veggie Lover's®, medium	1/8 pizza	230	9	28	2	3	9	3.5	500
Veggie Lover's®, small	1/8 small pizza	200	9	27	2	3	7	3.5	540
P'ZONE PIZZA									
Classic	1/2 order	630	28	77	3	3	23	11	1460
Marinara dipping sauce	3 oz	60	2	12	2	9	0	0	440

PIZZA HUT continued

Item	Serving Size	Calories	Protein	Carb	Fiber	Sugar	Total Fat	Sat Fat	Sodium
Meaty	1/2 order	710	32	76	2	3	31	14	1800
Pepperoni	1/2 order	630	29	76	2	3	24	11	1570
TUSCANI PASTAS									
Bacon mac N cheese	1/2 pan	520	24	54	4	4	22	12	1170
Chicken Alfredo	1/2 pan	630	27	56	4	5	33	11	1180
Lasagna	1/2 pan	600	31	43	5	11	33	14	1600
Meaty marinara	1/2 pan	520	26	50	6	10	24	10	1310
PERSONAL PANORMOUS PIZZA									
Personal pizza, cheese	each	1100	48	124	6	10	45	19	2400
Personal pizza, Dan's original	each	1270	55	124	7	10	62	23	2810
Personal pizza, ham & pineapple	each	1020	43	128	6	14	37	14	2330
Personal pizza, Hawaiian Luau	each	1150	49	129	6	14	49	18	2670
Personal pizza, Italian sausage & red onion	each	1210	50	128	7	12	56	21	2550
Personal pizza, Meat Lovers	each	1470	64	123	6	10	80	30	3670
Personal pizza, pepperoni	each	1100	47	121	6	9	48	18	2540
Personal pizza, pepperoni & mushroom	each	1050	45	123	7	10	42	16	2290
Personal pizza, Spicy Sicilian	each	1220	51	126	7	11	57	22	3150
Personal pizza, Supreme	each	1270	54	125	7	11	62	24	2920
Personal pizza, Triple Meat Italiano	each	1280	56	123	6	9	62	23	3070
personal pizza, V eggie Lovers	each	1010	42	127	8	12	38	14	2240
APPETIZERS									
Baked Hot wings	2 pieces	100	10	1	0	0	6	2	430
Baked mild wings	2 pieces	110	10	1	0	0	7	2	430
Breadsticks	each	150	5	19	1	2	7	2	250
Cheese breadsticks	each	180	7	20	1	2	7	3.5	370
Marinara dipping sauce	3 oz	60	2	12	2	9	0	0	440

PIZZA HUT continued

Item	Serving Size	Calories	Protein	Carb	Fiber	Sugar	Total Fat	Sat Fat	Sodium
Wing blue cheese dipping sauce	1.5 oz	230	1	2	0	2	24	4.5	420
Wing ranch dipping sauce	1.5 oz	220	0	2	0	1	23	3.5	420
DESSERTS & SIDES									
Apple pie	2 pies	330	2	40	2	20	17	5	190
Cinnamon stick	2 pieces	170	4	26	1	8	6	15	200
Fried cheese sticks	4 pieces	380	13	29	2	3	24	9	1020
Hershey's chocolate dunkers	2 pieces	200	5	26	1	9	9	4	210
Hershey's chocolate sauce	1.5 oz	120	1	24	1	18	2.5	1	75
Marinara dipping sauce	3 oz	60	2	12	2	9	0	0	440
Ranch dipping sauce	1.5 oz	220	0	2	0	1	23	3.5	420
Stuffed pizza rollers	as served	230	9	24	1	2	10	4.5	590
Wedge fries	1/2 order	320	4	35	3	0	18	3.5	530
White icing dipping cup	2 oz	170	0	44	0	38	0	0	5
WINGS									
All American bone out wings	2 pieces	150	10	11	1	0	8	1.5	490
All American crispy bone in wings	2 pieces	200	9	8	1	0	14	2.5	500
All American traditional wings	2 pieces	80	7	0	0	0	5	1.5	290
Buffalo Burnin' Hot bone-out wings	2 pieces	190	10	18	1	2	8	1.5	1000
Buffalo Burnin' Hot crispy bone-in wings	2 pieces	230	9	16	1	2	15	3	1020
Buffalo Burnin' Hot traditional wings	2 pieces	110	8	8	1	2	6	1.5	810
Buffalo medium bone-out wings	2 pieces	190	10	18	1	2	9	1.5	990
Buffalo medium crispy bone-in wings	2 pieces	230	9	16	2	2	15	3	1010
Buffalo medium traditional wings	2 pieces	110	8	8	1	2	6	1.5	800
Buffalo mild bone-out wings	2 pieces	190	10	18	1	2	9	1.5	1020

PIZZA HUT continued

Item	Serving Size	Calories	Protein	Carb	Fiber	Sugar	Total Fat	Sat Fat	Sodium
Buffalo mild crispy bone-in wings	2 pieces	230	9	16	1	2	15	3	1040
Buffalo mild traditional wings	2 pieces	110	8	8	1	2	6	1.5	830
Cajun bone-out wings	2 pieces	200	10	21	1	6	8	1.5	790
Cajun crispy bone-in wings	2 pieces	240	10	19	2	6	14	3	810
Cajun traditional wings	2 pieces	120	8	11	1	6	5	1.5	600
Garlic Parmesan bone-out wings	2 pieces	260	11	11	1	1	19	3.5	710
Garlic Parmesan crispy bone-in wings	2 pieces	300	10	9	1	1	25	5	730
Garlic Parmesan traditional wings	2 pieces	180	8	1	0	1	16	1.5	520
Honey BBQ bone-out wings	2 pieces	220	10	27	1	12	8	1.5	720
Honey BBQ crispy bone-in wings	2 pieces	260	10	24	1	12	14	3	740
Honey BBQ traditional wings	2 pieces	140	8	16	0	12	5	1.5	530
Spicy Asian bone-out wings	2 pieces	210	10	24	1	13	8	1.5	690
Spicy Asian crispy bone-in wings	2 pieces	250	10	21	1	13	14	2.5	710
Spicy Asian traditional wings	2 pieces	130	8	13	0	13	5	1.5	500
Spicy BBQ bone-out wings	2 pieces	200	10	21	1	11	8	1.5	940
Spicy BBQ crispy bone-in wings	2 pieces	240	9	19	1	11	14	2.5	950
Spicy BBQ traditional wings	2 pieces	120	8	11	0	11	5	1.5	750

POPEYES LOUISIANA KITCHEN

Item	Serving Size	Calories	Protein	Carb	Fiber	Sugar	Total Fat	Sat Fat	Sodium
Cajun chicken w/ rice	1 order	630	30	72	1	0	18	6	2229
Cajun chicken wings, fried	6 pieces	595	34	19	0	0	43	15	1274
Cajun-battered French fries	1 order	660	30	60	3	9	33	9	2280
Chicken deluxe sandwich w/ mayo	each	480	33	54	3	5	15	6	1290
Chicken sausage jambalaya	as served	220	10	20	1	3	11	3	760
Chicken strips	2 pieces	271	19	19	1	0	13	5.4	922
Étouffée Creole chicken w/ rice	1 order	480	36	18	6	3	30	9	2610
Fried chicken breast, mild	1 order	265	22	9	0	0	15.5	5.4	530
Fried chicken thigh, mild	1 order	313	19	11	1	0	22	7.4	595
Louisiana Travelers, mild tenders	3 pieces	375	33	24	0	0	17	7	1620
Louisiana Travelers, nuggets	6 pieces	220	15	13	<1	0	12	5	500
Louisiana Travelers, spicy tenders	3 pieces	405	33	30	0	0	17	7	2160
Naked chicken strips	3 pieces	220	30	2	0	0	10	15	1274
Red beans and rice	1 order	320	10	31	17	2	19	6	710
Shrimp, popcorn, batter-fried	as served	280	12	22	1	0	16	6	1110
Shrimp, popcorn, butterfly	as served	310	13	22	2	0	19	8	800

POTBELLY

Item	Serving Size	Calories	Protein	Carb	Fiber	Sugar	Total Fat	Sat Fat	Sodium
ORIGINALS									
A Wreck®	as served	468	18	56	6	3	14	5	1761
Big Jack's PB & J	as served	945	32	108	11	47	46	9	1050
Chicken salad	as served	530	35	61	6	2	22	3	1180
Italian	as served	585	27	54	6	3	29	11	1820
Meatball	as served	618	31	55	8	5	28	10	1051
Pizza w/ cheese	as served	395	23	56	7	5	9	4	818
Pizza w/ cheese & pepperoni	as served	536	29	54	7	5	22	10	1310
Roast beef	as served	403	31	55	6	4	6	2	1479
Smoked ham	as served	444	35	53	6	3	12	3	1886
Tuna salad	as served	490	29	54	6	2	15	3	1040
Turkey breast	as served	394	29	57	6	4	5	1	1550
Vegetarian	as served	550	30	55	7	3	22	12	1062
SKINNY									
T-K-Y	as served	272	20	41	4	2	4	0	1048
Hammie	as served	305	20	39	4	2	8	2	1269
Mushroom melt	as served	379	21	40	5	2	15	8	732
BIGS									
Pizza w/ cheese	as served	594	31	83	10	7	14	7	1270
Tuna salad	as served	684	47	80	8	4	19	4	1473
Meatball	as served	840	47	89	11	8	35	13	1499
Big Jack's PB & J	as served	1307	43	158	15	69	60	11	1501
Vegetarian	as served	784	42	81	9	5	30	17	1583
Chicken salad	as served	736	40	80	8	4	28	4	1653
Pizza w/ cheese & pepperoni	as served	769	37	83	10	7	30	15	1858
Roast beef	as served	572	42	82	8	7	8	2	2038
Turkey breast	as served	561	40	84	8	6	7	2	2129
A Wreck®	as served	641	37	81	8	5	19	6	2219
Italian	as served	810	38	81	8	5	38	14	2507
Smoked ham	as served	625	40	80	8	5	15	5	2561
SALADS W/O DRESSING									
Chicken salad	as served	460	22	46	6	34	22	5	652
A Wreck®	as served	423	35	9	4	5	27	13	1685

POTBELLY continued

Item	Serving Size	Calories	Protein	Carb	Fiber	Sugar	Total Fat	Sat Fat	Sodium
Chickpea veggie salad	as served	271	17	20	7	8	13	7	702
Farmhouse salad	as served	434	39	11	4	7	23	12	1504
Farmhouse salad, vegetarian	as served	203	13	9	4	6	12	7	478
Uptown salad	as served	508	29	42	9	33	25	9	1063
Uptown salad, vegetarian	as served	397	11	40	9	32	22	8	457
SALAD DRESSINGS									
Buttermilk ranch	2.5 oz	296	1	5	0	4	31	2	522
Creamy vinaigrette	2.5 oz	365	0	10	0	8	37	6	515
Non-fat vinaigrette	2.5 oz	50	0	12	0	12	0	0	400
Roasted garlic vinaigrette	2.5 oz	365	0	10	0	5	38	5	593
BOWL OF SOUP									
Loaded baked potato	as served	343	10	31	2	7	21	10	1029
Garden vegetable	as served	103	3	24	3	7	0	0	1097
Chili	as served	343	24	31	10	7	14	5	1200
Cream of tomato	as served	255	5	24	3	11	17	11	1230
Broccoli cheddar	as served	343	10	21	2	7	24	14	1406
Chicken noodle	as served	137	10	17	0	3	2	0	1646
SIDE STUFF									
Pickle	each	4	0	1	0	0	0	0	237
Coleslaw	as served	140	1	16	1	14	8	2	450
Macaroni salad	as served	240	5	23	1	4	14	5	650
Potato salad	as served	240	2	14	1	1	19	3	310
BAKED GOODS									
Chocolate brownie cookies	as served	460	6	61	3	43	22	9	250
Chocolate Mini cookies	as served	100	1	14	0	9	5	2	55
Oatmeal Mini cookies	as served	100	1	14	0	8	4	2	60
Oatmeal chocolate chip	as served	450	7	65	3	39	19	7	260
Sheila's Dream bar	as served	434	5	56	3	26	21	13	242

POTBELLY continued

Item	Serving Size	Calories	Protein	Carb	Fiber	Sugar	Total Fat	Sat Fat	Sodium
Sugar cookies	as served	550	7	80	1	42	22	14	530
BREAKFAST									
Bacon, egg, & cheese	as served	848	45	41	3	4	56	21	2345
Bacon, egg, lettuce & tomato	as served	847	39	42	4	5	59	17	2060
Banana nut muffin tops	as served	397	6	56	2	32	16	6	295
Blueberry muffin tops	as served	383	6	58	2	32	14	6	303
Egg & American cheese	as served	411	19	39	3	2	20	8	949
Ham, mushroom, egg, & cheese	as served	473	26	39	3	2	23	9	1489
Irish oatmeal	as served	229	3	55	3	37	1	0	13
Sausage, egg, & cheese	as served	631	27	39	3	2	40	15	1309
SHAKES									
Chocolate	each	684	15	89	1	74	31	22	272
Banana	each	635	15	78	1	63	31	22	263
Boysenberry	each	671	15	88	1	74	31	22	270
Coffee	each	625	12	75	0	61	34	22	263
Dreamsickle	each	685	15	88	1	74	31	22	266
Mocha	each	700	12	92	1	76	34	22	273
Oreo	each	740	16	92	1	71	36	23	415
Pineapple-coconut	each	684	17	88	2	73	33	23	271
Strawberry	each	641	15	80	1	67	31	22	268
Vanilla	each	610	15	72	0	60	31	22	262
MALTS									
Banana	each	757	18	99	1	77	34	23	398
Boysenberry	each	793	18	108	1	87	33	23	405
Chocolate	each	806	18	110	1	88	34	23	407
Coffee	each	747	14	95	0	75	36	23	398
Dreamsickle	each	807	18	109	1	88	33	23	401
Mocha	each	821	15	112	1	89	37	23	408
Oreo	each	861	19	112	1	85	39	25	550
Pineapple-coconut	each	806	19	109	2	87	35	24	406
Strawberry	each	762	17	100	1	80	33	23	403

POTBELLY continued

Item	Serving Size	Calories	Protein	Carb	Fiber	Sugar	Total Fat	Sat Fat	Sodium
Vanilla	each	732	17	92	0	73	33	23	397
SMOOTHIES									
Apple-Banana	each	500	12	97	1	91	6	4	330
Banana	each	475	15	82	1	79	9	6	363
Boysenberry	each	461	13	88	1	86	6	4	338
Chocolate	each	524	15	93	1	90	9	6	372
Pineapple-coconut	each	474	14	88	2	85	8	5	329
Strawberry	each	481	15	84	1	83	9	6	368
Vanilla	each	450	15	76	0	76	9	6	362

QUIZNOS

Item	Serving Size	Calories	Protein	Carb	Fiber	Sugar	Total Fat	Sat Fat	Sodium
SUBS									
Baja chicken sub w/ cheese, w/ dressing	small	480	23	41	2	8	21.5	8	460
Baja chicken sub w/ cheese, w/ dressing	regular	780	39	66	3	12	35	13.5	2090
Baja chicken sub w/ cheese, w/ dressing	large	1070	55	93	4	17	48	17.5	2940
Bourbon Grille steak sub w/ cheese, w/ dressing	small	575	35	50	2	12	26.5	6.5	1390
Bourbon Grille steak sub w/ cheese, w/ dressing	regular	880	53	79	3	21	40	10	2140
Bourbon Grille steak sub w/ cheese, w/ dressing	large	1190	71	109	5	28	53.5	13	3910
California club sub w/ cheese, w/ dressing	small	525	23	42	4	7	27.5	7.5	1520
California club sub w/ cheese, w/ dressing	regular	800	40	70	8	11	39	10.5	2640
California club sub w/ cheese, w/ dressing	large	1160	56	97	10	17	58	16.5	3710
Chicken carbenara sub w/ cheese, w/ dressing	small	525	24	39	2	4	27.5	8.5	1160
Chicken carbenara sub w/ cheese, w/ dressing	regular	860	41	63	3	7	44	14	1920
Chicken carbenara sub w/ cheese, w/ dressing	large	1200	57	87	4	11	61	19.5	2790

QUIZNOS continued

Item	Serving Size	Calories	Protein	Carb	Fiber	Sugar	Total Fat	Sat Fat	Sodium
Classic club sub w/ cheese, w/ dressing	small	550	24	40	2	6	32.5	9	1310
Classic club sub w/ cheese, w/ dressing	regular	860	41	66	4	10	49	13	2470
Classic club sub w/ cheese, w/ dressing	large	1240	56	91	6	14	72	20	3240
Classic sub w/ cheese, w/ dressing	small	475	19	42	3	6	26.5	9.5	1440
Classic sub w/ cheese, w/ dressing	regular	820	35	68	4	10	46	1	2610
Classic sub w/ cheese, w/ dressing	large	1100	45	94	6	14	61	23	3420
Double cheese cheesesteak sub w/ cheese, w/ dressing	small	700	35	43	2	5	42	5	1325
Double cheese cheesesteak sub w/ cheese, w/ dressing	regular	1070	54	67	4	8	67	8.5	2105
Double cheese cheesesteak sub w/ cheese, w/ dressing	large	1450	70	93	5	11	89	11	2890
Honey bacon club sub w/ cheese, w/ dressing	small	460	24	50	3	13	20	4	1410
Honey bacon club sub w/ cheese, w/ dressing	regular	760	35	81	4	22	32	7	2475
Honey bacon club sub w/ cheese, w/ dressing	large	1060	58	113	6	31	43	9	3545
Honey bourbon chicken sub w/ cheese, w/ dressing	small	315	16	48	2	12	4.5	1.5	860
Honey bourbon chicken sub w/ cheese, w/ dressing	regular	520	29	76	4	21	8	3	1470
Honey bourbon chicken sub w/ cheese, w/ dressing	large	730	41	107	5	28	11.5	4.5	2090
Honey mustard chicken sub w/ cheese, w/ dressing	small	500	24	43	2	8	25	6	1020
Honey mustard chicken sub w/ cheese, w/ dressing	regular	830	40	69	4	13	40	11	1715

QUIZNOS continued

Item	Serving Size	Calories	Protein	Carb	Fiber	Sugar	Total Fat	Sat Fat	Sodium
Honey mustard chicken sub w/ cheese, w/ dressing	large	1160	58	96	5	18	56	14.5	2415
Mesquite chicken sub w/ cheese, w/ dressing	small	490	24	40	2	6	23.5	8.5	1110
Mesquite chicken sub w/ cheese, w/ dressing	regular	790	39	64	4	8	38	14	1840
Mesquite chicken sub w/ cheese, w/ dressing	large	1100	57	89	5	12	51	18	2600
Prime rib & peppercorn sub w/ cheese, w/ dressing	small	624	30	43	2	6	35.5	5.5	1300
Prime rib & peppercorn sub w/ cheese, w/ dressing	regular	960	48	68	4	8	57	9.5	2020
Prime rib & peppercorn sub w/ cheese, w/ dressing	large	1320	63	94	5	12	78	13	2750
Prime rib mushroom & Swiss sub w/ cheese, w/ dressing	small	560	28	41	2	5	32	3.5	1075
Prime rib mushroom & Swiss sub w/ cheese, w/ dressing	regular	930	49	64	3	7	54	6	1815
Prime rib mushroom & Swiss sub w/ cheese, w/ dressing	large	1260	65	89	4	9	72	8.5	2465
Steakhouse prime rib dip sub w/ cheese, w/ dressing	small	560	33	44	2	5	29	3.5	1850
Steakhouse prime rib dip sub w/ cheese, w/ dressing	regular	860	49	67	3	8	44	5.5	2535
Steakhouse prime rib dip sub w/ cheese, w/ dressing	large	1170	65	93	4	11	58	7.5	3225
Tuna melt sub w/ cheese, w/ dressing	small	620	26	39	2	4	39.5	8.5	840
Tuna melt sub w/ cheese, w/ dressing	regular	1000	42	2	4	7	66	14	1350
Tuna melt sub w/ cheese, w/ dressing	large	1520	68	87	5	10	101	21	2020

QUIZNOS continued

Item	Serving Size	Calories	Protein	Carb	Fiber	Sugar	Total Fat	Sat Fat	Sodium
Turkey Cuban sub w/ cheese, w/ dressing	small	390	20	40	2	4	17	3	1270
Turkey Cuban sub w/ cheese, w/ dressing	regular	640	34	64	4	7	28	5.5	2235
Turkey Cuban sub w/ cheese, w/dressing	large	900	48	90	5	11	39	7.5	3205
Turkey, ranch & Swiss sub w/ cheese, w/ dressing	small	400	19	43	2	6	17	3	1130
Turkey, ranch & Swiss sub w/ cheese, w/ dressing	regular	650	33	69	4	9	28	5.5	2050
Turkey, ranch & Swiss sub w/ cheese, w/ dressing	large	920	48	98	6	14	38	7.5	2925
Veggie sub w/ cheese, w/ dressing	small	520	17	42	5	6	31	9	1260
Veggie sub w/ cheese, w/ dressing	regular	820	26	66	8	11	48	14	1950
Veggie sub w/ cheese, w/ dressing	large	1120	35	91	11	15	66	18.5	2670

TOASTED SUBS

Item	Serving Size	Calories	Protein	Carb	Fiber	Sugar	Total Fat	Sat Fat	Sodium
beef, bacon & cheddar Toasty Bullet w/ cheese, w/ dressing	each	405	19	42	2	7	17.5	5	1235
beef, bacon & cheddar Toasty Torpedo w/ cheese, w/ dressing	each	820	39	94	5	16	30.5	9	2480
Buffalo chicken sub w/ cheese, w/ dressing	large	1040	43	91	5	16	54	15	2520
Buffalo chicken toasted sub w/ cheese, w/ dressing	half	525	21	45	2	8	27.5	7	1260
French dip toasted sub w/ cheese, w/ dressing	half	500	19	45	2	9	28	6	1785
French dip toasted sub w/ cheese, w /dressing	large	980	37	86	4	19	54	11.5	2980
Honey-cured ham toasted sub w/ cheese, w/ dressing	half	505	21	40	3	10	28.5	7	1135
Honey-cured ham toasted sub w/ cheese, w/ dressing	large	1020	42	83	6	21	57	14.5	2260

QUIZNOS continued

Item	Serving Size	Calories	Protein	Carb	Fiber	Sugar	Total Fat	Sat Fat	Sodium
Italian Toasty Bullet w/ cheese, w/ dressing	each	435	16	40	2	7	23.5	6.5	1305
Italian Toasty Torpedo w/ cheese, w/ dressing	each	875	33	92	5	16	41.5	12	2550
Oven-roasted turkey toasted sub w/ cheese, w/ dressing	half	495	19	42	3	9	38.5	7	1235
Oven-roasted turkey toasted sub w/ cheese, w/ dressing	large	1010	40	86	5	18	57	14	2480
Pesto turkey Toasty Bullet w/ cheese, w/ dressing	each	345	16	41	2	7	13.5	3.5	1145
Pesto turkey Toasty Torpedo w/ cheese, w/ dressing	each	695	32	94	5	15	23.5	5	1230
Roast beef toasted sub w/ cheese, w/ dressing	half	505	21	43	2	10	27.5	6.5	1245
Roast beef toasted sub w/ cheese, w/ dressing	large	1020	43	87	4	20	55	14	2480
Tuna melt Toasty Bullet w/ cheese, w/ dressing	each	475	16	38	2	5	27.5	5.5	670
Tuna melt Toasty Torpedo w/ cheese, w/ dressing	each	920	32	88	4	12	48.5	10	1365
Turkey & ham toasted sub w/ cheese, w/ dressing	half	525	20	42	3	9	30.5	7.5	1205
Turkey & ham toasted sub w/ cheese, w/ dressing	large	1040	41	85	6	19	61	15	2410
Turkey club Toasty Bullet w/ cheese, w/ dressing	each	415	17	41	2	7	20.5	5	1235
Turkey club Toasty Bullet w/ cheese, w/ dressing	each	845	35	93	5	15	36.5	8.5	2470
FLATBREAD SAMMIES									
Bistro steak melt flatbread Sammie w/ cheese, w/ dressing	each	395	16	30	1	5	22.5	5.5	1020
Cantina chicken flatbread Sammie w/ cheese, w/ dressing	each	275	12	36	2	12	7	1.5	640

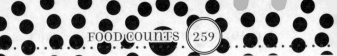

QUIZNOS continued

Item	Serving Size	Calories	Protein	Carb	Fiber	Sugar	Total Fat	Sat Fat	Sodium
Chicken bacon ranch flatbread Sammie w/ cheese, w/ dressing	each	380	20	28	1	4	19	4.5	780
Italian flatbread Sammie w/ cheese, w/ dressing	each	390	18	29	1	4	23	5	985
Roadhouse steak flatbread Sammie w/ cheese, w/ dressing	each	260	13	38	1	13	6	1	980
Smokey chipotle turkey flatbread Sammie w/ cheese, w/ dressing	each	380	15	29	1	4	23	5.5	1135
Veggie flatbread Sammie w/ cheese, w/ dressing	each	340	9	29	3	5	20	5	755
SOUPS & SALADS									
Broccoli cheese soup	1 bowl	260	9	18	1	3	17	12	1280
Broccoli cheese soup	1 cup	130	4	9	1	2	9	6	640
Chicken Caesar chopped salad	small	535	16	18	2	4	41	11.5	1235
Chicken Caesar chopped salad	regular	920	33	38	5	10	66	20	2110
Chicken noodle soup	1 bowl	110	7	17	1	2	2.5	0.5	1470
Chicken noodle soup	1 cup	60	4	16	1	1	2	0	880
Chicken taco chopped salad	small	530	14	14	3	3	42.5	8	1170
Chicken taco chopped salad	regular	880	27	19	5	7	72	14.5	2135
Chili	1 bowl	230	20	26	6	6	6	1.5	1050
Chili	1 cup	140	45	48	3	3	3.5	1	630
Classic Cobb chopped salad	small	445	13	19	2	4	33	9.5	995
Classic Cobb chopped salad	regular	780	28	38	4	9	56	18	1790
Honey mustard chicken chopped salad	small	530	15	25	2	12	38.5	10.5	895
Honey mustard chicken chopped salad	regular	910	31	46	5	18	64	19.5	1685
Raspberry vinaigrette chicken chopped salad	small	350	14	40	2	25	13	6.5	795
Raspberry vinaigrette chicken chopped salad	regular	700	33	70	5	40	29	15	1685

QUIZNOS continued

Item	Serving Size	Calories	Protein	Carb	Fiber	Sugar	Total Fat	Sat Fat	Sodium
Q-KIDZ									
Chicken toasted cheese sub w/ cheese, w/ dressing	kidz size	330	13	43	2	6	11	6	580
Ham melt Sammie w/ cheese, w/ dressing	kidz size	200	11	25	1	3	6	7.5	535
Just cheese Sammie w/ cheese, w/ dressing	kidz size	230	11	25	1	3	10	10	390
Kidz cheesy cheese pizza	kidz size	290	15	28	1	5	14	12	550
Kidz ham pizza	kidz size	210	11	27	1	5	7	8	560
Kidz pepperoni pizza	kidz size	265	11	27	1	4	12.5	10	680
Toasty ham & cheese sub w/ cheese, w/ dressing	kidz size	310	15	43	2	7	8.5	3.5	750
Toasty turkey & cheese sub w/ cheese, w/ dressing	kidz size	310	14	44	2	6	8	3.5	790
Toasty turkey Sammie w/ cheese, w/ dressing	kidz size	200	10	26	1	3	6	7.5	575

RED LOBSTER

Item	Serving Size	Calories	Protein	Carb	Fiber	Sugar	Total Fat	Sat Fat	Sodium
LIGHTHOUSE MENU									
Balsamic vinaigrette	as served	80	n/a	4	n/a	n/a	6	1	190
Chilled jumbo shrimp cocktail	as served	120	n/a	9	n/a	n/a	0.5	0	580
Cocktail sauce	as served	0	n/a	9	n/a	n/a	0	0	480
Fresh asparagus	as served	60	n/a	5	n/a	n/a	3	1.5	270
Fresh broccoli	as served	45	n/a	6	n/a	n/a	0.5	0	200
Garden salad, before dressing	as served	90	n/a	13	n/a	n/a	3	0	105
Live Maine lobster	1 1/4 lb	45	n/a	0	n/a	n/a	0	0	350
Petite shrimp salad topping	topping	15	n/a	0	n/a	n/a	0	0	125
Pico de gallo	as served	10	n/a	2	n/a	n/a	0	0	160
Rainbow trout, wood-grilled or broiled	as served	220	n/a	6	n/a	n/a	10	2.5	380

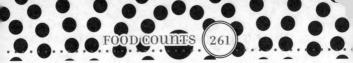
RED LOBSTER continued

Item	Serving Size	Calories	Protein	Carb	Fiber	Sugar	Total Fat	Sat Fat	Sodium
Salmon, wood-grilled or broiled	as served	270	n/a	6	n/a	n/a	9	2	310
Tilapia, wood-grilled or broiled	as served	210	n/a	9	n/a	n/a	3	1	230

FRESH FISH MENU

Item	Serving Size	Calories	Protein	Carb	Fiber	Sugar	Total Fat	Sat Fat	Sodium
Arctic char	1/2 portion	340	n/a	13	n/a	n/a	15	3	460
Arctic char	full portion	630	n/a	21	n/a	n/a	29	6	720
Barramundi	1/2 portion	230	n/a	8	n/a	n/a	5	1.5	270
Barramundi	full portion	420	n/a	11	n/a	n/a	10	2.5	350
Cobia	1/2 portion	400	n/a	6	n/a	n/a	26	8	250
Cobia	full portion	760	n/a	8	n/a	n/a	54	17	310
Cod	1/2 portion	170	n/a	8	n/a	n/a	2	0	500
Cod	full portion	300	n/a	10	n/a	n/a	3.5	0.5	810
Corvina	1/2 portion	180	n/a	7	n/a	n/a	1.5	0	300
Corvina	full portion	320	n/a	9	n/a	n/a	2.5	0.5	420
Flounder	1/2 portion	200	n/a	8	n/a	n/a	1.5	0	350
Flounder	full portion	350	n/a	11	n/a	n/a	2.5	0	500
Grouper	1/2 portion	210	n/a	6	n/a	n/a	1.5	0	280
Grouper	full portion	370	n/a	6	n/a	n/a	2.5	0.5	370
Haddock	1/2 portion	180	n/a	6	n/a	n/a	1.5	0	520
Haddock	full portion	310	n/a	6	n/a	n/a	3	0.5	850
Lake whitefish	1/2 portion	210	n/a	6	n/a	n/a	2.5	0.5	400
Lake whitefish	full portion	380	n/a	6	n/a	n/a	4.5	1	610
Mahi-mahi	1/2 portion	200	n/a	6	n/a	n/a	1.5	0	270
Mahi-mahi	full portion	360	n/a	7	n/a	n/a	2	0	360
Monchong	1/2 portion	190	n/a	7	n/a	n/a	1.5	0	290
Monchong	full portion	340	n/a	9	n/a	n/a	2.5	0.5	390
Opah	1/2 portion	280	n/a	8	n/a	n/a	12	3.5	280
Opah	full portion	510	n/a	11	n/a	n/a	24	7	380
Perch	1/2 portion	170	n/a	6	n/a	n/a	2	0	550
Perch	full portion	300	n/a	7	n/a	n/a	3.5	1	910
Pompano	1/2 portion	240	n/a	6	n/a	n/a	8	3.5	310
Pompano	full portion	430	n/a	7	n/a	n/a	16	7	430
Red rockfish	1/2 portion	170	n/a	6	n/a	n/a	2.5	0	580
Red rockfish	full portion	300	n/a	10	n/a	n/a	4	1	860
Salmon	1/2 portion	270	n/a	6	n/a	n/a	9	2	310

RED LOBSTER continued

Item	Serving Size	Calories	Protein	Carb	Fiber	Sugar	Total Fat	Sat Fat	Sodium
Salmon	full portion	490	n/a	6	n/a	n/a	17	3.5	440
Seabass	1/2 portion	230	n/a	6	n/a	n/a	6	1.5	450
Seabass	full portion	410	n/a	6	n/a	n/a	12	3	700
Snapper	1/2 portion	210	n/a	8	n/a	n/a	1.5	0	330
Snapper	full portion	370	n/a	11	n/a	n/a	2.5	0.5	470
Sole	1/2 portion	140	n/a	6	n/a	n/a	2	0	860
Sole	full portion	240	n/a	6	n/a	n/a	4	1	1530
Tilapia	1/2 portion	210	n/a	9	n/a	n/a	3	1	230
Tilapia	full portion	360	n/a	12	n/a	n/a	4.5	1	270
Trout, rainbow	1/2 portion	220	n/a	6	n/a	n/a	10	2.5	380
Trout, rainbow	full portion	410	n/a	7	n/a	n/a	19	5	580
Tuna	1/2 portion	200	n/a	7	n/a	n/a	1	0	42
Tuna	full portion	360	n/a	8	n/a	n/a	1.5	0	640
Wahoo	1/2 portion	220	n/a	8	n/a	n/a	2.5	0.5	340
Wahoo	full portion	400	n/a	10	n/a	n/a	4	1	490
Walleye	1/2 portion	170	n/a	7	n/a	n/a	2	0	400
Walleye	full portion	300	n/a	9	n/a	n/a	4	1	610
Wood-grilled seasonal selection, tilapia w/ spicy soy broth	as served	630	n/a	64	n/a	n/a	20	5	3480
Chef's Signature Toppings, New Orleans shrimp	Full or 1/2	250	n/a	3	n/a	n/a	19	10	800
Chef's Signature Toppings, shrimp bruschette	Full or 1/2	140	n/a	6	n/a	n/a	7	1.5	700

SEAFOOD STARTERS

Item	Serving Size	Calories	Protein	Carb	Fiber	Sugar	Total Fat	Sat Fat	Sodium
Buffalo chicken wings	as served	680	n/a	0	n/a	n/a	39	9	1750
Chilled jumbo shrimp cocktail	as served	120	n/a	9	n/a	n/a	0.5	0	580
Create Your Own Combo, stuffed mushrooms	Create your own combo	220	n/a	12	n/a	n/a	12	6	740
Create Your Own Combo, chicken breast strips	Create your own combo	410	n/a	28	n/a	n/a	24	2	1320

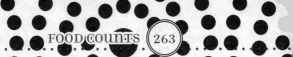

RED LOBSTER continued

Item	Serving Size	Calories	Protein	Carb	Fiber	Sugar	Total Fat	Sat Fat	Sodium
Create Your Own Combo, clam strips	Create your own combo	370	n/a	31	n/a	n/a	22	2	820
Create Your Own Combo, crispy calamari and vegetables	Create your own combo	760	n/a	58	n/a	n/a	49	6	1530
Create Your Own Combo, mozzarella cheesesticks	Create your own combo	340	n/a	24	n/a	n/a	20	7	950
Crispy calamari & vegetables	as served	1520	n/a	115	n/a	n/a	97	11	3050
Fried crawfish	as served	1190	n/a	104	n/a	n/a	69	7	2740
Fried oysters	as served	590	n/a	66	n/a	n/a	31	3	1220
Handshucked oysters	1 dozen	100	n/a	7	n/a	n/a	2.5	1	250
Lobster nachos	as served	1090	n/a	64	n/a	n/a	64	19	1680
Lobster pizza	as served	720	n/a	69	n/a	n/a	30	13	1390
Lobster, artichoke & seafood dip	as served	1200	n/a	101	n/a	n/a	74	20	1950
Lobster, crab & seafood stuffed mushrooms	as served	380	n/a	20	n/a	n/a	21	11	1050
Mozzarella cheesesticks	as served	680	n/a	49	n/a	n/a	39	14	1910
New England seafood sampler	as served	760	n/a	45	n/a	n/a	43	11	2050
Pan-seared crab cakes	as served	280	n/a	13	n/a	n/a	14	2.5	1110
Parrot Isle jumbo coconut shrimp	as served	590	n/a	54	n/a	n/a	33	7	1170
Peach-bourbon BBQ scallops	as served	430	n/a	21	n/a	n/a	27	5	121
Steamed clams	as served	430	n/a	10	n/a	n/a	15	3.5	1110
Wood-grilled shrimp bruschetta	as served	650	n/a	58	n/a	n/a	26	4.5	2380
SOUPS & SALADS									
Bayou seafood gumbo	1 cup	190	n/a	15	n/a	n/a	6	2	1130
Bayou seafood gumbo	1 bowl	380	n/a	31	n/a	n/a	12	3.5	2260
Creamy potato bacon soup	1 cup	220	n/a	19	n/a	n/a	15	9	790
Creamy potato bacon soup	1 bowl	450	n/a	37	n/a	n/a	3	17	1580

RED LOBSTER continued

Item	Serving Size	Calories	Protein	Carb	Fiber	Sugar	Total Fat	Sat Fat	Sodium
Hand-tossed Caesar salad w/ wood-grilled chicken	each	670	n/a	14	n/a	n/a	52	10	1750
Hand-tossed Caesar salad w/ wood-grilled shrimp	each	620	n/a	14	n/a	n/a	51	10	1370
Manhattan clam chowder	1 cup	80	n/a	12	n/a	n/a	1	0	690
Manhattan clam chowder	1 bowl	160	n/a	25	n/a	n/a	2	1	1420
New England clam chowder	1 cup	230	n/a	13	n/a	n/a	17	10	680
New England clam chowder	1 bowl	480	n/a	26	n/a	n/a	34	20	1390
Seafood gumbo	1 cup	230	n/a	25	n/a	n/a	8	2.5	160
Seafood gumbo	1 bowl	470	n/a	51	n/a	n/a	17	5	2370
Spicy shrimp Soup	1 cup	160	n/a	15	n/a	n/a	6	2.5	1010
Spicy shrimp Soup	1 bowl	320	n/a	31	n/a	n/a	12	5	2050
WOOD-FIRE GRILLED SHELLFISH									
Garlic-grilled jumbo shrimp	as served	370	n/a	40	n/a	n/a	9	2	2160
Maui Luau shrimp & salmon	as served	760	n/a	82	n/a	n/a	16	3.5	2640
Peach-bourbon BBQ shrimp & scallops	as served	540	n/a	36	n/a	n/a	27	4.5	1440
Wood-grilled lobster, shrimp & scallops	as served	500	n/a	42	n/a	n/a	11	2.5	3220
Wood-grilled scallops, shrimp & chicken	as served	600	n/a	42	n/a	n/a	13	3	3190
WOOD-GRILLED STEAK & CHICKEN									
Center-cut NY strip steak	14 oz	590	n/a	0	n/a	n/a	33	14	1420
Maple glazed chicken	as served	570	n/a	62	n/a	n/a	9	2.5	1950
Maple glazed shrimp add-on	skewer	110	n/a	11	n/a	n/a	1	0	780
NY Strip & Rock lobster tail	as served	690	n/a	0	n/a	n/a	35	14	1930
Steak lobster-&-shrimp Oscar	as served	1170	n/a	20	n/a	n/a	77	33	2770
Wood-grilled peppercorn sirloin & shrimp	as served	560	n/a	25	n/a	n/a	21	9	2210

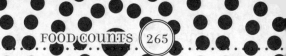

RED LOBSTER continued

Item	Serving Size	Calories	Protein	Carb	Fiber	Sugar	Total Fat	Sat Fat	Sodium
LOBSTER & CRAB									
Chef's Sig. lobster & shrimp pasta	Half Portion	510	n/a	43	n/a	n/a	25	11	1090
Chef's Sig. lobster & shrimp pasta	Full Portion	1020	n/a	86	n/a	n/a	50	21	2170
Live Maine lobster	1 1/4 lb	45	n/a	0	n/a	n/a	0	0	350
North Pacific King crab legs	as served	390	n/a	2	n/a	n/a	3.5	1	3520
Rock lobster tail	as served	90	n/a	0	n/a	n/a	1	0	490
Rockzilla	as served	130	n/a	0	n/a	n/a	1.5	0	690
Snow crab legs	1 lb	160	n/a	0	n/a	n/a	1	0	1960
Stuffed Maine lobster	as served	240	n/a	12	n/a	n/a	7	2.5	1150
SHRIMP									
Crunchy popcorn shrimp	as served	560	n/a	51	n/a	n/a	27	2.5	2100
Parrot Isle jumbo coconut shrimp	as served	980	n/a	90	n/a	n/a	55	12	1950
Add 5 More	5	590	n/a	54	n/a	n/a	33	7	1170
Shrimp linguini Alfredo	1/2 portion	550	n/a	41	n/a	n/a	29	10	150
Shrimp linguini Alfredo	full portion	1100	n/a	84	n/a	n/a	58	21	3200
Shrimp Your Way, Coconut shrimp bites	as served	290	n/a	19	n/a	n/a	18	3	830
Shrimp Your Way, Fried shrimp	as served	190	n/a	9	n/a	n/a	11	1	1010
Shrimp Your Way, Popcorn shrimp	as served	180	n/a	16	n/a	n/a	9	1	670
Shrimp Your Way, Scampi	as served	130	n/a	1	n/a	n/a	9	1.5	690
Walt's Favorite Shrimp	as served	700	n/a	52	n/a	n/a	39	3.5	2410
Add 1/2 Dozen More	1/2 dozen	350	n/a	26	n/a	n/a	20	1.5	1220
TRADITIONAL FAVORITES									
Bbroiled seafood platter	as served	280	n/a	11	n/a	n/a	8	2	1610
Cajun chicken linguini Alfredo	1/2 portion	630	n/a	45	n/a	n/a	27	10	1550
Cajun chicken linguini Alfredo	full portion	1260	n/a	91	n/a	n/a	53	19	3110

RED LOBSTER continued

Item	Serving Size	Calories	Protein	Carb	Fiber	Sugar	Total Fat	Sat Fat	Sodium
Flounder, broiled	as served	320	n/a	10	n/a	n/a	2	0	470
Flounder, fried	as served	440	n/a	5	n/a	n/a	16	1.5	560
Seafood, stuffed flounder	as served	320	n/a	13	n/a	n/a	11	3.5	1520
Walleye, beer battered	as served	700	n/a	24	n/a	n/a	42	4	1200
Walleye, blackened	as served	300	n/a	9	n/a	n/a	7	1	410
Walleye, broiled	as served	260	n/a	0	n/a	n/a	3.5	1	540
Walleye, fried	as served	600	n/a	35	n/a	n/a	29	2.5	990

CREATE YOUR OWN FEAST

Item	Serving Size	Calories	Protein	Carb	Fiber	Sugar	Total Fat	Sat Fat	Sodium
Fried crawfish	as served	750	n/a	49	n/a	n/a	47	4.5	1480
Fried oysters	as served	590	n/a	58	n/a	n/a	32	3.5	1100
Garlic shrimp scampi	as served	190	n/a	<1	n/a	n/a	13	2.5	1150
Garlic-grilled jumbo shrimp	as served	110	n/a	3	n/a	n/a	3	0.5	800
Parrot Isle jumbo coconut shrimp	as served	780	n/a	72	n/a	n/a	44	10	1560
Seafood-stuffed flounder	as served	160	n/a	6	n/a	n/a	5	1.5	760
Shrimp linguini Alfredo	as served	550	n/a	41	n/a	n/a	29	10	1580
Steamed snow crab legs	as served	0	n/a	0	n/a	n/a	0.5	0	940
Walt's Favorite Shrimp	as served	470	n/a	34	n/a	n/a	26	2.5	1610
Wood-grilled fresh salmon	as served	210	n/a	0	n/a	n/a	9	2	240
Wood-grilled peppercorn salmon	as served	280	n/a	0	n/a	n/a	10	4	850

SIGNATURE COMBINATIONS

Item	Serving Size	Calories	Protein	Carb	Fiber	Sugar	Total Fat	Sat Fat	Sodium
Admiral's Feast	as served	1500	n/a	110	n/a	n/a	87	7	4400
Seaside Shrimp Trio	as served	1030	n/a	68	n/a	n/a	57	14	3480
Ultimate Feast®	as served	620	n/a	29	n/a	n/a	30	3.5	3370

MONDAY & TUESDAY SPECIALS

Item	Serving Size	Calories	Protein	Carb	Fiber	Sugar	Total Fat	Sat Fat	Sodium
Cocount shrimp bites	as served	290	n/a	19	n/a	n/a	18	3	830
Fried shrimp	as served	190	n/a	9	n/a	n/a	11	1	1010
Popcorn shrimp	as served	180	n/a	16	n/a	n/a	9	1	670

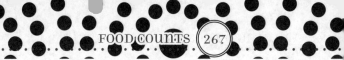

RED LOBSTER continued

Item	Serving Size	Calories	Protein	Carb	Fiber	Sugar	Total Fat	Sat Fat	Sodium
Scampi	as served	130	n/a	1	n/a	n/a	9	1.5	690
ADD TO ANY MEAL									
Maine lobster tail	each	60	n/a	0	n/a	n/a	0.5	0	490
North Pacific King crab legs	1/2 lb	130	n/a	<1	n/a	n/a	1	0	1190
Snow crab legs	1/2 lb	80	n/a	0	n/a	n/a	0.5	0	940
ENDLESS SHRIMP (seasonal)									
Garlic shrimp scampi	Initial Order	190	n/a	1	n/a	n/a	13	2.5	1150
Garlic shrimp scampi	Refill Order	130	n/a	1	n/a	n/a	9	1.5	690
Garlic-grilled shrimp	Initial Order	150	n/a	18	n/a	n/a	2.5	0.5	900
Garlic-grilled shrimp	Refill Order	150	n/a	18	n/a	n/a	2.5	0.5	900
Hand-breaded shrimp	Initial Order	290	n/a	14	n/a	n/a	17	1.5	1520
Hand-breaded shrimp	Refill Order	190	n/a	9	n/a	n/a	11	1	1010
Parmesan shrimp	Initial Order	250	n/a	19	n/a	n/a	12	5	1050
Parmesan shrimp	Refill Order	250	n/a	19	n/a	n/a	12	5	1050
Seaport lobster & shrimp	Initial Order	560	n/a	40	n/a	n/a	18	3.5	3860
Shrimp linguini Alfredo	Initial Order	550	n/a	41	n/a	n/a	29	10	1580
Shrimp linguini Alfredo	Refill Order	550	n/a	41	n/a	n/a	29	10	1580
ACCOMPANIMENTS									
Baked potato	each	190	n/a	40	n/a	n/a	1	0	900
w/ butter	as served	90	n/a	1	n/a	n/a	10	6	80
w/ sour cream	as served	30	n/a	1	n/a	n/a	2.5	1.5	10
Caesar salad	each	270	n/a	13	n/a	n/a	21	4.5	560
w/ petite shrimp	as served	15	n/a	0	n/a	n/a	0	0	125
Cheddar Bay biscuit	each	150	n/a	16	n/a	n/a	8	2.5	350
Coleslaw	as served	200	n/a	13	n/a	n/a	15	2.5	250
Creamy Langostino lobster baked potato	each	370	n/a	48	n/a	n/a	12	7	1110

RED LOBSTER continued

Item	Serving Size	Calories	Protein	Carb	Fiber	Sugar	Total Fat	Sat Fat	Sodium
Creamy Langostino lobster mashed potatoes	as served	360	n/a	23	n/a	n/a	22	12	1110
Fresh asparagus	as served	60	n/a	5	n/a	n/a	3	1.5	270
Fresh broccoli	as served	45	n/a	6	n/a	n/a	0.5	0	200
Freshly cooked potato chips	as served	300	n/a	28	n/a	n/a	19	1.5	580
Fries	as served	330	n/a	40	n/a	n/a	17	1.5	740
Garden salad	each	90	n/a	13	n/a	n/a	3	0	105
w/ petite shrimp	as served	15	n/a	0	n/a	n/a	0	0	125
Home-style mashed potatoes	as served	180	n/a	22	n/a	n/a	9	4	610
Wild rice pilaf	as served	180	n/a	34	n/a	n/a	3	0.5	650
DRESSINGS									
Balsamic vinaigrette	1.5 oz	80	n/a	4	n/a	n/a	6	1	190
Blue cheese	1.5 oz	240	n/a	2	n/a	n/a	26	4.5	260
Caesar	1.5 oz	280	n/a	1	n/a	n/a	30	5	560
French	1.5 oz	160	n/a	9	n/a	n/a	14	2	390
Honey mustard	1.5 oz	190	n/a	8	n/a	n/a	17	2.5	250
Ranch	1.5 oz	160	n/a	3	n/a	n/a	16	2.5	380
Ranch, fat-free	1.5 oz	60	n/a	5	n/a	n/a	0	0	250
Thousand Island	1.5 oz	200	n/a	6	n/a	n/a	20	3	180
DIPPING SAUCES									
100% pure melted butter	1.5 oz	350	n/a	2	n/a	n/a	38	23	30
Cocktail sauce	1.5 oz	40	n/a	9	n/a	n/a	0	0	480
Honey mustard dipping sauce	1.5 oz	280	n/a	12	n/a	n/a	26	4	360
Ketchup	1.5 oz	50	n/a	11	n/a	n/a	0	0	460
Marinara sauce	1.5 oz	25	n/a	4	n/a	n/a	1	0	170
Pico de gallo	1.5 oz	10	n/a	2	n/a	n/a	0	0	160
Piña colada sauce	1.5 oz	80	n/a	12	n/a	n/a	4	3	20
Rémoulade	1.5 oz	230	n/a	6	n/a	n/a	22	3.5	220
Sweet & spicy glaze	1.5 oz	100	n/a	24	n/a	n/a	0	0	290
Tartar sauce	1.5 oz	190	n/a	6	n/a	n/a	16	3	170

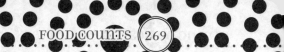

RED LOBSTER continued

Item	Serving Size	Calories	Protein	Carb	Fiber	Sugar	Total Fat	Sat Fat	Sodium
LUNCH MENU									
SEASIDE STARTERS									
Buffalo chicken wings	as served	680	n/a	0	n/a	n/a	39	9	1750
Chilled jumbo shrimp cocktail	as served	120	n/a	9	n/a	n/a	0.5	2	580
Create Your Own Combo, stuffed mushrooms	Create your own combo	220	n/a	12	n/a	n/a	12	6	740
Create Your Own Combo, chicken breast strips	Create your own combo	410	n/a	28	n/a	n/a	24	2	1320
Create Your Own Combo, clam strips	Create your own combo	370	n/a	31	n/a	n/a	22	2	820
Create Your Own Combo, crispy calamari & vegetables	Create your own combo	760	n/a	58	n/a	n/a	49	6	1530
Create Your Own Combo, mozzarella cheesesticks	Create your own combo	340	n/a	24	n/a	n/a	20	7	950
Crispy calamari & vegetables	as served	1520	n/a	115	n/a	n/a	97	11	3050
Fried crawfish	as served	1190	n/a	104	n/a	n/a	69	7	2740
Fried oysters	as served	590	n/a	66	n/a	n/a	31	3	1220
Handshucked oysters	1 dozen	100	n/a	7	n/a	n/a	2.5	1	250
Lobster nachos	as served	1090	n/a	64	n/a	n/a	64	19	1680
Lobster pizza	as served	720	n/a	69	n/a	n/a	30	13	1390
Lobster, artichoke, & seafood dip	as served	1200	n/a	101	n/a	n/a	74	20	1950
Lobster, crab, & seafood stuffed mushrooms	as served	380	n/a	20	n/a	n/a	21	11	1050
Mango-jalapeño shrimp skewers	as served	560	n/a	58	n/a	n/a	22	3	1030
Mozzarella cheesesticks	as served	680	n/a	49	n/a	n/a	39	14	1910
New England seafood sample	as served	760	n/a	45	n/a	n/a	43	11	2050
Pan-seared crab cakes	as served	280	n/a	13	n/a	n/a	14	2.5	1110
Parrot Isle jumbo coconut shrimp	as served	590	n/a	54	n/a	n/a	33	7	1170

RED LOBSTER continued

Item	Serving Size	Calories	Protein	Carb	Fiber	Sugar	Total Fat	Sat Fat	Sodium
Peach-bourbon BBQ scallops	as served	430	n/a	21	n/a	n/a	27	5	121
Steamed clams	as served	430	n/a	10	n/a	n/a	15	3.5	1110
Wood-grilled shrimp bruschetta	as served	650	n/a	58	n/a	n/a	26	4.5	2380
LUNCH SOUPS									
Bayou seafood gumbo	1 cup	190	n/a	15	n/a	n/a	6	2	1130
Bayou seafood gumbo	1 bowl	380	n/a	31	n/a	n/a	12	3.5	2260
Creamy potato bacon	1 cup	220	n/a	19	n/a	n/a	15	9	790
Creamy potato bacon	1 bowl	450	n/a	37	n/a	n/a	3	17	1580
Manhattan clam chowder	1 cup	80	n/a	12	n/a	n/a	1	0	690
Manhattan clam chowder	1 bowl	160	n/a	25	n/a	n/a	2	1	1420
New England clam chowder	1 cup	230	n/a	13	n/a	n/a	17	10	680
New England clam chowder	1 bowl	480	n/a	26	n/a	n/a	34	20	1390
Seafood gumbo	1 cup	230	n/a	25	n/a	n/a	8	2.5	160
Seafood gumbo	1 bowl	470	n/a	51	n/a	n/a	17	5	2370
Spicy shrimp	1 cup	160	n/a	15	n/a	n/a	6	5	1010
Spicy shrimp	1 bowl	320	n/a	31	n/a	n/a	12		2050
WOOD-FIRE GRILLED SHELLFISH									
Garlic-grilled jumbo shrimp	as served	370	n/a	40	n/a	n/a	9	3.5	2160
Maui Luau shrimp & salmon	as served	760	n/a	82	n/a	n/a	16	4.5	2640
Peach-bourbon BBQ shrimp & scallops	as served	540	n/a	36	n/a	n/a	27	2.5	1440
Wood-grilled lobster, shrimp & scallops	as served	500	n/a	42	n/a	n/a	11	3	3220
Wood-grilled scallops, shrimp & chicken	as served	600	n/a	42	n/a	n/a	13		3190
WOOD-GRILLED STEAK & CHICKEN									
Center-cut NY strip steak	14 oz	590	n/a	0	n/a	n/a	33	2.5	1420
Maple glazed chicken	as served	570	n/a	62	n/a	n/a	9	0	1950
Maple glazed shrimp add-on	skewer	110	n/a	11	n/a	n/a	1	14	780
NY strip & rock lobster tail	as served	690	n/a	0	n/a	n/a	35	33	1930

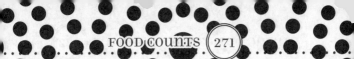

RED LOBSTER continued

Item	Serving Size	Calories	Protein	Carb	Fiber	Sugar	Total Fat	Sat Fat	Sodium
Steak lobster-&-shrimp Oscar	as served	1170	n/a	20	n/a	n/a	77	9	2770
Wood-grilled peppercorn sirloin & shrimp	as served	560	n/a	25	n/a	n/a	21	n/a	2210
QUICK CATCHES FOR LUNCH									
Beer-battered shrimp & chips	as served	540	n/a	40	n/a	n/a	35	3	1170
Coastal soup & salad (bread wedges only)	as served	n/a	n/a	n/a	n/a	n/a	n/a	n/a	n/a
w/ Bayou seafood gumbo	as served	660	n/a	81	n/a	n/a	20	4.5	2120
w/ creamy potato bacon soup	as served	700	n/a	84	n/a	n/a	29	11	1780
w/ New England Clam Chowder	as served	710	n/a	79	n/a	n/a	30	12	1670
w/ seafood gumbo	as served	680	n/a	87	n/a	n/a	22	4.5	1950
w/ spicy shrimp soup	as served	630	n/a	81	n/a	n/a	20	5	2010
Crunch-fried fish sandwich	as served	730	n/a	67	n/a	n/a	37	9	1540
Hand-tossed Caesar salad w/ wood-grilled chicken	each	670	n/a	14	n/a	n/a	52	10	1750
Hand-tossed Caesar salad w/ wood-grilled shrimp	each	620	n/a	14	n/a	n/a	51	10	1370
Shrimp & wood-grilled chicken	as served	n/a	n/a	n/a	n/a	n/a	n/a	n/a	n/a
Shrimp jambalaya	as served	590	n/a	47	n/a	n/a	34	10	1860
w/ garlic shrimp scampi	as served	380	n/a	36	n/a	n/a	8	2	1720
w/ hand-breaded shrimp	as served	520	n/a	43	n/a	n/a	18	2.5	2340
w/ wood-grilled shrimp skewer	as served	380	n/a	34	n/a	n/a	8	2	1490
Wood-grilled chicken BLT, w/ freshly-cooked chips	as served	1030	n/a	68	n/a	n/a	55	11	2760
Wood-grilled salmon BLT, w/ freshly-cooked chips	as served	1100	n/a	68	n/a	n/a	59	12	2380

RED LOBSTER continued

Item	Serving Size	Calories	Protein	Carb	Fiber	Sugar	Total Fat	Sat Fat	Sodium
Wood-grilled shrimp skewers	as served	360	n/a	47			7	1.5	1290
FAVORITES									
Cajun chicken linguini Alfredo	lunch portion	630	n/a	45	n/a	n/a	27	10	1550
Cajun chicken linguini Alfredo	full portion	1260	n/a	91	n/a	n/a	53	19	3110
Chef's Sig. lobster & shrimp pasta	lunch portion	510	n/a	43	n/a	n/a	25	11	1090
Chef's Sig. lobster & shrimp pasta	full portion	102	n/a	86	n/a	n/a	50	21	2170
Crab linguini Alfredo	lunch portion	560	n/a	47	n/a	n/a	25	12	1310
Crab linguini Alfredo	full portion	1120	n/a	95	n/a	n/a	50	24	2650
Crunchy popcorn shrimp	as served	280	n/a	26	n/a	n/a	14	1.5	1050
Farm-raised catfish, blackened	as served	190	n/a	0	n/a	n/a	9	1.5	150
Farm-raised catfish, fried	as served	220	n/a	3	n/a	n/a	12	1.5	280
Flounder, broiled	as served	150	n/a	0	n/a	n/a	1	0	150
Flounder, fried	as served	210	n/a	2	n/a	n/a	8	0.5	260
Garlic shrimp scampi	as served	130	n/a	1	n/a	n/a	9	1.5	690
Hand-breaded shrimp	as served	230	n/a	11	n/a	n/a	13	1	1240
Maple-glazed chicken	as served	410	n/a	55	n/a	n/a	7	1.5	143
Maple-glazed shrimp add-on	skewer	110	n/a	11	n/a	n/a	1	0	780
Sailor's Platter	as served	300	n/a	9	n/a	n/a	7	1	1040
Seafood-stuffed flounder	as served	160	n/a	6	n/a	n/a	5	1.5	760
Shrimp linguini Alfredo	lunch portion	550	n/a	41	n/a	n/a	29	10	1580
Shrimp linguini Alfredo	full portion	1100	n/a	84	n/a	n/a	58	21	3200
Walleye, beer battered	as served	350	n/a	12	n/a	n/a	21	2	600
Walleye, blackened	as served	150	n/a	5	n/a	n/a	3.5	0.5	200
Walleye, broiled	as served	130	n/a	0	n/a	n/a	1.5	0	270
Walleye, fried	as served	300	n/a	18	n/a	n/a	15	1.5	500

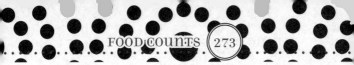

RED LOBSTER continued

Item	Serving Size	Calories	Protein	Carb	Fiber	Sugar	Total Fat	Sat Fat	Sodium
CREATE YOUR OWN LUNCH									
Bay Scallops, broiled	as served	70	n/a	2	n/a	n/a	1	0	490
Bay Scallops, fried	as served	140	n/a	9	n/a	n/a	7	0.5	760
Chicken breast strips	as served	410	n/a	28	n/a	n/a	24	2	1320
Crunch-fried fish	as served	410	n/a	27	n/a	n/a	24	2	1200
Fried crawfish	as served	420	n/a	28	n/a	n/a	26	2.5	830
Garlic shrimp scampi	as served	90	n/a	4	n/a	n/a	2	0	670
Hand-breaded Shrimp	as served	130	n/a	7	n/a	n/a	8	0.5	720
Lightly breaded clam strips	as served	370	n/a	31	n/a	n/a	22	2	820
LOBSTER, CRAB & SHRIMP									
North Pacific King crab legs	as served	390	n/a	2	n/a	n/a	3.5	1	3520
Parrot Isle jumbo coconut shrimp	as served	980	n/a	90	n/a	n/a	55	12	1950
Add 5 More	5 pieces	590	n/a	54	n/a	n/a	33	7	1170
Rock lobster tail	as served	90	n/a	0	n/a	n/a	1	0	490
Shrimp Your Way, coconut shrimp bites	as served	290	n/a	19	n/a	n/a	18	3	830
Shrimp Your Way, fried shrimp	as served	190	n/a	9	n/a	n/a	11	1	1010
Shrimp Your Way, popcorn shrimp	as served	180	n/a	16	n/a	n/a	9	1	670
Shrimp Your Way, scampi	as served	130	n/a	1	n/a	n/a	9	1.5	690
Walt's Favorite Shrimp	as served	700	n/a	52	n/a	n/a	39	3.5	2410
add 1/2 dozen more	1/2 dozen	350	n/a	26	n/a	n/a	20	1.5	1220
CREATE YOUR OWN FEAST									
Fried crawfish	as served	750	n/a	49	n/a	n/a	47	4.5	1480
Fried oysters	as served	590	n/a	58	n/a	n/a	32	3.5	1100
Garlic shrimp scampi	as served	190	n/a	<1	n/a	n/a	13	2.5	1150
Garlic-grilled jumbo shrimp	as served	110	n/a	3	n/a	n/a	3	0.5	800
Parrot Isle jumbo coconut shrimp	as served	780	n/a	72	n/a	n/a	44	10	1560
Seafood-stuffed flounder	as served	160	n/a	6	n/a	n/a	5	1.5	760

RED LOBSTER continued

Item	Serving Size	Calories	Protein	Carb	Fiber	Sugar	Total Fat	Sat Fat	Sodium
Shrimp linguini Alfredo	as served	550	n/a	41	n/a	n/a	29	10	1580
Steamed Snow Crab legs	as served	80	n/a	0	n/a	n/a	0.5	0	940
Walt's Favorite Shrimp	as served	470	n/a	34	n/a	n/a	26	2.5	1610
Wood-grilled fresh salmon	as served	210	n/a	0	n/a	n/a	9	2	240
Wood-grilled peppercorn sirloin	as served	280	n/a	0	n/a	n/a	10	4	850
SIGNATURE COMBINATIONS									
Admiral's Feast	as served	1500	n/a	110	n/a	n/a	87	7	4400
Broiled Seafood Platter	as served	280	n/a	11	n/a	n/a	8	2	1610
Seaside Shrimp Trio	as served	1030	n/a	68	n/a	n/a	57	14	3480
Ultimate Feast	as served	620	n/a	29	n/a	n/a	30	3.5	3370
MONDAY & TUESDAY SPECIALS									
Cocount shrimp bites	as served	290	n/a	19	n/a	n/a	18	3	830
Fried shrimp	as served	190	n/a	9	n/a	n/a	11	1	1010
Popcorn shrimp	as served	180	n/a	16	n/a	n/a	9	1	670
Scampi	as served	130	n/a	1	n/a	n/a	9	1.5	690
ADD TO ANY MEAL									
Maine lobster tail	each	60	n/a	0	n/a	n/a	0.5	0	490
North Pacific King Crab legs	1/2 lb	130	n/a	<1	n/a	n/a	1	0	1190
Snow Crab legs	1/2 lb	80	n/a	0	n/a	n/a	0.5	0	940
ACCOMPANIMENTS									
Baked potato	each	190	n/a	40	n/a	n/a	1	0	900
add butter	as served	90	n/a	1	n/a	n/a	10	6	80
add sour cream	as served	30	n/a	1	n/a	n/a	2.5	1.5	10
Caesar salad	each	270	n/a	13	n/a	n/a	21	4.5	560
add petite shrimp	as served	15	n/a	0	n/a	n/a	0	0	125
Cheddar Bay biscuit	each	150	n/a	16	n/a	n/a	8	2.5	350
Coleslaw	as served	200	n/a	13	n/a	n/a	15	2.5	250
Creamy Langostino lobster baked potato	each	370	n/a	48	n/a	n/a	12	7	1110

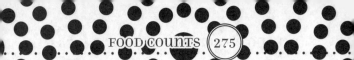

RED LOBSTER continued

Item	Serving Size	Calories	Protein	Carb	Fiber	Sugar	Total Fat	Sat Fat	Sodium
Creamy Langostino lobster mashed potatoes	as served	360	n/a	23	n/a	n/a	22	12	1110
Fresh asparagus	as served	60	n/a	5	n/a	n/a	3	1.5	270
Fresh broccoli	as served	45	n/a	6	n/a	n/a	0.5	0	200
Freshly cooked potato chips	as served	300	n/a	28	n/a	n/a	19	1.5	580
Fries	as served	330	n/a	40	n/a	n/a	17	1.5	740
Garden salad	each	90	n/a	13	n/a	n/a	3	0	105
add petite shrimp	as served	15	n/a	0	n/a	n/a	0	0	125
Home-Style mashed potatoes	as served	180	n/a	22	n/a	n/a	9	4	610
Wild rice pilaf	as served	180	n/a	34	n/a	n/a	3	0.5	650

DRESSINGS

Item	Serving Size	Calories	Protein	Carb	Fiber	Sugar	Total Fat	Sat Fat	Sodium
Balsamic vinaigrette	1.5 oz	80	n/a	4	n/a	n/a	6	1	190
Blue cheese	1.5 oz	240	n/a	2	n/a	n/a	26	4.5	260
Caesar	1.5 oz	280	n/a	1	n/a	n/a	30	5	560
French	1.5 oz	160	n/a	9	n/a	n/a	14	2	390
Honey mustard	1.5 oz	190	n/a	8	n/a	n/a	17	2.5	250
Ranch	1.5 oz	160	n/a	3	n/a	n/a	16	2.5	380
Ranch, fat-free	1.5 oz	60	n/a	5	n/a	n/a	0	0	250
Thousand Island	1.5 oz	200	n/a	6	n/a	n/a	20	3	180

DIPPING SAUCES

Item	Serving Size	Calories	Protein	Carb	Fiber	Sugar	Total Fat	Sat Fat	Sodium
Cocktail sauce	1.5 oz	40	n/a	9	n/a	n/a	0	0	480
Honey mustard dipping sauce	1.5 oz	280	n/a	12	n/a	n/a	26	4	360
Ketchup	1.5 oz	50	n/a	11	n/a	n/a	0	0	460
Marinara sauce	1.5 oz	25	n/a	4	n/a	n/a	1	0	170
Pico de gallo	1.5 oz	10	n/a	2	n/a	n/a	0	0	160
Pina colada sauce	1.5 oz	80	n/a	12	n/a	n/a	4	3	20
Rémoulade	1.5 oz	230	n/a	6	n/a	n/a	22	3.5	220
Sweet & spicy glaze	1.5 oz	100	n/a	24	n/a	n/a	0	0	290
Tartar sauce	1.5 oz	190	n/a	6	n/a	n/a	16	3	170
100% pure melted butter	1.5 oz	350	n/a	2	n/a	n/a	38	23	30

RED LOBSTER continued

Item	Serving Size	Calories	Protein	Carb	Fiber	Sugar	Total Fat	Sat Fat	Sodium
KIDS' COVE MENU									
ENTRÉES									
Broiled fish	kids' portion	150	n/a	3	n/a	n/a	1	0	150
Chicken fingers	kids' portion	410	n/a	28	n/a	n/a	24	2	1320
Grilled chicken	kids' portion	210	n/a	14	n/a	n/a	4	1	710
Macaroni & cheese	kids' portion	280	n/a	42	n/a	n/a	7	2	590
Popcorn shrimp	kids' portion	140	n/a	13	n/a	n/a	7	0.5	530
Chicken fingers	kids' portion	80	n/a	0	n/a	n/a	0.5	0	940
ACCOMPANIMENTS									
Baked potato	each	190	n/a	40	n/a	n/a	1	0	900
w/ butter	as served	90	n/a	1	n/a	n/a	10	6	80
w/ sour cream	as served	30	n/a	1	n/a	n/a	2.5	1.5	10
Caesar Salad	each	270	n/a	13	n/a	n/a	21	4.5	560
Cheddar Bay biscuit	each	150	n/a	16	n/a	n/a	8	2.5	350
Fresh broccoli	as served	45	n/a	6	n/a	n/a	0.5	0	200
Fries	as served	330	n/a	40	n/a	n/a	17	1.5	740
Garden salad	each	90	n/a	13	n/a	n/a	3	0	105
Home-style mashed potatoes	as served	180	n/a	22	n/a	n/a	9	4	610
Wild rice pilaf	as served	180	n/a	34	n/a	n/a	3	0.5	650
KID'S DESSERTS & DRINKS									
Banana berry chocolate smoothie	each	460	n/a	78	n/a	n/a	14	9	10
Berry strawberry banana smoothie	each	340	n/a	63	n/a	n/a	9	6	85
Cherry Wave slushy	each	290	n/a	73	n/a	n/a	0	0	10
Sunset Strawberry smoothie	each	250	n/a	47	n/a	n/a	3	4	45
Juice	as served	140	n/a	30	n/a	n/a	0	0	25
Milk	as served	130	n/a	13	n/a	n/a	5	3	125
Raspberry lemonade	each	180	n/a	30	n/a	n/a	0	0	20
Red Rockin' Shirley T	each	170	n/a	43	n/a	n/a	0	0	0
Surf's Up sundae	each	170	n/a	20	n/a	n/a	9	6	45

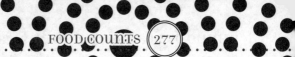

RED LOBSTER continued

Item	Serving Size	Calories	Protein	Carb	Fiber	Sugar	Total Fat	Sat Fat	Sodium
DESSERTS									
Chocolate Wave	as served	1490	n/a	172	n/a	n/a	81	25	950
Key lime pie	as served	580	n/a	88	n/a	n/a	22	12	450
New York–style cheesecake w/ strawberries	as served	520	n/a	39	n/a	n/a	36	21	270
Warm apple crumble à la Mode	as served	770	n/a	117	n/a	n/a	31	13	200
Warm chocolate chip Lava Cookie	as served	1070	n/a	142	n/a	n/a	51	23	470
BEVERAGES									
Bahama Mama	each	230	n/a	57	n/a	n/a	0	0	25
Berry mango daiquiri	each	210	n/a	52	n/a	n/a	0	0	20
Classic margarita, frozen	each	280	n/a	69	n/a	n/a	0	0	510
Classic margarita, on the rocks	each	150	n/a	22	n/a	n/a	0	0	750
Piña Colada	each	280	n/a	52	n/a	n/a	7	6	20
Raspberry margarita	each	330	n/a	81	n/a	n/a	0	0	0
Sail Away smoothie, banana bay chocolate	each	460	n/a	78	n/a	n/a	14	9	10
Sail Away smoothie, berry strawberry banana	each	340	n/a	63	n/a	n/a	9	6	85
Sail Away smoothie, Sunset strawberry	each	250	n/a	47	n/a	n/a	6	4	45
Strawberry daquiri	each	230	n/a	56	n/a	n/a	0	0	5
Strawberry margarita	each	340	n/a	85	n/a	n/a	0	0	10
Sunset Passion Colada	each	330	n/a	62	n/a	n/a	8	7	25
Tropical Freeze, orange	each	250	n/a	49	n/a	n/a	6	5	20
Tropical Freeze, pineapple	each	250	n/a	50	n/a	n/a	5	4.5	180
DRAFT BEER									
Blue Moon	16 oz	220	n/a	20	n/a	n/a	0	0	20
Bud Light	16 oz	160	n/a	19	n/a	n/a	0	0	20
Fat Tire	16 oz	210	n/a	20	n/a	n/a	0	0	20
Sam Adams	16 oz	210	n/a	24	n/a	n/a	0	0	15
Shiner Bock	16 oz	190	n/a	16	n/a	n/a	0	0	15
Yuengling	16 oz	190	n/a	16	n/a	n/a	0	0	15

RED LOBSTER continued

Item	Serving Size	Calories	Protein	Carb	Fiber	Sugar	Total Fat	Sat Fat	Sodium
CLASSIC COCKTAILS									
Amaretto Sour	each	170	n/a	30	n/a	n/a	0	0	0
Biscayne Bay Breeze	each	240	n/a	46	n/a	n/a	0	0	10
Bloody Mary	each	140	n/a	16	n/a	n/a	0	0	1170
Malibu Hurricane	each	200	n/a	35	n/a	n/a	0	0	15
Screwdriver	each	100	n/a	8	n/a	n/a	0	0	10
Tequila Sunrise	each	170	n/a	24	n/a	n/a	0	0	10
Top-Shelf Long Island iced tea	each	190	n/a	21	n/a	n/a	0	0	0
MARTINIS									
Caramel Appletini	each	160	n/a	18	n/a	n/a	0	0	10
Classic martini w/ gin	each	140	n/a	0	n/a	n/a	1.5	0	330
Classic martini w/ vodka	each	150	n/a	0	n/a	n/a	0.5	0	170
Cosmopolitan	each	220	n/a	15	n/a	n/a	0	0	0
Manhattan w/ bourbon	each	150	n/a	5	n/a	n/a	0	0	0
Rob Roy	each	160	n/a	3	n/a	n/a	0	0	10
SPECIALTY DRINKS									
Alotta Colada	each	700	n/a	95	n/a	n/a	16	14	55
Bahama Mama	each	350	n/a	51	n/a	n/a	0	0	20
Berry Mango daiquiri	each	350	n/a	62	n/a	n/a	0	0	30
Big Berry daiquiri	each	350	n/a	65	n/a	n/a	0	0	20
Mango Mai Tai	each	190	n/a	34	n/a	n/a	0	0	5
Mudslide	each	520	n/a	52	n/a	n/a	21	13	160
Piña colada	each	320	n/a	55	n/a	n/a	6	5	35
Red Passion Colada	each	310	n/a	55	n/a	n/a	4.5	4	35
Strawberry daiquiri	each	250	n/a	46	n/a	n/a	0	0	10
Sunset Passion Colada	each	360	n/a	63	n/a	n/a	8	7	15
Triple berry sangria	each	200	n/a	35	n/a	n/a	0	0	30

RED LOBSTER continued

Item	Serving Size	Calories	Protein	Carb	Fiber	Sugar	Total Fat	Sat Fat	Sodium
MARGARITAS									
Classic margarita, frozen	each	470	n/a	96	n/a	n/a	0	0	590
Classic margarita, on the rocks	each	250	n/a	22	n/a	n/a	0	0	770
Frozen raspberry margarita	each	320	n/a	61	n/a	n/a	0	0	0
Frozen strawberry margarita	each	350	n/a	68	n/a	n/a	0	0	20
Lobsterita, strawberry	each	700	n/a	135	n/a	n/a	0	0	55
Lobsterita, traditional	each	890	n/a	183	n/a	n/a	0	0	860
Lobsterita-raspberry	each	690	n/a	131	n/a	n/a	0	0	50
Top-Shelf margarita, frozen	each	520	n/a	97	n/a	n/a	0	0	640
Top-Shelf margarita, on the rocks	each	300	n/a	25	n/a	n/a	0	0	810
AFTER DINNER DRINKS									
Baileys & Coffee	each	180	n/a	15	n/a	n/a	8	5	50
Baileys Irish Cream	each	270	n/a	6	n/a	n/a	4.5	0	0
Coffee Nudge	each	130	n/a	13	n/a	n/a	2	1.5	15
Disaronno Amaretto	each	80	n/a	12	n/a	n/a	0	0	0
Frangelico	each	70	n/a	12	n/a	n/a	0	0	0
Grand marnier	each	80	n/a	6	n/a	n/a	0	0	0
Irish Coffee	each	90	n/a	4	n/a	n/a	2	1	25
Kahlúa	each	90	n/a	15	n/a	n/a	0	0	0

RED ROBIN

Item	Serving Size	Calories	Protein	Carb	Fiber	Sugar	Total Fat	Sat Fat	Sodium
A.1.® peppercorn burger	each	1025	51	70	3	15	59	n/a	2032
All-American patty melt	each	1315	48	60	3	12	98	n/a	2064
Banzai Burger®	each	1033	47	68	3	25	62	n/a	1922
Bleu Ribbon cheeseburger	each	1042	47	69	4	21	57	6	2076
Burnin' Love Burger™	each	936	45	55	3	10	60	n/a	2198
Chili Chili™ Cheeseburger	each	923	55	59	5	10	50	20	1601
Gardenburger	each	561	10	73	6	9	23	4	1724
Gourmet cheeseburger	each	931	45	53	3	9	60	n/a	1818
Guacamole bacon burger	each	1046	61	54	4	10	64	n/a	1515
Natural burger	each	569	37	51	3	9	24	n/a	989
Pub burger	each	957	54	57	4	14	55	n/a	1310
Red Robin bacon cheeseburger	each	1030	51	51	3	8	69	n/a	1930
Royal Red Robin Burger®	each	1196	59	52	3	9	83	n/a	2113
Sautéed 'Shroom burger	each	961	59	58	6	10	56	n/a	1352
Teriyaki chicken sandwich	each	905	56	64	3	20	48	n/a	1616
Whiskey River® BBQ burger	each	1114	48	72	4	16	68	n/a	1815

ROMANO'S MACARONI GRILL

Item	Serving Size	Calories	Protein	Carb	Fiber	Sugar	Total Fat	Sat Fat	Sodium
FRESH ANTIPASTI									
Calamari fritti	as served	650	n/a	42	n/a	n/a	n/a	8	1880
Crab-stuffed mushrooms	as served	310	n/a	4	n/a	n/a	n/a	6	910
Fresh mozzarella fritta	as served	680	n/a	39	n/a	n/a	n/a	15	740
Mediterranean olives	as served	150	n/a	4	n/a	n/a	n/a	3	910
Mozzarella alla Caprese	as served	370	n/a	12	n/a	n/a	n/a	13	340
Roasted vegetables	as served	330	n/a	32	n/a	n/a	n/a	3	440
Romano's Sampler	as served	1330	n/a	90	n/a	n/a	n/a	23	2300
Spinach artichoke dip	as served	850	n/a	83	n/a	n/a	n/a	22	1530
Tomato bruschette	as served	690	n/a	81	n/a	n/a	n/a	8	2220
PIZZA									
Italian sausage	as served	970	n/a	95	n/a	n/a	n/a	18	2430

ROMANO'S MACARONI GRILL continued

Item	Serving Size	Calories	Protein	Carb	Fiber	Sugar	Total Fat	Sat Fat	Sodium
Margherita	as served	720	n/a	95	n/a	n/a	n/a	11	1490
Pepperoni	as served	920	n/a	102	n/a	n/a	n/a	17	2200
Roasted vegetali	as served	800	n/a	102	n/a	n/a	n/a	13	1550
SOUPS & SALADS									
Amalfi chicken soup	as served	420	n/a	45	n/a	n/a	n/a	7	1380
Caesar	as served	260	n/a	14	n/a	n/a	n/a	4	480
Chicken Caesar	as served	650	n/a	29	n/a	n/a	n/a	9	1450
Fresh greens	as served	320	n/a	20	n/a	n/a	n/a	5	300
Insalata blu	as served	640	n/a	22	n/a	n/a	n/a	13	1420
Insalata blu w/ chicken	as served	730	n/a	15	n/a	n/a	n/a	11	1840
Parmesan-crusted chicken	as served	880	n/a	41	n/a	n/a	n/a	16	1650
Pasta e fagioli soup	as served	330	n/a	39	n/a	n/a	n/a	3	790
Scallops & spinach salad	as served	340	n/a	11	n/a	n/a	n/a	6	820
Warm spinach salad	as served	330	n/a	13	n/a	n/a	n/a	8	1030
ENTRÉES									
Antonio's beef rigatoni	as served	770	n/a	80	n/a	n/a	n/a	10	1320
Capellini pomodoro	as served	490	n/a	76	n/a	n/a	n/a	2	960
Chicken Marsala	lunch portion	750	n/a	60	n/a	n/a	n/a	12	1050
Chicken Marsala	dinner portion	810	n/a	61	n/a	n/a	n/a	12	1110
Chicken Parmigiana	as served	890	n/a	70	n/a	n/a	n/a	15	1280
Chicken scaloppine	lunch portion	1030	n/a	47	n/a	n/a	n/a	39	1230
Chicken scaloppine	dinner portion	1090	n/a	48	n/a	n/a	n/a	39	1290
Cramela's chicken rigatoni	as served	930	n/a	75	n/a	n/a	n/a	26	950
Eggplant Parmigiana	as served	910	n/a	73	n/a	n/a	n/a	15	1230
Fettuccine Alfredo	as served	770	n/a	63	n/a	n/a	n/a	27	1180
Fettuccine Alfredo w/ chicken	as served	1050	n/a	66	n/a	n/a	n/a	31	1830
Fettuccine Alfredo w/ shrimp	as served	950	n/a	64	n/a	n/a	n/a	30	1630
Lasagna al forno	as served	690	n/a	40	n/a	n/a	n/a	19	1160

ROMANO'S MACARONI GRILL continued

Item	Serving Size	Calories	Protein	Carb	Fiber	Sugar	Total Fat	Sat Fat	Sodium
Lobster ravioli	as served	710	n/a	39	n/a	n/a	n/a	25	1010
Mama's Trio	as served	1520	n/a	93	n/a	n/a	n/a	36	2870
Mushroom ravioli	as served	960	n/a	57	n/a	n/a	n/a	35	1230
Pasta Milano	as served	750	n/a	93	n/a	n/a	n/a	10	1730
Penne rustica	as served	980	n/a	94	n/a	n/a	n/a	17	2830
Pollo Caprese	as served	550	n/a	45	n/a	n/a	n/a	5	1660
Pollo limone rustica	as served	990	n/a	79	n/a	n/a	n/a	24	2140
Roasted chicken cannelloni	as served	790	n/a	37	n/a	n/a	n/a	20	2200
Sausage Vesuvio	as served	1190	n/a	72	n/a	n/a	n/a	24	2500
Seafood linguine	as served	650	n/a	75	n/a	n/a	n/a	4	1280
Shrimp portofino	lunch portion	770	n/a	57	n/a	n/a	n/a	26	710
Shrimp portofino	dinner portion	780	n/a	58	n/a	n/a	n/a	26	730
Spaghetti Bolognese	as served	710	n/a	69	n/a	n/a	n/a	8	1470
Spaghetti e meatballs, w/ Bolognese sauce	as served	1230	n/a	95	n/a	n/a	n/a	21	3040
Spaghetti e meatballs, w/ tomato sauce	as served	970	n/a	90	n/a	n/a	n/a	15	2520
MEAT, FISH, & SEAFOOD									
Aged beef tenderloin	as served	410	n/a	27	n/a	n/a	n/a	4	620
Calabrese strip	as served	990	n/a	34	n/a	n/a	n/a	23	1120
Center-cut filet	as served	710	n/a	29	n/a	n/a	n/a	16	500
Center-cut lamb	as served	490	n/a	29	n/a	n/a	n/a	5	750
Corvina	as served	1010	n/a	71	n/a	n/a	n/a	21	1150
Crusted sole	as served	1120	n/a	21	n/a	n/a	n/a	45	870
Gilled chicken	as served	390	n/a	31	n/a	n/a	n/a	1.5	970
Grilled halibut	as served	1040	n/a	96	n/a	n/a	n/a	23	1670
Grilled salmon	as served	660	n/a	29	n/a	n/a	n/a	11	610
Honey balsamic chicken	lunch portion	900	n/a	74	n/a	n/a	n/a	7	1290
Honey balsamic chicken	dinner portion	990	n/a	74	n/a	n/a	n/a	7	1380
Jumbo shrimp	as served	320	n/a	31	n/a	n/a	n/a	1	1380
King salmon	as served	1160	n/a	72	n/a	n/a	n/a	25	1240
Prime pork loin	as served	670	n/a	57	n/a	n/a	n/a	6	1820
Snapper	as served	400	n/a	24	n/a	n/a	n/a	2.5	1420

RUBY TUESDAY

Item	Serving Size	Calories	Protein	Carb	Fiber	Sugar	Total Fat	Sat Fat	Sodium
SMART EATING CHOICES									
Baked Potato, plain	each	282	n/a	46	9	n/a	2	n/a	113
Brown-rice pilaf	as served	230	n/a	27	9	n/a	9	n/a	981
Chicken bella	as served	397	n/a	9	9	n/a	15	n/a	1526
Creamy mashed cauliflower	as served	136	n/a	10	9	n/a	8	n/a	714
Creole Catch	as served	196	n/a	1	9	n/a	8	n/a	383
Fresh steamed broccoli	as served	91	n/a	5	9	n/a	6	n/a	227
Grilled chicken salad	as served	701	n/a	35	9	n/a	22	n/a	1216
Grilled chicken wrap	as served	459	n/a	46	9	n/a	17	n/a	1369
New Orleans seafood	as served	316	n/a	3	9	n/a	18	n/a	945
Plain grilled chicken	as served	240	n/a	0	9	n/a	4	n/a	75
Plain grilled petite sirloin	as served	200	n/a	0	9	n/a	6	n/a	240
Plain grilled salmon	as served	245	n/a	0	99	n/a	11	n/a	129
Plain grilled top sirloin	as served	290	n/a	0	9	n/a	12	n/a	420
Sautéed baby portabella mushrooms	as served	98	n/a	10	9	n/a	4	n/a	353
Sugar snap peas	as served	113	n/a	6	9	n/a	6	n/a	202
Turkey burger wrap	as served	590	n/a	45	9	n/a	27	n/a	2656
White bean chicken chili	as served	229	n/a	21	9	n/a	8	n/a	1441
White Cheddar mashed potatoes	as served	169	n/a	19	9	n/a	10	n/a	520
APPETIZERS (note: 4 servings per item)									
Asian dumplings	1 serving	114	n/a	11	1	n/a	5	n/a	295
Buffalo shrimp	1 serving	126	n/a	11	1	n/a	6	n/a	580
California club quesadilla	1 serving	362	n/a	10	2	n/a	23	n/a	684
Cheddar fries	1 serving	335	n/a	25	3	n/a	20	n/a	826
Chicken quesadilla	1 serving	294	n/a	10	0	n/a	18	n/a	568
Chicken strips, Buffalo	1 serving	114	n/a	4	1	n/a	6	n/a	375
Chicken strips, Thai Phoon	1 serving	179	n/a	4	0	n/a	13	n/a	297
Chicken strips, traditional	1 serving	94	n/a	3	0	n/a	4	n/a	222

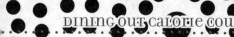

RUBY TUESDAY continued

Item	Serving Size	Calories	Protein	Carb	Fiber	Sugar	Total Fat	Sat Fat	Sodium
Chicken strips, Boston barbecue	1 serving	115	n/a	8	0	n/a	4	n/a	367
Fire wings	1 serving	178	n/a	3	1	n/a	11	n/a	603
Four Way Sampler	1 serving	301	n/a	16	2	n/a	15	n/a	816
Fresh avocado quesadilla	1 serving	266	n/a	11	2	n/a	19	n/a	346
Fresh guacamole dip	1 serving	358	n/a	22	10	n/a	24	n/a	429
Fried mozzarella	1 serving	145	n/a	12	1	n/a	6	n/a	428
Jumbo lump crab cake	1 serving	68	n/a	3	1	n/a	4	n/a	200
Lobster mac 'n cheese	1 serving	159	n/a	8	0	n/a	9	n/a	356
Queso & chips	1 serving	317	n/a	26	3	n/a	20	n/a	535
Shrimp Sampler	1 serving	224	n/a	17	3	n/a	12	n/a	767
Southwestern spring rolls	1 serving	173	n/a	14	1	n/a	10	n/a	324
Spinach Artichoke dip	1 serving	310	n/a	23	3	n/a	19	n/a	470
Thai Phoon shrimp	1 serving	191	n/a	11	1	n/a	13	n/a	502

PETITE LUNCH SALADS

Item	Serving Size	Calories	Protein	Carb	Fiber	Sugar	Total Fat	Sat Fat	Sodium
Petite Carolina chicken salad	as served	436	n/a	20	6	n/a	16	n/a	629
Petite creole shrimp salad	as served	248	n/a	20	5	n/a	8	n/a	492
Petite grilled chicken salad	as served	362	n/a	20	5	n/a	11	n/a	629
Petite grilled salmon salad	as served	322	n/a	20	5	n/a	8	n/a	492

PERFECT LUNCH COMBINATION

Item	Serving Size	Calories	Protein	Carb	Fiber	Sugar	Total Fat	Sat Fat	Sodium
Broccoli & cheese soup	as served	378	n/a	13	1	n/a	32	n/a	1438
Buffalo chicken minis	as served	619	n/a	64	5	n/a	23	n/a	1703
Clam chowder	as served	318	n/a	16	2	n/a	20	n/a	635
Ruby minis	as served	635	n/a	48	2	n/a	35	n/a	1418
Salmon cake minis	as served	702	n/a	62	5	n/a	33	n/a	1231
Tortilla soup	as served	286	n/a	29	2	n/a	13	n/a	1592
Turkey minis	as served	551	n/a	51	3	n/a	28	n/a	1703
Vegetarian minis	as served	682	n/a	92	3	n/a	27	n/a	1182
White bean chicken chili	as served	229	n/a	21	8	n/a	8	n/a	1441

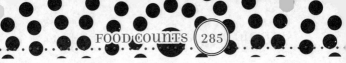

RUBY TUESDAY continued

Item	Serving Size	Calories	Protein	Carb	Fiber	Sugar	Total Fat	Sat Fat	Sodium
GARDEN FRESH SALADS									
Carolina chicken	as served	707	n/a	22	8	n/a	24	n/a	826
Creole shrimp	as served	447	n/a	35	9	n/a	17	n/a	942
Garden	as served	396	n/a	39	10	n/a	17	n/a	985
Garden add-on	as served	186	n/a	18	4	n/a	8	n/a	470
Grilled chicken	as served	701	n/a	35	9	n/a	22	n/a	1216
Grilled salmon	as served	621	n/a	35	9	n/a	17	n/a	942
SAUCES & DRESSINGS									
Balsamic vinaigrette dressing	1 oz	35	n/a	4	0	n/a	3	n/a	550
BBQ sauce	1 oz	50	n/a	13	0	n/a	0	n/a	330
Blue cheese dressing	1 oz	180	n/a	1	0	n/a	19	n/a	250
Boston BBQ sauce	1 oz	42	n/a	10	0	n/a	0	n/a	289
Caramel sauce	1 oz	100	n/a	25	0	n/a	0	n/a	110
Chocolate sauce	1 oz	120	n/a	21	1	n/a	3	n/a	60
French dressing	1 oz	120	n/a	6	0	n/a	11	n/a	260
Honey mustard dressing	1 oz	90	n/a	5	0	n/a	8	n/a	150
Italian dressing	1 oz	60	n/a	2	0	n/a	6	n/a	330
Lemon butter sauce	1 oz	88	n/a	1	0	n/a	9	n/a	160
Lite ranch dressing	1 oz	50	n/a	1	0	n/a	5	n/a	300
Marinara sauce	1 oz	17	n/a	1	1	n/a	1	n/a	43
Orange peanut sauce	1 oz	88	n/a	11	0	n/a	4	n/a	422
Parmesan cream sauce	1 oz	64	n/a	2	0	n/a	6	n/a	181
Ranch dressing	1 oz	100	n/a	1	0	n/a	11	n/a	300
Salsa	1 oz	8	n/a	1	0	n/a	0	n/a	170
Sesame-peanut sauce	1 oz	83	n/a	8	0	n/a	5	n/a	355
Signature Parmesan dressing	1 oz	150	n/a	1	0	n/a	16	n/a	230
Sour cream	1 oz	35	n/a	3	0	n/a	2	n/a	16
Sriracha ranch	1 oz	75	n/a	1	0	n/a	8	n/a	273
Sweet chili sauce	1 oz	170	n/a	2	0	n/a	17	n/a	150
Thousand Island dressing	1 oz	70	n/a	3	0	n/a	7	n/a	220
PASTA CLASSICS									
Chicken & broccoli pasta	as served	1564	n/a	87	7	n/a	96	n/a	2811

RUBY TUESDAY continued

Item	Serving Size	Calories	Protein	Carb	Fiber	Sugar	Total Fat	Sat Fat	Sodium
Chicken & mushroom Alfredo	as served	1220	n/a	81	8	n/a	59	n/a	3007
Parmesan chicken pasta	as served	1418	n/a	104	7	n/a	77	n/a	3187
Parmesan shrimp pasta	as served	1050	n/a	84	5	n/a	57	n/a	3270
Shrimp carbonara	as served	1368	n/a	74	7	n/a	96	n/a	3766
Vegetarian pasta marinara	as served	487	n/a	71	10	n/a	10	n/a	1303

SANDWICHES & BURGERS

Item	Serving Size	Calories	Protein	Carb	Fiber	Sugar	Total Fat	Sat Fat	Sodium
Alpine Swiss burger	as served	1048	n/a	65	5	n/a	62	n/a	1976
Avocado turkey burger	as served	886	n/a	48	9	n/a	54	n/a	2712
Bacon cheeseburger	as served	1059	n/a	61	5	n/a	66	n/a	2209
Boston blue burger	as served	1201	n/a	81	6	n/a	71	n/a	2653
Buffalo chicken burger	as served	788	n/a	60	3	n/a	41	n/a	2009
Chicken BLT	as served	798	n/a	60	3	n/a	40	n/a	1759
Classic cheeseburger	as served	999	n/a	61	5	n/a	61	n/a	1999
Fresh grilled chicken sandwich	as served	869	n/a	46	5	n/a	41	n/a	1841
Ruby's classic burger	as served	929	n/a	60	5	n/a	55	n/a	1759
Smokehouse burger	as served	1219	n/a	83	5	n/a	73	n/a	2539
Triple prime bacon Cheddar burger	as served	1332	n/a	45	4	n/a	101	n/a	2163
Triple prime burger	as served	1112	n/a	45	4	n/a	82	n/a	1673
Triple prime Cheddar burger	as served	1272	n/a	45	4	n/a	96	n/a	1953
Turkey burger	as served	699	n/a	47	3	n/a	39	n/a	2459

SEAFOOD

Item	Serving Size	Calories	Protein	Carb	Fiber	Sugar	Total Fat	Sat Fat	Sodium
Asian glazed salmon	as served	349	n/a	12	3	n/a	26	n/a	972
Chesapeake Catch	as served	426	n/a	8	2	n/a	25	n/a	1055
Crab cake dinner	as served	271	n/a	10	3	n/a	17	n/a	800
Creole catch	as served	196	n/a	1	1	n/a	8	n/a	383
Grilled salmon	as served	249	n/a	0	0	n/a	11	n/a	110
Herb-crusted tilapia	as served	402	n/a	9	2	n/a	24	n/a	944
New Orleans seafood	as served	316	n/a	3	1	n/a	18	n/a	945

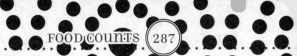

RUBY TUESDAY continued

Item	Serving Size	Calories	Protein	Carb	Fiber	Sugar	Total Fat	Sat Fat	Sodium
Salmon cakes	as served	540	n/a	18	3	n/a	33	n/a	930
Salmon florentine	as served	492	n/a	5	2	n/a	31	n/a	1282
Trout almondine	as served	468	n/a	3	2	n/a	30	n/a	640
RIBS & PLATTERS									
Asian sesame glazed	1/2 rack	542	n/a	18	1	n/a	32	n/a	628
Chicken strips add-on	as served	377	n/a	11	0	n/a	17	n/a	888
Chicken tender dinner	as served	377	n/a	11	0	n/a	17	n/a	888
Classic barbecue	1/2 rack	485	n/a	26	0	n/a	24	n/a	590
Fried shrimp add-on	as served	426	n/a	38	2	n/a	17	n/a	1709
Louisiana Fried Shrimp	as served	423	n/a	38	2	n/a	17	n/a	1709
Memphis dry rub	1/2 rack	460	n/a	6	0	n/a	29	n/a	150
Rib add-on	as served	485	n/a	26	0	n/a	24	n/a	590
Wing add-on	as served	350	n/a	5	0	n/a	20	n/a	1000
STEAKS & CHICKEN									
Barbecue grilled chicken	as served	290	n/a	11	0	n/a	4	n/a	1314
Chef's Cut 12-ounce sirloin	as served	741	n/a	1	0	n/a	50	n/a	1555
Chicken bella	as served	397	n/a	9	1	n/a	15	n/a	1526
Chicken florentine	as served	391	n/a	6	2	n/a	14	n/a	1692
Chicken fresco	as served	409	n/a	9	1	n/a	19	n/a	1549
Cowboy sirloin	as served	569	n/a	22	1	n/a	29	n/a	1633
Lobster mac 'n cheese add-on	as served	637	n/a	32	2	n/a	37	n/a	1426
Lobster tail add-on	as served	113	n/a	0	0	n/a	3	n/a	608
Peppercorn mushroom sirloin	as served	461	n/a	12	0	n/a	22	n/a	2149
Petite sirloin	as served	301	n/a	1	0	n/a	16	n/a	1285
Rib eye	as served	821	n/a	1	0	n/a	63	n/a	1495
Scampi add-on	as served	681	n/a	3	1	n/a	67	n/a	1674
Top sirloin	as served	391	n/a	1	0	n/a	22	n/a	1465
FEATURE MENU									
Double chocolate cake	as served	897	n/a	124	0	n/a	40	n/a	614
Fresh guacamole dip	as served	358	n/a	22	10	n/a	24	n/a	429

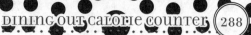
RUBY TUESDAY continued

Item	Serving Size	Calories	Protein	Carb	Fiber	Sugar	Total Fat	Sat Fat	Sodium
Jumbo lump crab cake (app)	as served	68	n/a	3	1	n/a	4	n/a	200
Lobster carbonara	as served	1426	n/a	75	7	n/a	94	n/a	3613
New Orleans seafood	as served	316	n/a	3	1	n/a	18	n/a	945
New York cheesecake	as served	736	n/a	82	2	n/a	60	n/a	740
Salmon Florentine	as served	492	n/a	5	2	n/a	31	n/a	1282
Spinach artichoke dip	as served	310	n/a	23	3	n/a	19	n/a	470
Steak & lobster tail	7 oz steak	413	n/a	1	0	n/a	20	n/a	1893
Steak & lobster tail	9 oz steak	503	n/a	1	0	n/a	26	n/a	2073
Steak & lobster mac 'n cheese	as served	938	n/a	33	2	n/a	53	n/a	2711
Tiramisu	as served	545	n/a	66	0	n/a	29	n/a	60

BRUNCH MENU

Item	Serving Size	Calories	Protein	Carb	Fiber	Sugar	Total Fat	Sat Fat	Sodium
Bacon slices	5 slices	285	n/a	24	5	n/a	13	n/a	420
Bella chicken crepe	as served	1052	n/a	53	7	n/a	56	n/a	2528
Bella chicken omelet	as served	1162	n/a	20	5	n/a	75	n/a	2668
Berry Good yogurt parfait	as served	162	n/a	26	1	n/a	3	n/a	127
Crabacado omelet	as served	808	n/a	8	5	n/a	61	n/a	1392
Cranapple crepes	as served	1151	n/a	180	12	n/a	36	n/a	1282
French toast	as served	1795	n/a	44	9	n/a	117	n/a	3395
Garlic cheese biscuit	as served	90	n/a	10	0	n/a	4	n/a	260
Grapes	1 oz	200	n/a	0	0	n/a	18	n/a	700
Kids' Eggscellent Combo	as served	570	n/a	48	10	n/a	26	n/a	840
Kids' French toast	5 each	511	n/a	52	2	n/a	27	n/a	883
Kids Patty cakes	as served	170	n/a	1	1	n/a	12	n/a	330
Mini Benedicts, crispy Southern chicken	as served	639	n/a	42	4	n/a	33	n/a	1526
Pancake syrup	as served	30	n/a	8	0	n/a	0	n/a	0
Seasoned potatoes	as served	109	n/a	27	0	n/a	0	n/a	9
Spinach & mushroom omelet	as served	979	n/a	20	4	n/a	65	n/a	2201
Steak & eggs	as served	548	n/a	3	2	n/a	30	n/a	1850
Sunrise quesadilla, bacon avocado	as served	483	n/a	28	2	n/a	26	n/a	1261

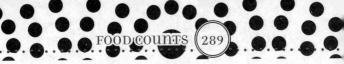

RUBY TUESDAY continued

Item	Serving Size	Calories	Protein	Carb	Fiber	Sugar	Total Fat	Sat Fat	Sodium
Sunrise quesadilla, California club	as served	1595	n/a	44	8	n/a	114	n/a	2983
Western omelet	as served	1051	n/a	10	1	n/a	75	n/a	2309
ZERO PROOF BEVERAGES									
Berry Fusion	each	148	n/a	28	1	n/a	0	n/a	2
Freshly Made lemonade, blackberry	each	190	n/a	46	2	n/a	0	n/a	13
Freshly Made lemonade, pomegranate	each	236	n/a	59	0	n/a	0	n/a	24
Freshly Made lemonade, raspberry	each	187	n/a	37	2	n/a	0	n/a	13
Freshly Made lemonade, strawberry	each	192	n/a	48	1	n/a	0	n/a	13
Freshly Made lemonade, wild berry	each	190	n/a	46	1	n/a	0	n/a	13
Handcrafted fruit tea, blackberry	each	162	n/a	39	2	n/a	0	n/a	15
Handcrafted fruit tea, mango	each	104	n/a	26	1	n/a	0	n/a	10
Handcrafted fruit tea, peach	each	157	n/a	41	0	n/a	0	n/a	15
Handcrafted fruit tea, raspberry	each	159	n/a	30	2	n/a	0	n/a	15
Handcrafted fruit tea, wild berry	each	162	n/a	39	1	n/a	0	n/a	15
Peach Splash	each	152	n/a	38	0	n/a	0	n/a	8
POM Tea	each	115	n/a	29	0	n/a	0	n/a	16
RT Palmer	each	124	n/a	31	0	n/a	0	n/a	18
Tropical Sunrise	each	193	n/a	4	1	n/a	0	n/a	6
SIGNATURE SIDES									
Baked mac 'n cheese	as served	570	n/a	31	2	n/a	37	n/a	1067
Baked potato, plain	as served	282	n/a	46	10	n/a	2	n/a	113
Baked potato, w/ butter & sour cream	as served	441	n/a	48	10	n/a	17	n/a	228
Blue cheese coleslaw	as served	329	n/a	8	3	n/a	32	n/a	371
Brown rice pilaf	as served	230	n/a	27	3	n/a	9	n/a	981
Creamy mashed cauliflower	as served	136	n/a	10	3	n/a	8	n/a	714

RUBY TUESDAY continued

Item	Serving Size	Calories	Protein	Carb	Fiber	Sugar	Total Fat	Sat Fat	Sodium
French fries	as served	396	n/a	50	5	n/a	18	n/a	1389
Fresh grilled asparagus	as served	49	n/a	2	9	n/a	3	n/a	136
Fresh grilled green beans	as served	45	n/a	2	9	n/a	2	n/a	145
Fresh steamed broccoli	as served	91	n/a	5	3	n/a	6	n/a	227
Garlic cheese biscuit	as served	90	n/a	10	0	n/a	4	n/a	260
Loaded baked potato	as served	591	n/a	48	10	n/a	29	n/a	545
Onion rings	as served	350	n/a	35	0	n/a	21	n/a	350
Sauteed baby portabella mushrooms	as served	98	n/a	10	0	n/a	4	n/a	353
Sugar snap peas	as served	113	n/a	6	3	n/a	6	n/a	202
White Cheddar mashed potatoes	as served	169	n/a	19	2	n/a	10	n/a	520

DESSERTS

Item	Serving Size	Calories	Protein	Carb	Fiber	Sugar	Total Fat	Sat Fat	Sodium
Berry Good yogurt parfait	as served	162	n/a	26	1	n/a	3	n/a	127
Blondie for One	each	625	n/a	86	2	n/a	27	n/a	219
Blondie for Two	as served	1053	n/a	148	3	n/a	44	n/a	374
Chocolate chip cookie	each	180	n/a	23	1	n/a	9	n/a	190
Double chocolate cake	as served	897	n/a	124	0	n/a	40	n/a	614
Italian ice cream cake	as served	990	n/a	108	2	n/a	56	n/a	550
New York cheesecake	as served	736	n/a	82	2	n/a	60	n/a	740
Tiramisu	as served	545	n/a	66	0	n/a	29	n/a	60
White chocolate macadamia nut cookie	each	200	n/a	22	1	n/a	12		190

KIDS' MENU

Item	Serving Size	Calories	Protein	Carb	Fiber	Sugar	Total Fat	Sat Fat	Sodium
Beef minis	as served	599	n/a	47	2	n/a	31	n/a	1245
Butter pasta	as served	567	n/a	70	4	n/a	24	n/a	943
Chicken breast	as served	124	n/a	1	0	n/a	2	n/a	513
Chicken tenders	as served	226	n/a	7	0	n/a	10	n/a	533
Chop steak	as served	264	n/a	1	0	n/a	20	n/a	545
Cookies	as served	360	n/a	46	2	n/a	18	n/a	380
Fried shrimp	as served	211	n/a	19	1	n/a	9	n/a	855

RUBY TUESDAY continued

Item	Serving Size	Calories	Protein	Carb	Fiber	Sugar	Total Fat	Sat Fat	Sodium
Grilled cheese	as served	500	n/a	56	2	n/a	22	n/a	1180
Mac & cheese	as served	680	n/a	58	3	n/a	37	n/a	1565
Pasta marinara	as served	469	n/a	78	8	n/a	7	n/a	978
Sundae	as served	574	n/a	70	1	n/a	29	n/a	193
Turkey minis	as served	539	n/a	47	2	n/a	27	n/a	1675

SKYLINE CHILI

Item	Serving Size	Calories	Protein	Carb	Fiber	Sugar	Total Fat	Sat Fat	Sodium
FRESH SELECT SALADS W/O DRESSINGS									
Buffalo chicken salad	as served	150	17	7	2	4	7	n/a	640
Classic chicken salad	as served	150	17	8	2	4	7	n/a	480
Garden salad	as served	80	5	6	2	3	5	n/a	105
Greek chicken salad	as served	170	18	9	8	5	8	n/a	2830
Greek salad	as served	60	3	5	2	3	3.5	n/a	210
Southwest chicken salad w/ tortilla chips	as served	760	25	66	8	5	44	n/a	1570
FRESH SELECT WRAPS W/O DRESSINGS									
Buffalo chicken wrap	as served	520	31	55	3	3	21	n/a	1460
Classic chicken wrap	as served	510	31	55	3	3	21	n/a	1300
Greek chicken wrap	as served	510	29	54	7	7	21	n/a	2070
Southwest chicken wrap	as served	670	34	65	6	6	30	n/a	2040
DRESSINGS									
Buttermilk ranch	as served	230	1	2	0	2	24	n/a	390
Chili ranch	as served	275	0	0	0	2	29	n/a	606
Dijon honey mustard	as served	180	1	8	0	7	17	n/a	240
Greek salad	as served	250	0	1	0	0	28	n/a	470
Honey French	as served	210	0	14	0	13	18	n/a	310
Light Italian	as served	20	0	2	0	2	1	n/a	770
Light ranch	as served	70	1	8	0	3	4	n/a	310
BURRITOS									
All chili	as served	560	34	37	3	4	30	n/a	1100
All chili deluxe	as served	650	37	45	6	9	35	n/a	1200
Black bean	as served	600	25	67	9	4	25	n/a	1090

SKYLINE CHILI continued

Item	Serving Size	Calories	Protein	Carb	Fiber	Sugar	Total Fat	Sat Fat	Sodium
Black bean deluxe	as served	690	27	75	11	9	30	n/a	1190
Chili bean mix	as served	610	30	54	8	4	30	n/a	960
Chili bean mix deluxe	as served	700	33	62	10	10	36	n/a	1060
Chili cheese Melt	as served	350	17	33	2	2	16	n/a	390
STEAMED POTATOES									
3-way potato	as served	870	33	75	7	6	49	n/a	1140
4-way potato	as served	890	33	78	7	7	49	n/a	1150
5-way potato	as served	950	37	90	12	9	50	n/a	1150
Cheddar potato	as served	740	21	72	6	5	41	n/a	590
Chili potato	as served	440	19	74	7	6	8	n/a	580
Plain potato	as served	310	7	72	6	5	0	n/a	25
Sour cream potato	as served	570	7	72	6	5	27	n/a	290
BOWLS									
Chili bean bowl	as served	270	23	17	6	3	12	n/a	840
Chili bowl	as served	270	25	6	1	3	16	n/a	1110
Chili cheese bowl	as served	440	35	6	1	3	30	n/a	1380
Coney bowl	as served	870	54	9	2	4	69	n/a	2170
Loaded chili bowl	as served	580	38	18	4	5	40	n/a	1450
Vegetarian black beans	as served	320	12	46	8	3	9	n/a	1090
CONEYS									
Cheese Coney	as served	340	18	17	1	3	22	n/a	730
Chili cheese sandwich	as served	290	19	17	1	3	17	n/a	760
Regular chili w/o cheese	as served	180	12	17	1	3	7	n/a	580
Regular w/o cheese	as served	220	11	17	1	3	12	n/a	560
CHILI SPAGHETTI DISHES									
3-way	large	1070	65	58	5	5	64	n/a	3880
3-way	medium	760	46	43	3	4	44	n/a	2850
3-way	small	380	23	22	2	2	22	n/a	1420
4-way bean	large	1230	76	61	12	7	67	n/a	4070
4-way bean	medium	850	52	59	9	5	45	n/a	2880
4-way bean	small	420	26	29	4	2	23	n/a	1440
4-way onion	large	1090	66	62	5	7	64	n/a	3890
4-way onion	medium	770	47	46	4	5	44	n/a	2850

SKYLINE CHILI continued

Item	Serving Size	Calories	Protein	Carb	Fiber	Sugar	Total Fat	Sat Fat	Sodium
4-way onion	small	390	23	23	2	2	22	n/a	1420
5-way	large	1230	73	87	13	9	65	n/a	4130
5-way	medium	840	51	58	9	6	45	n/a	2850
5-way	small	420	25	29	4	3	22	n/a	1420
Black bean & rice spaghetti	small	250	8	40	5	2	6	n/a	1280
Black bean & rice spaghetti	medium	490	16	79	9	3	12	n/a	2550
Black bean & rice spaghetti	large	680	23	110	13	4	16	n/a	3570
Black bean 3-way	small	420	19	40	5	2	20	n/a	1540
Black bean 3-way	medium	800	36	74	9	4	40	n/a	2830
Black bean 3-way	large	1160	53	105	12	5	58	n/a	4110
Black bean 4-way	small	430	19	44	5	4	20	n/a	1540
Black bean 4-way	medium	810	37	77	9	5	40	n/a	2830
Black bean 4-way	large	1170	54	109	13	7	58	n/a	4110
Black bean 5-way	small	470	21	50	8	4	20	n/a	1540
Black bean 5-way	medium	880	41	89	14	6	40	n/a	2830
Black bean 5-way	large	1240	59	121	20	8	58	n/a	3860
Chili spaghetti bean	small	260	16	28	4	2	9	n/a	1230
Chili spaghetti bean	medium	520	30	61	9	4	17	n/a	2570
Chili spaghetti bean	large	730	42	87	13	6	23	n/a	3590
Chili spaghetti bean & onion	small	270	15	32	5	3	9	n/a	1280
Chili spaghetti bean & onion	medium	530	31	64	9	6	17	n/a	2570
Chili spaghetti bean & onion	large	750	42	92	14	8	24	n/a	3590
Chili spaghetti	small	230	14	22	2	2	9	n/a	1230
Chili spaghetti	medium	450	28	43	4	4	18	n/a	2460
Chili spaghetti	large	620	40	58	5	5	26	n/a	3370
Chili spaghetti onion	small	230	14	23	2	2	9	n/a	1230
Chili spaghetti onion	medium	470	26	51	4	5	17	n/a	2570
Chili spaghetti onion	large	640	40	62	5	7	26	n/a	3370

KIDS' MEALS

Item	Serving Size	Calories	Protein	Carb	Fiber	Sugar	Total Fat	Sat Fat	Sodium
3-way special	as served	380	23	22	2	2	22	n/a	1420
Coney special	as served	210	10	15	1	3	12	n/a	480

SKYLINE CHILI continued

Item	Serving Size	Calories	Protein	Carb	Fiber	Sugar	Total Fat	Sat Fat	Sodium
Coney special w/ cheese	as served	330	17	16	1	3	22	n/a	650
Double Weiner Hot Doggy	as served	250	8	15	0	3	17	n/a	430
Double Weiner Hot Doggy w/cheese	as served	360	15	16	0	3	26	n/a	600
P'sghetti special	as served	280	14	19	1	1	16	n/a	1010
Single Weiner Hot Doggy	as served	160	5	14	0	2	9	n/a	260
Single Weiner Hot Doggy w/ cheese	as served	270	12	15	0	2	18	n/a	430

SIDES

Item	Serving Size	Calories	Protein	Carb	Fiber	Sugar	Total Fat	Sat Fat	Sodium
Bowl of crackers	as served	100	3	20	1	0	3	n/a	300
Cheddar bread	full	520	12	32	0	0	39	n/a	650
Cheddar bread	1/2	260	6	16	0	0	20	n/a	320
Garlic bread	full	410	5	31	0	0	30	n/a	470
Garlic bread	1/2	200	3	16	0	0	15	n/a	240
Side of cheese	side	230	14	1	0	0	19	n/a	350
Side of chili	side	130	12	3	1	1	8	n/a	560

SONIC DRIVE-IN

Item	Serving Size	Calories	Protein	Carb	Fiber	Sugar	Total Fat	Sat Fat	Sodium
BREAKFAST TOASTER® w/ bacon, egg & cheese	each	530	20	40	2	7	32	10	1440
CroisSONIC® breakfast sandwich w/ bacon	each	510	18	29	0	5	36	15	1400
CroisSONIC® breakfast sandwich w/ ham	each	430	21	25	1	4	27	12	1510
CroisSONIC® breakfast sandwich w/ sausage	each	600	19	29	0	5	46	18	1340
French toast sticks	4 sticks	500	7	49	2	9	31	5	490
Sausage Biscuit Dippers™ w/ gravy	1 order	690	16	57	0	7	44	18	1770
Steak & egg breakfast burrito	each	590	28	47	5	3	34	12	1370
SuperSONIC® breakfast burrito	each	570	19	48	3	3	36	12	1650

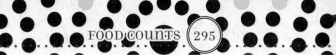

SONIC DRIVE-IN continued

Item	Serving Size	Calories	Protein	Carb	Fiber	Sugar	Total Fat	Sat Fat	Sodium
BURGERS & SANDWICHES									
Bacon cheeseburger Toaster®	each	670	29	52	3	13	39	14	1440
BLT Toaster®	each	500	17	45	2	7	29	7	950
Breaded pork fritter sandwich	each	640	22	66	7	11	33	6	840
California cheeseburger	each	690	29	57	5	13	39	13	1060
Chicken club Toaster®	each	740	29	55	4	7	46	11	1740
Chili cheeseburger	each	660	31	56	5	11	35	14	990
Country-fried steak Toaster®	each	670	14	71	4	6	37	10	1370
Fish sandwich	each	650	22	71	7	12	31	5	1160
Green chili cheeseburger	each	630	29	56	5	12	31	12	1070
Hickory cheeseburger	each	640	28	61	5	17	31	12	1170
Jalapeño burger	each	550	25	53	5	10	26	9	880
Sonic® bacon cheeseburger	each	780	33	57	5	12	48	16	1300
Sonic® burger	each	650	26	55	5	11	37	10	720
Sonic® cheeseburger	each	720	29	56	5	12	42	14	1040
Thousand Island burger	each	610	26	56	5	13	32	10	810
SHAKES, MALTS, & SLUSHES									
Banana cream pie shake	regular	640	9	87	1	77	29	20	330
Banana malt	regular	510	8	62	1	55	26	18	290
Banana shake	regular	500	8	60	1	54	26	18	280
Barq's Root Beer Float / blended float	regular	340	4	51	0	50	14	10	170
Blue Coconut CreamSlush® treat	regular	350	4	53	0	51	14	10	170
Butterfinger Sonic Blast®	regular	730	11	87	0	75	38	26	410
Caramel malt	regular	570	8	75	0	68	27	19	430
Cherry CreamSlush® treat	regular	350	4	54	0	53	14	10	170
Chocolate cream pie shake	regular	700	8	101	0	88	29	20	410
Chocolate malt	regular	580	8	76	0	66	26	18	370
Chocolate shake	regular	560	8	74	0	65	26	18	360

SONIC DRIVE-IN continued

Item	Serving Size	Calories	Protein	Carb	Fiber	Sugar	Total Fat	Sat Fat	Sodium
Coca-Cola float/ blended float	regular	330	4	49	0	47	14	10	160
Coconut cream pie shake	regular	600	8	78	0	72	29	20	330
Diet Coke float/ blended float	regular	260	4	29	0	27	14	10	160
Diet Dr Pepper float/ blended float	regular	260	4	28	0	27	14	10	190
Dr Pepper float/ blended float	regular	320	4	48	0	46	14	10	180
Grape CreamSlush® treat	regular	350	4	53	0	52	14	10	170
Hot fudge malt	regular	610	8	72	1	63	31	23	350
Hot fudge shake	regular	590	8	70	1	62	31	22	340
Java chiller, caramel	regular	500	7	64	0	58	25	18	360
Java chiller, chocolate	regular	500	7	64	0	56	24	17	320
Lemon CreamSlush® treat	regular	350	4	54	0	51	14	10	170
Lemon real fruit slush w/ Wacky Pack®	regular	170	0	46	0	44	0	0	25
Lemon-berry CreamSlush® treat	regular	400	5	66	1	58	14	10	180
Lime CreamSlush® treat	regular	350	4	54	0	50	14	10	170
M&M'S SONIC Blast®	regular	750	11	86	1	81	40	28	380
Orange CreamSlush® treat	regular	350	4	54	0	51	14	10	170
Oreo® SONIC Blast®	regular	680	11	78	1	70	37	25	460
Peanut butter malt	regular	690	12	63	0	56	45	22	420
Peanut butter shake	regular	660	12	60	0	54	44	21	400
Pineapple malt	regular	510	8	67	0	58	26	18	300
Pineapple shake	regular	520	8	65	0	57	26	18	290
Reese's peanut butter cups SONIC Blast®	regular	710	13	88	1	77	35	25	430
Snickers SONIC Blast®	regular	770	11	96	0	88	38	25	530
Sprite float/ blended float	regular	330	4	48	0	47	14	10	170
Sprite Zero float/ blended float	regular	260	4	28	0	27	14	10	160
Strawberry cream pie shake	regular	670	9	95	1	83	29	20	340

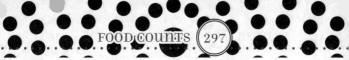

SONIC DRIVE-IN continued

Item	Serving Size	Calories	Protein	Carb	Fiber	Sugar	Total Fat	Sat Fat	Sodium
Strawberry CreamSlush® treat	regular	400	5	65	1	58	14	10	180
Strawberry malt	regular	540	9	70	1	61	26	18	300
Strawberry shake	regular	530	8	68	1	59	26	18	290
Vanilla malt	regular	480	8	53	0	50	26	18	290
Vanilla shake	regular	460	8	51	0	49	26	18	280
Watermelon CreamSlush® treat	regular	350	4	54	0	51	14	10	170

SIDES

Item	Serving Size	Calories	Protein	Carb	Fiber	Sugar	Total Fat	Sat Fat	Sodium
Apple slices	1 order	35	0	9	2	7	0	0	0
Apple slices w/ fat-free caramel dipping sauce	1 order	120	0	27	2	23	0	0	60
Ched 'R' Bites®	12 pieces	280	13	22	1	0	15	6	740
Ched 'R' Peppers®	4 pieces	330	8	36	2	2	17	6	1110
French fries	small	200	2	30	2	0	8	1.5	270
French fries w/ cheese	small	270	5	32	2	1	13	5	590
French fries w/ chili & cheese	small	300	8	33	3	1	16	6	540
Mozzarella sticks	1 order	440	19	40	2	1	22	9	1050
Pickle-O's®	1 order	310	5	36	2	2	16	3	1020

STARBUCKS COFFEE

Item	Serving Size	Calories	Protein	Carb	Fiber	Sugar	Total Fat	Sat Fat	Sodium
BREAKFAST									
Bacon, Gouda cheese, & egg frittata on artisan roll	as served	350	17	30	0	n/a	18	n/a	n/a
Black Forest ham, parmesan frittata, & Cheddar on artisan roll	as served	370	23	32	0	n/a	16	n/a	n/a
Brown sugar Topping for Starbucks® Perfect Oatmeal	as served	50	0	13	0	n/a	0	n/a	n/a
Chicken & vegetable wrap	as served	290	19	36	4	n/a	9	n/a	n/a

STARBUCKS COFFEE continued

Item	Serving Size	Calories	Protein	Carb	Fiber	Sugar	Total Fat	Sat Fat	Sodium
Chicken Santa Fe panini	as served	400	27	47	2	n/a	11	n/a	n/a
Dark cherry yogurt parfait	as served	310	10	61	3	n/a	4	n/a	n/a
Dried fruit topping for Starbucks® Perfect Oatmeal	as served	100	<1	24	2	n/a	0	n/a	n/a
Egg white, spinach & feta wrap	as served	280	18	33	6	n/a	10	n/a	n/a
Greek yogurt honey parfait	as served	290	8	43	<1	n/a	12	n/a	n/a
Huevos rancheros wrap	as served	330	16	35	8	n/a	15	n/a	n/a
Nut medley topping for Starbucks® Perfect Oatmeal	as served	100	2	2	<1	n/a	9	n/a	n/a
Roasted vegetable panini	as served	350	13	48	4	n/a	12	n/a	n/a
Roma tomato & mozzarella sandwich	as served	380	16	40	2	n/a	18	n/a	n/a
Sausage, egg & cheese on English muffin	as served	500	19	41	<1	n/a	28	n/a	n/a
Starbucks® Perfect Oatmeal	as served	140	5	25	4	n/a	2.5	n/a	n/a
Strawberry & blueberry yogurt parfait	as served	300	7	60	3	n/a	3.5	n/a	n/a
Tarragon chicken salad sandwich	as served	480	35	62	3	n/a	11	n/a	n/a
Tuna melt panini	as served	390	22	49	3	n/a	12	n/a	n/a
Turkey & Swiss sandwich	as served	390	34	36	2	n/a	13	n/a	n/a
Cappuccino w/ nonfat milk	tall	80	8	11	0	10	0	0	110
Iced Latte w/ nonfat milk	tall	70	7	10	0	9	0	0	100
Mocha w/ nonfat milk	tall	180	12	33	1	28	2	0.5	150
Mocha Frappuccino® w/ nonfat milk	tall	230	6	44	0	36	3	2	180

SIDES & SNACKS

Item	Serving Size	Calories	Protein	Carb	Fiber	Sugar	Total Fat	Sat Fat	Sodium
8-grain roll	as served	350	10	67	5	n/a	8	n/a	n/a

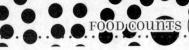

STARBUCKS COFFEE continued

Item	Serving Size	Calories	Protein	Carb	Fiber	Sugar	Total Fat	Sat Fat	Sodium
Apple bran muffin	as served	350	6	64	7	n/a	9	n/a	n/a
Apple fritter	as served	420	5	59	<1	n/a	20	n/a	n/a
Asiago bagel	as served	310	13	54	2	n/a	4.5	n/a	n/a
Banana nut loaf	as served	490	7	75	4	n/a	19	n/a	n/a
Birthday cake mini doughnut	as served	130	<1	17	0	n/a	6	n/a	n/a
Blueberry oat bar	as served	370	6	47	5	n/a	14	n/a	n/a
Blueberry scone	as served	460	7	61	2	n/a	22	n/a	n/a
Blueberry streusel muffin	as served	360	7	59	2	n/a	11	n/a	n/a
Butter croissant	as served	310	5	32	<1	n/a	18	n/a	n/a
Cheese Danish	as served	420	7	39	<1	n/a	25	n/a	n/a
Chicken on flatbread w/ hummus artisan snack plate	as served	250	17	27	5	n/a	9	n/a	n/a
Chocolate chunk cookie	as served	360	4	50	2	n/a	17	n/a	n/a
Chocolate croissant	as served	300	5	34	2	n/a	17	n/a	n/a
Chocolate old-fashioned doughnut	as served	420	5	57	2	n/a	21	n/a	n/a
Chonga bagel	as served	310	12	52	3	n/a	5	n/a	n/a
Cinnamon chip scone	as served	480	7	70	3	n/a	18	n/a	n/a
Cranberry orange scone	as served	490	8	73	2	n/a	18	n/a	n/a
Double chocolate brownie	as served	410	6	46	3	n/a	24	n/a	n/a
Double fudge mini doughnut	as served	130	<1	16	0	n/a	7	n/a	n/a
Double iced cinnamon roll	as served	490	7	70	3	n/a	20	n/a	n/a
Fruit, nut & cheese artisan snack plate	as served	460	19	33	6	n/a	29	n/a	n/a
Ginger molasses cookie	as served	360	3	58	<1	n/a	12	n/a	n/a
Hawaiian bagel	as served	360	12	60	2	n/a	8	n/a	n/a
Iced lemon pound cake	as served	490	5	68	<1	n/a	23	n/a	n/a

STARBUCKS COFFEE continued

Item	Serving Size	Calories	Protein	Carb	Fiber	Sugar	Total Fat	Sat Fat	Sodium
Lowfat red raspberry muffin	as served	340	7	65	2	n/a	6	n/a	n/a
Mallorca sweet bread	as served	420	7	42	<1	n/a	25	n/a	n/a
Maple oat pecan scone	as served	440	8	59	3	n/a	18	n/a	n/a
Protein artisan snack plate	as served	370	13	36	4	n/a	19	n/a	n/a
BREWED COFFEE									
Bold pick of the day	Grande, 16 oz	5	<1	0	0	n/a	0	n/a	n/a
Clover brewed coffee	Grande, 16 oz	5	<1	0	0	n/a	0	n/a	n/a
Pike Place Roast, regular / decaf	Grande, 16 oz	5	<1	0	0	n/a	0	n/a	n/a
SPECIALTY BEVERAGES MADE WITH 2% MILK									
Caffe latte	Grande, 16 oz	190	12	18	2	n/a	7	n/a	n/a
Caffe mocha	Grande, 16 oz	260	13	41	0	n/a	8	n/a	n/a
Cappuccino	Grande, 16 oz	120	8	12	0	n/a	4	n/a	n/a
Caramel brulee latte	Grande, 16 oz	300	7	59	0	n/a	3.5	n/a	n/a
Caramel macchiato	Grande, 16 oz	240	10	34	0	n/a	7	n/a	n/a
Cinnamon dolce latte	Grande, 16 oz	260	11	40	0	n/a	6	n/a	n/a
Eggnog latte	Grande, 16 oz	470	16	53	0	n/a	21	n/a	n/a
Flavored latte	Grande, 16 oz	250	12	36	0	n/a	6	n/a	n/a
Ginergerbread latte	Grande, 16 oz	250	11	37	0	n/a	6	n/a	n/a
Hot chocolate	Grande, 16 oz	300	14	47	2	n/a	9	n/a	n/a
Iced caffe latte	Grande, 16 oz	130	8	13	0	n/a	4.5	n/a	n/a
Iced caffe mocha	Grande, 16 oz	200	9	35	2	n/a	6	n/a	n/a
Iced caramel macchiato	Grande, 16 oz	230	10	33	0	n/a	6	n/a	n/a
Iced cinnamon dolce latte	Grande, 16 oz	200	7	34	0	n/a	4	n/a	n/a
Iced flavored latte	Grande, 16 oz	250	12	36	0	n/a	6	n/a	n/a
Iced gingerbread latte	Grande, 16 oz	190	7	32	0	n/a	4	n/a	n/a

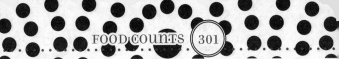

STARBUCKS COFFEE continued

Item	Serving Size	Calories	Protein	Carb	Fiber	Sugar	Total Fat	Sat Fat	Sodium
Iced peppermint mocha	Grande, 16 oz	260	8	52	2	n/a	6	n/a	n/a
Iced peppermint white chocolate mocha	Grande, 16 oz	400	10	72	0	n/a	9	n/a	n/a
Iced pumpkin spice latte	Grande, 16 oz	250	10	44	0	n/a	4	n/a	n/a
Iced skinny flavored latte	Grande, 16 oz	110	7	12	0	n/a	4	n/a	n/a
Iced toffee mocha	Grande, 16 oz	280	12	51	2	n/a	3.5	n/a	n/a
Iced white chocolate mocha	Grande, 16 oz	340	10	55	0	n/a	9	n/a	n/a
Peppermint mocha	Grande, 16 oz	330	12	58	2	n/a	8	n/a	n/a
Peppermint mocha hot chocolate	Grande, 16 oz	360	13	63	2	n/a	9	n/a	n/a
Peppermint while chocolate mocha	Grande, 16 oz	470	14	78	0	n/a	12	n/a	n/a
Pumpkin spice latte	Grande, 16 oz	310	14	49	0	n/a	6	n/a	n/a
Salted caramel hot chocolate	Grande, 16 oz	360	13	66	2	n/a	9	n/a	n/a
Skinny caramel macchiato	Grande, 16 oz	140	11	21	0	18	1	.5	150
Skinny cinnamon dolce latte	Grande, 16 oz	180	12	18	0	n/a	6	n/a	n/a
Skinny flavored latte	Grande, 16 oz	180	12	18	0	n/a	6	n/a	n/a
Toffee mocha	Grande, 16 oz	350	17	58	2	n/a	7	n/a	n/a
White chocolate mocha	Grande, 16 oz	400	15	61	0	n/a	11	n/a	n/a
White hot chocolate	Grande, 16 oz	410	16	61	0	n/a	12	n/a	n/a

FRAPPUCCINO

Item	Serving Size	Calories	Protein	Carb	Fiber	Sugar	Total Fat	Sat Fat	Sodium
Caramel Brulee Frappuccino	Grande, 16 oz	300	6	63	0	n/a	3.5	n/a	n/a
Double Chocolaty Chip Frappuccino	Grande, 16 oz	500	14	98	0	n/a	9	n/a	n/a
Peppermint Mocha Frappuccino	Grande, 16 oz	220	4	45	0	n/a	3	n/a	n/a

STARBUCKS COFFEE continued

Item	Serving Size	Calories	Protein	Carb	Fiber	Sugar	Total Fat	Sat Fat	Sodium
Peppermint Mocha Frappuccino, light	Grande, 16 oz	150	5	30	3	n/a	1	n/a	n/a
Pumpkin Spice Frappuccino	Grande, 16 oz	290	6	59	0	n/a	3.5	n/a	n/a
Pumpkin Spice Frappuccino, light	Grande, 16 oz	150	6	31	3	n/a	0.5	n/a	n/a
White Chocolate Crème Frappuccino	Grande, 16 oz	480	15	89	0	n/a	0	n/a	n/a

SUBWAY

Item	Serving Size	Calories	Protein	Carb	Fiber	Sugar	Total Fat	Sat Fat	Sodium
SUBS & SANDWICHES									
Beef steak & cheese	6"	390	24	48	5	7	14	5	1210
Black Forest ham w/o cheese	6"	290	18	47	5	7	4.5	1	1200
Breakfast egg, & bacon, deli style	as served	320	14	34	3	3	16	4.5	520
Breakfast egg, & cheese, deli style	as served	320	14	34	3	3	15	5	550
Cold cut trio	6"	440	21	47	4	6	21	7	1680
Footlong ham	12"	570	35	94	10	14	9	2.5	2400
Footlong oven roasted chicken	12"	640	46	97	11	14	9	2.5	1490
Footlong roast beef	12"	630	52	91	11	12	9	3	1600
Footlong Subway Club®	12"	640	52	96	11	12	10	3	2270
Footlong sweet onion chicken teriyaki	12"	760	51	120	10	34	9	2	2020
Footlong turkey breast	12"	570	35	94	10	11	7	1.5	1830
Footlong turkey breast & ham	12"	590	38	95	10	13	8	2	2280
Footlong Veggie Delite®	12"	460	17	90	10	10	4.5	1	830
Ham mini sub	each	180	10	31	3	4	2.5	0.5	670
Ham w/ honey mustard	6"	310	18	52	4	12	5	1.5	1260
Italian BMT®	6"	480	23	46	4	6	24	9	1900
Meatball	6"	530	24	53	6	7	26	10	1360
Oven roasted chicken	6"	320	23	49	5	7	4.5	1.5	750

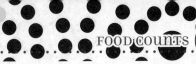

SUBWAY continued

Item	Serving Size	Calories	Protein	Carb	Fiber	Sugar	Total Fat	Sat Fat	Sodium
Roast beef	6"	310	26	45	5	6	4.5	1.5	800
Roast beef mini sub	each	200	15	30	4	4	3	1	480
Southwest turkey bacon	6"	410	21	48	4	7	17	4.5	1230
Subway Club®	6"	320	26	47	5	6	5	1.5	1140
Sweet onion chicken teriyaki	6"	380	26	60	5	17	4.5	1	1010
Tuna w/ light mayonnaise	6"	450	20	46	4	5	22	6	1190
Turkey breast	6"	280	18	47	5	6	3.5	1	910
Turkey breast & ham	6"	300	19	47	5	6	4	1	1140
Turkey breast mini sub	each	190	12	31	3	4	2.5	0.5	610
Veggie Delite®	6"	230	8	45	5	5	2.5	0.5	410
Veggie Delite® mini sub	each	150	6	30	3	3	1.5	0	280
SOUPS									
Black bean	1 cup	180	9	27	15	4	4.5	2	1160
Chicken noodle	1 cup	90	7	7	1	1	4	1	1180
Cream of broccoli	1 cup	130	5	15	2	0	6	0	860
Cream of potato w/ bacon	1 cup	210	5	20	4	3	12	4	970
Minestrone	1 cup	70	3	11	2	2	1	0	610
Rice w/ chicken	1 cup	190	6	17	2	3	11	4.5	990
Tomato bisque	1 cup	90	1	15	3	7	2.5	0.5	750
Vegetable beef	1 cup	90	5	14	2	4	1.5	0.5	1340
COOKIES									
Chocolate chip	each	210	2	30	1	18	10	6	150
Chocolate chunk	each	200	2	30	1	17	10	5	100
Double chocolate	each	210	2	30	1	20	10	5	170
M&M'S	each	210	2	32	1	18	10	5	100
Oatmeal raisin	each	200	3	30	1	17	8	4	170
Peanut butter	each	220	4	26	1	16	12	5	200
Sugar	each	220	2	28	0	14	12	6	140
White macadamia nut	each	220	2	29	1	18	11	5	160

TACO BELL

Item	Serving Size	Calories	Protein	Carb	Fiber	Sugar	Total Fat	Sat Fat	Sodium
DRINKS									
Cherry limeade sparkler	16 oz	180	0	43	0	43	0	0	105
Cherry limeade sparkler	20 oz	270	0	66	0	65	0	0	160
Classic limeade sparkler	16 oz	150	0	39	0	38	0	0	80
Classic limeade sparkler	20 oz	230	0	60	0	59	0	0	125
Classic margarita Frutista Freeze®	16 oz	220	0	55	0	51	0	0	0
Classic margarita Frutista Freeze®	20 oz	280	0	69	0	63	0	0	0
Mango strawberry Frutista Freeze®	16 oz	250	0	62	0	59	0	0	10
Mango strawberry Frutista Freeze®	20 oz	280	0	70	0	69	0	0	65
Strawberry Frutista Freeze®	16 oz	230	0	57	0	57	0	0	55
Strawberry Frutista Freeze®	20 oz	230	0	70	0	69	0	0	65
Strawberry Frutista Freeze®	16 oz	250	0	63	0	58	0	0	0
Strawberry Frutista Freeze®	20 oz	310	0	77	0	70	0	0	0
BURRITOS									
1/2 lb.* cheesy potato burrito	1 burrito	530	19	57	7	5	25	8	1690
1/2 lb.* Combo burrito	1 burrito	450	22	52	10	3	18	7	1640
1/2 lb.* nacho crunch burrito	1 burrito	520	19	54	6	5	25	8	1400
7-Layer burrito	1 burrito	510	18	68	12	5	18	6	1420
Bean burrito	1 burrito	370	14	55	11	3	10	3.5	1270
Beefy 5-layer burrito	1 burrito	550	20	69	9	6	22	8	1640
Burrito Supreme®, beef	1 burrito	420	17	52	9	5	15	7	1380
Burrito Supreme®, chicken	1 burrito	390	21	51	7	5	12	5	1420
Burrito Supreme®, steak	1 burrito	380	18	51	7	5	12	5	1340
Cheesy bean and rice burrito	1 burrito	480	13	60	8	5	21	5	1380

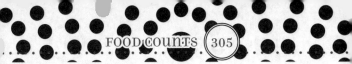

TACO BELL continued

Item	Serving Size	Calories	Protein	Carb	Fiber	Sugar	Total Fat	Sat Fat	Sodium
Cheesy double beef burrito	1 burrito	470	18	54	6	4	20	6	1580
Chili cheese burrito	1 burrito	370	16	40	4	3	16	8	1080
Fresco bean burrito	1 burrito	340	12	56	11	4	8	2.5	1290
Grilled chicken burrito	1 burrito	430	18	48	3	3	18	5	1280
Grilled Stuft burrito, beef	1 burrito	700	27	79	12	6	30	10	2110
Grilled Stuft burrito, chicken	1 burrito	650	34	77	9	5	24	7	2180
Grilled Stuft burrito, steak	1 burrito	640	28	76	9	6	24	8	2040

CHALUPAS

Item	Serving Size	Calories	Protein	Carb	Fiber	Sugar	Total Fat	Sat Fat	Sodium
Chalupa Baja, beef	1 chalupa	410	13	31	5	4	26	5	730
Chalupa Baja, chicken	1 chalupa	390	16	29	3	4	23	4	760
Chalupa Baja, steak	1 chalupa	380	13	29	3	4	23	4	690
Chalupa nacho cheese, beef	1 chalupa	370	12	31	4	4	22	3.5	730
Chalupa nacho cheese, chicken	1 chalupa	340	15	30	3	4	18	2	770
Chalupa nacho cheese, steak	1 chalupa	330	12	30	3	4	19	2.5	700
Chalupa Supreme, chicken	1 chalupa	350	17	30	3	4	18	4	640
Chalupa Supreme, steak	1 chalupa	340	14	29	3	4	18	4	570
Chalupa Supreme, beef	1 chalupa	370	13	31	4	4	21	5	600
XXL chalupa	1 chalupa	650	23	53	7	6	39	9	1300

CONDIMENTS &SAUCES

Item	Serving Size	Calories	Protein	Carb	Fiber	Sugar	Total Fat	Sat Fat	Sodium
Border sauce, fire	1 sauce	0	0	0	0	0	0	0	60
Border sauce, hot	1 sauce	0	0	0	0	0	0	0	45
Border sauce, mild	1 sauce	0	0	0	0	0	0	0	35
Creamy jalapeño sauce	1 sauce	70	0	1	0	1	7	1	50
Fiesta salsa	1 sauce	5	0	1	1	1	0	0	60
Green tomatillo sauce	1 sauce	10	0	2	0	1	0	0	170
Guacamole	1 sauce	35	0	2	1	0	3	0	85
Pepper Jack sauce	1 sauce	70	0	1	0	1	7	1	85

TACO BELL continued

Item	Serving Size	Calories	Protein	Carb	Fiber	Sugar	Total Fat	Sat Fat	Sodium
Pizza sauce	1 sauce	10	0	2	0	1	0	0	90
Red sauce	1 sauce	10	0	2	0	0	0	0	240
Reduced fat sour cream	1 sauce	30	1	2	0	1	2	1	20
Salsa	1 sauce	5	0	1	0	1	0	0	80
Spicy avocado ranch dressing	1 sauce	80	0	1	0	0	8	1	120
Zesty dressing	1 sauce	200	1	3	0	1	20	3.5	250
FRESCO MENU									
Fresco bean burrito	1 burrito	340	12	56	11	4	8	2.5	1290
Fresco Burrito Supreme®, chicken	1 burrito	340	18	50	8	4	8	2.5	1410
Fresco Burrito Supreme®, steak	1 burrito	330	16	49	8	4	8	3	1340
Fresco crunchy taco	1 taco	150	7	13	3	1	7	2.5	350
Fresco grilled steak soft taco	1 taco	160	9	21	2	3	4.5	1.5	600
Fresco ranchero chicken soft taco	1 taco	170	12	22	2	3	4	1.5	740
Fresco soft taco	1 taco	180	8	22	3	2	7	3	640
GORDITAS									
Cheesy gordita crunch	1 gordita	500	20	40	5	6	28	10	880
Gordita Baja®, beef	1 gordita	340	13	30	4	6	18	5	710
Gordita Baja®, chicken	1 gordita	320	16	29	3	6	15	3.5	750
Gordita Baja®, steak	1 gordita	310	14	28	3	6	15	3.5	680
Gordita nacho cheese, beef	1 gordita	290	12	31	4	6	14	3	720
Gordita nacho cheese, chicken	1 gordita	270	15	30	2	6	10	1.5	760
Gordita nacho cheese, steak	1 gordita	260	12	29	2	6	11	2	690
Gordita Supreme®, beef	1 gordita	300	13	31	4	6	13	5	590
Gordita Supreme®, chicken	1 gordita	270	17	29	2	6	10	3.5	630
Gordita Supreme®, steak	1 gordita	270	14	29	2	6	11	4	550

TACO BELL continued

Item	Serving Size	Calories	Protein	Carb	Fiber	Sugar	Total Fat	Sat Fat	Sodium
NACHOS									
Cheesy nachos	as served	280	4	28	2	1	17	1.5	300
Nachos	as served	330	4	31	2	2	21	2	520
Nachos BellGrande®	as served	770	20	78	15	5	42	7	1300
Nachos supreme	as served	440	13	42	8	3	24	5	800
Triple-layer nachos	as served	350	7	39	7	2	18	1.5	740
Volcano nachos	as served	1000	22	89	16	6	62	9	1930
SIDES									
Caramel apple empanada	as served	310	3	39	2	13	15	2.5	310
Cheesy fiesta potatoes	as served	270	4	28	3	2	16	2.5	840
Cinnamon twists	as served	170	1	26	1	10	7	0	200
Mexican rice	as served	130	2	21	1	1	3.5	0	410
Pintos 'n cheese	as served	170	10	19	9	1	6	2.5	750
OTHER SPECIALITIES									
Cheese quesadilla	as served	470	19	40	4	3	26	11	1120
Cheese roll-up	as served	200	9	19	2	1	10	5	540
Chicken flatbread sandwich	as served	290	15	23	2	5	15	3.5	720
Chicken quesadilla	as served	520	28	41	4	3	28	12	1440
Crunchwrap Supreme®	as served	540	16	71	6	7	21	7	1400
Enchirito®, beef	as served	370	19	35	8	2	17	8	1430
Enchirito®, chicken	as served	350	22	34	7	2	14	7	1470
Enchirito®, steak	as served	340	19	33	7	2	14	7	1400
Express taco salad w/ chips	as served	660	25	67	11	7	34	10	1520
Grilled chicken taquitos	as served	320	18	37	2	2	11	4.5	1000
Grilled steak taquitos	as served	310	15	37	2	3	11	5	930
Mexican pizza	as served	540	21	47	8	2	30	8	1030
MexiMelt®	as served	280	15	23	4	2	14	7	880
Mini quesadilla	as served	190	9	17	2	1	9	5	510
Steak quesadilla	as served	510	25	40	4	3	28	12	1370
Tostada	as served	250	11	29	10	1	10	3.5	730

TACO BELL continued

Item	Serving Size	Calories	Protein	Carb	Fiber	Sugar	Total Fat	Sat Fat	Sodium
TACO SALADS									
Chicken ranch taco salad	1 salad	910	35	71	9	6	54	10	1660
Chipotle steak taco salad	1 salad	900	28	70	8	7	57	11	1700
Express taco salad w/ chips	1 salad	660	25	67	11	7	34	10	1520
Fiesta taco salad	1 salad	770	27	75	12	8	41	10	1650
TACOS									
Chicken soft taco	1 taco	190	13	20	1	1	6	2.5	660
Crispy potato soft taco	1 taco	260	6	31	3	2	13	3	690
Crunchy taco	1 taco	170	8	12	3	1	10	3.5	330
Double Decker® taco	1 taco	330	14	38	8	2	13	5	820
Double Decker® taco Supreme®	1 taco	360	15	41	8	3	15	6	840
Fresco crunchy taco	1 taco	150	7	13	3	1	7	2.5	350
Grilled steak soft taco	1 taco	250	11	20	2	2	14	4	710
Ranchero chicken soft taco	1 taco	270	14	21	2	2	14	4	840
Soft Taco Supreme®, beef	1 taco	240	11	24	3	3	11	5	650
Soft taco, beef	1 taco	210	10	21	3	2	9	4	620
Taco Supreme®	1 taco	200	9	15	3	2	12	5	350
VOLCANO MENU									
Volcano burrito	1 burrito	800	24	81	8	6	42	12	2010
Volcano nachos	as served	1000	22	89	16	6	62	9	1930
Volcano taco	1 taco	240	8	14	3	1	17	5	470
WHY PAY MORE!® MENU									
Bean burrito	1 burrito	370	14	55	11	3	10	3.5	1270
Beefy 5-layer burrito	1 burrito	550	20	69	9	6	22	8	1640
Caramel apple empanada	as served	310	3	39	2	13	15	2.5	310
Cheese roll-up	as served	200	9	19	2	1	10	5	540
Cheesy nachos	as served	280	4	28	2	1	17	1.5	300
Cinnamon twists	as served	170	1	26	1	10	7	0	200
Crispy potato soft taco	1 taco	260	6	31	3	2	13	3	690
Crunchy taco	1 taco	170	8	12	3	1	10	3.5	330

TACO BELL continued

Item	Serving Size	Calories	Protein	Carb	Fiber	Sugar	Total Fat	Sat Fat	Sodium
Fresco bean burrito	1 burrito	340	12	56	11	4	8	2.5	1290
Fresco crunchy taco	1 taco	150	7	13	3	1	7	2.5	350
Grilled chicken burrito	1 burrito	430	18	48	3	3	18	5	1280
Mini quesadilla	as served	190	9	17	2	1	9	5	510
Soft taco, beef	1 taco	210	10	21	3	2	9	4	620
Triple-layer nachos	as served	350	7	39	7	2	18	1.5	740

TGI FRIDAY'S

Item	Serving Size	Calories	Protein	Carb	Fiber	Sugar	Total Fat	Sat Fat	Sodium
APPETIZERS									
Bruschetta chicken pasta	as served	1172	42	191	27	7	29	5.6	1260
Buffalo wings	1 box	574	38	6	0	2	38	10	3542
Chicken quesadilla rolls	1 box	821	26	67	6	3	38	12	1172
French fries	1 order	140	2	14	0	1	8	2	370
Honey BBQ wings	3 pieces	190	11	5	0	6	12	3	630
Mozzarella cheese sticks	1 stick	110	4	7	0	1	6	2	260
Potato skins w/ Cheddar & bacon	3 pieces	211	8	19	2	1	12	4	382
Shrimp, medium, breaded, fried	1 shrimp	27	2	1	0	0	1.4	0.3	54
Spinach, cheese & artichoke dip	1 oz	50	2	2	2	1	3.5	2	150
ENTRÉES									
Cedar-seared salmon pasta	as served	500	30	55	9	34	12	6	400
Complete Skillet Meals, Cajun-style Alfredo chicken & shrimp	as served	280	21	34	2	4	7	3	760
Complete Skillet Meals, chicken & broccoli Alfredo	as served	270	19	28	3	2	9	4	520
Gourmet mac 'n' five cheese	as served	792	38	76	2	12	35	20.5	800
Sirloin beef steak	as served	185	31	0	0	0	7	2.8	194
Spicy Cajun chicken pasta	as served	1100	53	144	8	8	32	16	1760

WENDY'S

Item	Serving Size	Calories	Protein	Carb	Fiber	Sugar	Total Fat	Sat Fat	Sodium
SALADS, DRESSINGS, & SIDES									
Apple pecan chicken salad	full size	350	37	29	5	20	12	7	1210
Apple pecan chicken salad	1/2 size	180	18	15	3	10	6	3.5	610
Baja salad	full size	550	33	36	12	12	33	14	1610
Baja salad	1/2 size	280	17	19	6	7	17	7	820
BLT Cobb salad	full size	460	46	12	3	4	26	12	1490
BLT Cobb salad	1/2 size	230	23	7	2	2	13	6	750
Caesar side salad	side	60	4	5	2	2	3.5	2	95
Chili	large	330	28	32	8	10	10	4	1310
Chili	small	220	18	22	6	6	7	3	870
Classic ranch dressing	as served	110	1	1	0	1	11	2	190
Fat free French dressing	as served	40	0	9	0	8	0	0	95
Garden side salad	side	25	1	5	2	3	0	0	30
Gourmet croutons	as served	80	2	12	0	0	3	0	220
Italian vinaigrette dressing	as served	70	0	4	0	3	6	1	180
Lemon garlic Caesar dressing	as served	110	2	2	0	1	11	2	180
Light classic ranch dressing	as served	50	1	2	0	1	4.5	1	200
Mandarin orange cup	each	90	1	21	1	18	0	0	10
Natural-cut fries	value	220	3	29	3	0	11	2	270
Natural-cut fries	small	320	4	41	5	0	15	3	380
Natural-cut fries	medium	420	5	54	6	0	20	3.5	500
Natural-cut fries	large	520	6	67	7	0	25	4.5	630
Plain baked potato	each	270	7	61	7	3	0	0	25
Sour cream & chives baked potato	each	320	8	63	7	4	3.5	2	50
Spicy chicken Caesar salad	full size	450	32	25	6	3	25	11	1290
Spicy chicken Caesar salad	1/2 size	230	17	14	4	3	13	6	650
Thousand Island dressing	as served	160	0	5	0	4	15	2.5	290

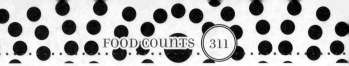

WENDY'S continued

Item	Serving Size	Calories	Protein	Carb	Fiber	Sugar	Total Fat	Sat Fat	Sodium
BONELESS WINGS & CHICKEN NUGGESTS									
Chicken nuggets	kids'	180	9	10	0	1	12	2.5	340
Chicken nuggets	5 piece	230	12	13	0	1	14	3	430
Chicken nuggets	10 piece	450	23	25	0	1	29	6	850
Honey BBQ boneless wings	one order	570	33	69	3	34	18	3.5	1950
Spicy chipotle boneless wings	one order	500	33	48	3	10	20	4	1640
Sweet & spicy Asian boneless wings	one order	540	33	62	3	27	18	3.5	2490
SANDWICHES									
Bacon deluxe double	each	870	53	46	2	11	52	22	1550
Bacon deluxe single	each	650	34	46	2	11	37	15	1380
Baconator® double	each	980	58	46	2	9	63	27	1830
Baconator® single	each	610	32	43	2	9	34	14	1170
Chicken club sandwich	each	630	34	55	3	8	31	10	1410
Crispy chicken sandwich regular		350	15	38	2	4	15	3	830
Double jr. bacon cheeseburger	each	440	25	28	2	5	25	11	730
Double stack	each	360	23	27	1	6	18	8	760
Double w/ everything & cheese	each	750	49	44	2	10	42	18	1370
Grilled Chicken Go Wrap	each	260	20	25	1	3	10	3.5	750
Homestyle chicken fillet sandwich	each	470	26	52	3	7	18	3.5	1160
Homestyle Chicken Go Wrap	each	320	15	29	1	1	16	4.5	770
Jr. bacon cheeseburger	each	350	17	28	2	5	19	8	660
Jr. cheeseburger	each	270	15	27	1	6	11	5	690
Jr. cheeseburger deluxe	each	300	15	29	2	7	14	6	720
Jr. hamburger	each	230	12	26	1	6	8	3	480
Single, w/ everything	each	470	26	43	2	10	21	8	880
Spicy chicken fillet sandwich	each	460	26	54	3	7	16	3	1330
Spicy Chicken Go Wrap	each	310	15	30	2	1	15	4.5	860
Triple w/ everything & cheese	each	1030	71	44	2	11	63	29	1860

WENDY'S continued

Item	Serving Size	Calories	Protein	Carb	Fiber	Sugar	Total Fat	Sat Fat	Sodium
Ultimate Chicken Grill Sandwich	each	370	34	42	2	9	7	1.5	1150
FROSTY TREATS									
Chocolate Frosty™	small	310	8	52	0	44	8	5	140
Chocolate fudge Frosty™ shake	small	410	8	69	1	58	11	7	190
Chocolate fudge Frosty™ shake	large	540	11	94	1	80	13	8	270
Coffee toffee twisted Frosty™, chocolate	each	540	9	83	1	69	20	15	230
Coffee toffee twisted Frosty™, vanilla	each	540	8	83	1	70	20	15	230
Frosty™-cino	small	380	7	63	0	53	11	7	140
Frosty™-cino	large	510	9	87	0	72	13	8	180
M&M's twisted Frosty™, chocolate	each	550	10	86	1	75	19	12	170
M&M's twisted Frosty™, vanilla	each	560	10	87	1	76	19	12	170
Nestlé Toll House cookie dough twisted Frosty™, chocolate	each	480	9	77	1	60	16	10	200
Nestlé Toll House cookie dough twisted Frosty™, vanilla	each	480	9	77	1	61	16	10	210
Oreo twisted Frosty™, chocolate	each	440	9	72	1	54	14	7	290
Oreo twisted Frosty™, vanilla	each	440	9	72	1	55	14	7	290
Strawberry Frosty™ shake	small	390	7	66	0	59	11	7	140
Strawberry Frosty™ shake	large	510	9	89	0	81	13	8	180
Vanilla Frosty™	small	310	8	52	0	45	8	5	150
Vanilla Frosty™ float w/ Coca-Cola	each	390	7	75	0	69	7	5	130
Vanilla Frosty™ shake	small	380	7	64	0	57	11	7	140
Vanilla Frosty™ shake	large	510	9	88	0	78	13	8	180

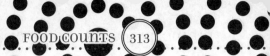

WHATABURGER

Item	Serving Size	Calories	Protein	Carb	Fiber	Sugar	Total Fat	Sat Fat	Sodium
Biscuit	each	300	5	32	1	2	17	8	644
Biscuit & gravy	as served	560	9	54	1	4	33	16	1960
Biscuit sandwich w/ bacon, egg, & cheese	as served	500	16	33	1	2	32	14	1231
Biscuit sandwich w/ egg & cheese	as served	450	13	33	1	2	28	13	1028
Biscuit sandwich w/ sausage, egg & cheese	as served	690	26	33	1	2	49	21	1553
Biscuit w/ sausage	as served	540	18	32	1	2	37	17	1169
Breakfast On A Bun® w/ bacon	as served	360	15	25	1	4	21	6	807
Breakfast On A Bun® w/ sausage	as served	550	25	25	1	4	38	14	1129
Breakfast platter w/ bacon	as served	730	24	93	1	3	45	14	1376
Breakfast platter w/ sausage	as served	920	34	93	1	3	63	21	1698
Chicken strip	1 piece	150	9	11	1	0	8	3	296
Chicken strips	2 pieces	300	18	22	1	1	16	6	593
Chicken strips	3 pieces	450	26	33	2	1	24	9	889
Chicken strips w/ gravy	4 pieces	680	35	53	2	1	35	14	1665
Chocolate brownie pie	as served	280	2	41	1	16	12	6	240
Cinnamon roll	each	390	7	71	3	35	9	3.5	390
Cookie, sugar	each	210	2	31	0	16	9	4.5	180
French fries	large	640	6	73	10	1	36	6	463
French fries	medium	480	5	55	7	1	27	4.5	347
French fries	small	320	3	36	5	1	18	3	231
Fruit chew	as served	80	1	19	0	15	0	0	10
Gravy, white peppered	as served	80	0	9	0	1	3.5	2	479
Grilled chicken sandwich	as served	470	27	49	3	9	19	4	1018
Hash brown sticks	4 pieces	200	2	60	0	0	12	0.5	280
Honey butter chicken biscuit	as served	560	14	50	2	9	34	13	1008
Hot apple pie	as served	250	3	31	2	7	12	2.5	292
Jalepeño, sliced	each	0	0	0	1	0	0	0	168

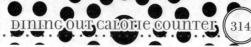

WHATABURGER continued

Item	Serving Size	Calories	Protein	Carb	Fiber	Sugar	Total Fat	Sat Fat	Sodium
Justaburger®	as served	290	13	26	1	4	15	4.5	727
Kids' Meal chicken strips	as served	300	18	22	1	1	16	6	593
Kids' Meal Justaburger®	as served	290	13	25	1	4	15	4.5	727
Malt, chocolate	small	1460	29	264	5	246	35	24	642
Malt, chocolate	medium	1050	21	188	3	175	25	18	460
Malt, chocolate	large	670	13	123	2	115	15	11	297
Malt, chocolate	kids'	520	11	94	2	88	13	9	230
Malt, strawberry	small	1450	26	263	0	250	33	23	548
Malt, strawberry	medium	1040	19	188	0	178	24	17	397
Malt, strawberry	large	670	12	123	0	117	15	10	250
Malt, strawberry	kids'	520	10	94	0	89	12	9	199
Malt, vanilla	small	1300	29	215	0	201	37	26	569
Malt, vanilla	medium	940	21	155	0	144	27	19	409
Malt, vanilla	large	600	13	98	0	92	17	12	259
Malt, vanilla	kids'	470	11	77	0	72	13	9	205
Onion rings	large	600	8	56	4	7	38	12	1182
Onion rings	medium	400	5	37	3	5	25	8	787
Pancakes, w/ bacon	as served	580	18	104	3	21	11	4	2153
Pancakes, w/ sausage	as served	780	28	104	3	21	28	11	2475
Pancakes, plain	as served	540	15	104	3	21	7	3	1950
Ranch sauce	as served	480	1	4	0	3	51	7	731
Salad, chicken strips	as served	350	19	33	5	7	16	6	606
Salad, garden	as served	50	1	11	5	6	0	0	13
Salad, grilled chicken	as served	220	21	18	4	6	7	1.5	633
Salad, side salad	as served	25	0	5	3	3	0	0	6
Taquito w/ bacon & egg	as served	380	17	27	3	2	21	7	932
Taquito w/ bacon, egg, & cheese	as served	420	19	27	3	2	24	9	1157
Taquito w/ potato & egg	as served	430	15	57	3	2	23	6	869
Taquito w/ potato, egg, & cheese	as served	470	17	57	3	2	27	8	1094
Taquito w/ sausage & egg	as served	410	17	27	3	2	24	8	909

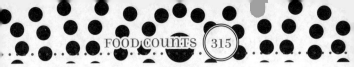

WHATABURGER continued

Item	Serving Size	Calories	Protein	Carb	Fiber	Sugar	Total Fat	Sat Fat	Sodium
Taquito w/ sausage, egg, & cheese	as served	450	19	27	3	2	28	11	1134
Texas toast	1 slice	150	3	20	1	3	7	1	170
Whataburger®	as served	620	26	58	2	13	30	10	1262
Whataburger® double meat	as served	870	43	58	2	13	49	18	1510
Whataburger® Jr.	as served	300	13	28	1	5	15	4.5	730
Whataburger® w/ bacon & cheese	as served	780	36	89	2	13	43	16	1997
Whataburger®, triple meat	as served	1120	61	58	2	13	68	26	1759
Whatacatch® dinner	as served	1630	30	181	12	92	89	16	1975
Whatacatch® sandwich	as served	450	16	44	3	7	24	4	881
Whatachick'n® sandwich	as served	550	23	57	4	12	27	6	968

WHITE CASTLE

Item	Serving Size	Calories	Protein	Carb	Fiber	Sugar	Total Fat	Sat Fat	Sodium
SANDWICHES									
A.1. slider	each	140	7	16	1	3	6	2.5	430
A.1. slider w/ cheese	each	170	8	16	1	4	9	4	570
Bacon cheeseburger	each	190	9	13	1	2	11	5	550
Bacon jalapeño cheeseburger	each	190	9	14	1	2	12	5	560
Cheeseburger	each	170	8	15	1	3	9	4	550
Chicken breast sandwich	each	360	11	20	1	1	26	3.5	510
Chicken breast sandwich w/ cheese	each	390	13	20	1	2	28	5	650
Chicken ring sandwich	each	350	8	16	1	1	28	4.5	320
Chicken ring sandwich w/ cheese	each	380	10	16	1	2	30	6	460
Double A.1. slider	each	260	12	25	1	6	12	5	800
Double A.1. slider w/ cheese	each	310	15	26	1	6	17	8	1070
Double bacon cheeseburger	each	350	18	21	1	2	22	10	1050

WHITE CASTLE continued

Item	Serving Size	Calories	Protein	Carb	Fiber	Sugar	Total Fat	Sat Fat	Sodium
Double cheeseburger	each	300	15	20	1	3	17	8	940
Double fish w/ cheese	each	610	19	25	23	2	48	9	700
Double fish w/o cheese	each	550	17	24	23	1	43	6	420
Double garlic cheese & mushroom slider	each	300	15	23	2	2	17	8	1060
Double garlic cheeseburger	each	290	15	21	1	2	16	7	910
Double jalapeño cheeseburger	each	280	15	21	1	2	17	8	860
Double White Castle®	each	240	12	21	1	2	12	5	660
Fish sandwich	each	310	9	18	12	1	22	3	270
Fish sandwich w/ cheese	each	340	11	18	12	2	24	4.5	410
Garlic cheese & chicken marinara slider	each	390	13	22	1	2	23	5	740
Garlic cheese & mushroom slider	each	170	8	14	1	2	9	4	560
Garlic cheeseburger	each	160	8	14	1	2	8	3.5	490
Jalapeño cheeseburger	each	160	8	14	1	2	9	4	460
Pulled pork BBQ sandwich	each	170	9	25	1	12	4.5	1	460
Surf and Turf w/ cheese	each	540	22	27	13	2	38	11	990
Surf and Turf w/o cheese	each	480	19	226	13	2	33	8	720
Traditional bun w/ cheese	each	90	4	12	1	2	3	1.5	260
White Castle	each	140	7	13	1	1	6	2.5	360

BREAKFAST SANDWICHES ON A BUN

Item	Serving Size	Calories	Protein	Carb	Fiber	Sugar	Total Fat	Sat Fat	Sodium
Bacon	each	130	5	12	1	1	6	2	330
Bacon & cheese	each	150	7	12	1	2	9	3.5	460
Bacon & egg	each	200	12	12	1	2	11	3.5	400
Bacon, egg, & cheese	each	190	12	13	1	2	11	4	430
Egg	each	140	9	12	1	2	6	2	190
Egg & cheese	each	160	10	13	1	2	8	3	330
Hamburger & egg	each	200	13	12	1	2	11	4	210
Hamburger, egg, & cheese	each	230	14	13	1	2	14	6	350
Sausage	each	220	8	12	1	1	15	6	430
Sausage & cheese	each	250	9	13	1	2	17	7	570
Sausage, egg, & cheese	each	320	15	13	1	2	22	9	640
Sausage, egg, & cheese	each	290	14	13	1	2	20	7	500

WHITE CASTLE continued

Item	Serving Size	Calories	Protein	Carb	Fiber	Sugar	Total Fat	Sat Fat	Sodium
BREAKFAST SIDES									
Awrey apple Danish	each	450	6	52	1	22	24	6	390
Awrey cheese Danish	each	450	6	52	1	22	24	6	390
Awrey cinnamon roll	each	420	6	56	2	22	20	8	460
Awrey strawberry Danish	each	480	6	67	2	34	21	8	400
French toast sticks	each	460	5	39	2	10	31	4.5	410
Haas apple Danish	each	470	6	62	1	29	22	10	520
Haas cheese Danish	each	490	6	62	1	28	25	11	550
Haas chocolate fried donuts	each	460	12	120	4	52	24	12	760
Haas cinnamon Danish	each	490	6	60	2	26	25	6	380
Haas French twist Donuts	twin pack	460	6	58	2	34	24	10	580
Haas plain old-fashioned donut	Single	385	5	51	2	23	21	9	403
Hash rounds/hash bites	Saver	360	2	25	2	0	28	3.5	460
Hash rounds/hash bites	Medium	600	4	42	4	0	46	6	760
Hash rounds/hash bites	Sack	1440	10	101	10	0	110	14	1830
SIDES									
Chicken rings	3 rings	260	9	6	0	0	24	4	300
Chicken rings	6 rings	530	18	12	0	0	47	10	610
Chicken rings	9 rings	790	26	18	1	0	71	12	910
Chicken rings	20 rings	1760	58	41	2	1	158	27	2020
Clam strips	regular	210	8	5	0	1	17	2	620
Clam strips	sack	410	16	9	0	2	34	4	1250
French fries	saver	350	3	32	3	2	24	4	50
French fries	medium	370	3	33	3	2	25	4	50
French fries	sack	850	8	76	8	4	57	9	115
Mozzarella cheese sticks	3 Sticks	440	12	22	1	1	33	8	850
Mozzarella cheese sticks	5 Sticks	740	21	36	2	2	55	14	1420
Mozzarella cheese sticks	10 Sticks	1470	41	73	4	4	111	28	2850
Nibblers	regular	320	16	28	1	1	16	2.5	700

WHITE CASTLE continued

Item	Serving Size	Calories	Protein	Carb	Fiber	Sugar	Total Fat	Sat Fat	Sodium
Nibblers	sack	1100	55	95	3	3	53	8	2390
Onion chips	kids'	510	4	35	6	4	38	6	730
Onion rings	saver	220	1	21	2	3	14	2.5	190
CONDIMENTS									
BBQ sauce	1 pkt	10	0	1	0	2	0	0	130
Fat free honey mustard	1 pkt	20	0	2	0	3	0	0	50
Hot sauce	1 pkt	5	0	0	1	0	0	0	170
Ketchup	1 pkt	10	0	1	0	2	0	0	100
Lemon juice	1 pkt	5	0	0	0	0	0	0	0
Mayonnaise	1 pkt	60	0	0	0	0	7	1	55
Mustard	1 pkt	5	0	0	0	0	0	0	85
Tartar sauce	1 pkt	25	1	0	0	1	1.5	0	85
DESSERTS									
Chocolate chunk cookie	each	170	2	8	1	13	8	4	130
Oatmeal raisin cookie	each	160	2	8	1	12	6	2.5	115
White chocolate macadamia cookie	each	180	2	7	1	14	9	4	125

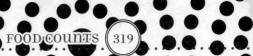

MISC BEVERAGES, SOFT DRINKS

Item	Serving Size	Calories	Protein	Carb	Fiber	Sugar	Total Fat	Sat Fat	Sodium
7UP	16 fl oz	200	0	52	0	52	0	0	50
7UP	20 fl oz	250	0	65	0	65	0	0	65
7UP	32 fl oz	400	0	104	0	104	0	0	100
7UP	64 fl oz	800	0	208	0	208	0	0	200
Coca-Cola Classic	16 oz	198	0	54	0	54	0	0	12
Code Red Mountain Dew	16 fl oz	220	0	62	0	62	0	0	70
Code Red Mountain Dew	20 fl oz	280	0	78	0	78	0	0	90
Code Red Mountain Dew	32 fl oz	440	0	124	0	124	0	0	140
Code Red Mountain Dew	64 fl oz	880	0	248	0	248	0	0	280
Diet Coke	16 oz	0	0	0	0	0	0	0	20
Diet Dr Pepper	16 fl oz	0	0	0	0	0	0	0	70
Diet Dr Pepper	20 fl oz	0	0	0	0	0	0	0	90
Diet Dr Pepper	32 fl oz	0	0	0	0	0	0	0	140
Diet Dr Pepper	64 fl oz	0	0	0	0	0	0	0	280
Diet Mountain Dew	16 fl oz	0	0	0	0	0	0	0	80
Diet Mountain Dew	20 fl oz	0	0	0	0	0	0	0	100
Diet Mountain Dew	32 fl oz	0	0	0	0	0	0	0	160
Diet Mountain Dew	64 fl oz	0	0	0	0	0	0	0	320
Diet Pepsi	16 fl oz	0	0	0	0	0	0	0	50
Diet Pepsi	20 fl oz	0	0	0	0	0	0	0	65
Diet Pepsi	32 fl oz	0	0	0	0	0	0	0	100
Diet Pepsi	64 fl oz	0	0	0	0	0	0	0	200
Diet Sierra Mist	16 fl oz	0	0	0	0	0	0	0	50
Diet Sierra Mist	20 fl oz	0	0	0	0	0	0	0	65
Diet Sierra Mist	32 fl oz	0	0	0	0	0	0	0	100
Diet Sierra Mist	64 fl oz	0	0	0	0	0	0	0	200
Dr Pepper	16 fl oz	200	0	54	0	54	0	0	70
Dr Pepper	20 fl oz	250	0	68	0	68	0	0	90
Dr Pepper	32 fl oz	400	0	108	0	108	0	0	140
Dr Pepper	64 fl oz	800	0	216	0	216	0	0	280
Lipton Brisk Green with Peach Tea	16 fl oz	0	0	0	0	0	0	0	140
Lipton Brisk Green with Peach Tea	20 fl oz	0	0	0	0	0	0	0	180

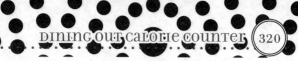

MISC BEVERAGES, SOFT DRINKS continued

Item	Serving Size	Calories	Protein	Carb	Fiber	Sugar	Total Fat	Sat Fat	Sodium
Lipton Brisk Green with Peach Tea	32 fl oz	0	0	0	0	0	0	0	280
Lipton Brisk Green with Peach Tea	64 fl oz	0	0	0	0	0	0	0	560
Lipton Brisk Lemon Tea	16 fl oz	160	0	44	0	44	0	0	130
Lipton Brisk Lemon Tea	20 fl oz	200	0	55	0	55	0	0	160
Lipton Brisk Lemon Tea	32 fl oz	320	0	88	0	88	0	0	260
Lipton Brisk Lemon Tea	64 fl oz	640	0	176	0	176	0	0	520
Lipton Brisk Peach Tea	16 fl oz	160	0	42	0	42	0	0	50
Lipton Brisk Peach Tea	20 fl oz	200	0	53	0	53	0	0	65
Lipton Brisk Peach Tea	32 fl oz	320	0	84	0	84	0	0	100
Lipton Brisk Peach Tea	64 fl oz	640	0	168	0	168	0	0	200
Lipton Brisk Raspberry Tea	16 fl oz	160	0	42	0	42	0	0	50
Lipton Brisk Raspberry Tea	20 fl oz	200	0	53	0	53	0	0	65
Lipton Brisk Raspberry Tea	32 fl oz	320	0	84	0	84	0	0	100
Lipton Brisk Raspberry Tea	64 fl oz	640	0	168	0	168	0	0	200
Lipton Brisk Tea	16 fl oz	0	0	0	0	0	0	0	60
Lipton Brisk Tea	20 fl oz	0	0	0	0	0	0	0	75
Lipton Brisk Tea	32 fl oz	0	0	0	0	0	0	0	120
Lipton Brisk Tea	64 fl oz	0	0	0	0	0	0	0	240
Manzanita Sol	16 fl oz	220	0	58	0	56	0	0	50
Manzanita Sol	20 fl oz	280	0	73	0	70	0	0	65
Manzanita Sol	32 fl oz	440	0	116	0	112	0	0	100
Manzanita Sol	64 fl oz	880	0	232	0	224	0	0	200
Milk, 2%	10 fl oz	170	12	17	0	16	6	4	180
Miranda Strawberry	16 fl oz	220	0	58	0	58	0	0	100
Miranda Strawberry	20 fl oz	280	0	73	0	73	0	0	125
Miranda Strawberry	32 fl oz	440	0	116	0	116	0	0	200
Miranda Strawberry	64 fl oz	880	0	232	0	232	0	0	400
Mountain Dew	16 fl oz	220	0	58	0	58	0	0	70
Mountain Dew	20 fl oz	280	0	73	0	73	0	0	90
Mountain Dew	32 fl oz	440	0	116	0	116	0	0	140
Mountain Dew	64 fl oz	880	0	232	0	232	0	0	280

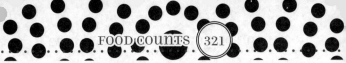

MISC BEVERAGES, SOFT DRINKS continued

Item	Serving Size	Calories	Protein	Carb	Fiber	Sugar	Total Fat	Sat Fat	Sodium
Mug Root Beer	16 fl oz	200	0	52	0	52	0	0	30
Mug Root Beer	20 fl oz	250	0	65	0	65	0	0	40
Mug Root Beer	32 fl oz	400	0	104	0	104	0	0	60
Mug Root Beer	64 fl oz	800	0	208	0	208	0	0	120
Pepsi	16 fl oz	200	0	56	0	54	0	0	50
Pepsi	20 fl oz	250	0	70	0	68	0	0	65
Pepsi	32 fl oz	400	0	112	0	108	0	0	100
Pepsi	64 fl oz	800	0	224	0	216	0	0	200
Sierra Mist	16 fl oz	200	0	54	0	54	0	0	40
Sierra Mist	20 fl oz	250	0	68	0	68	0	0	50
Sierra Mist	32 fl oz	400	0	108	0	108	0	0	80
Sierra Mist	64 fl oz	800	0	216	0	216	0	0	160
Tropicana Fruit Punch	16 fl oz	220	0	60	0	60	0	0	50
Tropicana Fruit Punch	20 fl oz	280	0	75	0	75	0	0	65
Tropicana Fruit Punch	32 fl oz	440	0	120	0	120	0	0	100
Tropicana Fruit Punch	64 fl oz	880	0	240	0	240	0	0	200
Tropicana Lemonade	16 fl oz	200	0	54	0	54	0	0	210
Tropicana Lemonade	20 fl oz	250	0	68	0	68	0	0	260
Tropicana Lemonade	32 fl oz	400	0	108	0	108	0	0	420
Tropicana Lemonade	64 fl oz	800	0	216	0	216	0	0	840
Tropicana Pink Lemonade	16 fl oz	200	0	54	0	54	0	0	210
Tropicana Pink Lemonade	20 fl oz	250	0	68	0	68	0	0	268
Tropicana Pink Lemonade	32 fl oz	400	0	108	0	108	0	0	420
Tropicana Pink Lemonade	64 fl oz	800	0	216	0	216	0	0	840
Tropicana Sugar Free Lemonade	16 fl oz	16	0	4	0	4	0	0	130
Tropicana Sugar Free Lemonade	20 fl oz	20	0	5	0	5	0	0	160
Tropicana Sugar Free Lemonade	32 fl oz	32	0	8	0	8	0	0	260
Tropicana Sugar Free Lemonade	64 fl oz	64	0	16	0	16	0	0	520
Tropicana Twister Orange	16 fl oz	220	0	62	0	62	0	0	50

MISC BEVERAGES, SOFT DRINKS continued

Item	Serving Size	Calories	Protein	Carb	Fiber	Sugar	Total Fat	Sat Fat	Sodium
Tropicana Twister Orange	20 fl oz	280	0	78	0	78	0	0	65
Tropicana Twister Orange	32 fl oz	440	0	124	0	124	0	0	100
Tropicana Twister Orange	64 fl oz	880	0	248	0	248	0	0	200
Wild Cherry Pepsi	16 fl oz	200	0	56	0	56	0	0	40
Wild Cherry Pepsi	20 fl oz	250	0	70	0	70	0	0	50
Wild Cherry Pepsi	32 fl oz	400	0	112	0	112	0	0	80
Wild Cherry Pepsi	64 fl oz	800	0	224	0	224	0	0	160

ADULT BEVERAGES

Item	Serving Size	Calories	Carb	Total Fat	Sat Fat	Sodium
DRAFT BEER						
Blue Moon	16 oz	220	20	0	0	20
Bud Light	16 oz	160	19	0	0	20
Fat Tire	16 oz	210	20	0	0	20
Sam Adams	16 oz	210	24	0	0	15
Shiner Bock	16 oz	190	16	0	0	15
Yuengling	16 oz	190	16	0	0	15
CLASSIC COCKTAILS & SPIRITS						
80 proof distilled spirits	each	100	0	0	0	0
Amaretto Sour	each	170	30	0	0	0
Baileys and Coffee	each	180	15	8	5	50
Baileys Irish Cream	each	270	6	4.5	0	0
Bloody Mary	each	140	16	0	0	1170
Classic martini w/ gin	each	140	0	1.5	0	330
Classic martini w/ vodka	each	150	0	0.5	0	170
Cognac	each	70	0	0	0	0
Cosmopolitan	each	220	15	0	0	0
Disaronno Amaretto	each	80	12	0	0	0
Frangelico	each	70	12	0	0	0
Grand Marnier	each	80	6	0	0	0
Irish Coffee	each	90	4	2	1	25
Kahlúa	each	90	15	0	0	0
Manhattan w/ bourbon	each	150	5	0	0	0

ADULT BEVERAGES continued

Item	Serving Size	Calories	Carb	Total Fat	Sat Fat	Sodium
Mudslide	each	520	52	21	13	160
Piña Colada	each	320	55	6	5	35
Rob Roy	each	160	3	0	0	10
Screwdriver	each	100	8	0	0	0

WINES

Item	Serving Size	Calories	Carb	Total Fat	Sat Fat	Sodium
Red, Cabernet Sauvignon	5 oz	122	3.8	0	0	n/a
Red, Merlot	5 oz	122	3.7	0	0	6
Red, Pinot Noir	5 oz	121	3.4	0	0	n/a
White, Pinot Gris (Grigio)	5 oz	122	3	0	0	n/a
White, Riesling	5 oz	118	5.54	0	0	n/a
White, Sauvignon Blanc	5 oz	119	3	0	0	n/a